Children with School Problems

Children with School Problems

A Physician's Manual

Canadian Paediatric Society

Debra Andrews, MD, FRCPC
William Mahoney, MD, FRCPC
Editors

2nd edition

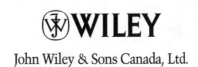

John Wiley & Sons Canada, Ltd.

Library and Archives Canada Cataloguing in Publication Data
Children with school problems: a physician's manual / Canadian Paediatric Society. --2nd ed.

Includes bibliographical references and index.
ISBN 978-1-118-30251-4

1. Learning disabilities--Handbooks, manuals, etc. 2. Learning disabilities--Diagnosis--Handbooks, manuals, etc. 3. Learning disabled children--Handbooks, manuals, etc. 4. Learning disabled children--Education--Handbooks, manuals, etc. 5. Pediatrics--Handbooks, manuals, etc. I. Canadian Paediatric Society

LC4704.C55 2012   678.92'85889   C2012-902324-8
978-1-118-45710-8 (ebk); 978-1-118-45274-5 (ebk); 978-1-118-45275-2 (ebk)

Production Credits
Cover design: Adrian So
Typesetting: Laserwords
Cover image: iStockphoto
Printer: Friesens

Editorial Credits
Executive editor: Robert Hickey
Managing editor: Alison Maclean
Production editor: Jeremy Hanson-Finger

John Wiley & Sons Canada, Ltd.
6045 Freemont Blvd.
Mississauga, Ontario
L5R 4J3

Printed in Canada

1 2 3 4 5 FP 16 15 14 13 12

Contents

List of Tools

About the Canadian Paediatric Society

OUR MISSION

The Canadian Paediatric Society is the national association of paediatricians, committed to working together to advance the health of children and youth by nurturing excellence in health care, advocacy, education, research, and support of its membership.

WHO WE ARE

As a voluntary professional association, the CPS represents more than 3,000 paediatricians, paediatric subspecialists, paediatric residents, and other professionals who work with and care for children and youth.

WHAT WE DO

- **Advocacy**: The CPS works to improve public policy that affects the health of children and youth.
- **Public education:** The CPS helps parents and caregivers make informed decisions about their children's health by producing reliable and accessible health information.
- **Professional education:** The CPS supports the continuing learning needs of paediatricians and other child and youth health professionals through position statements, a peer-reviewed journal, and educational events.
- **Surveillance and research:** The CPS monitors rare diseases and conditions, and ensures continued research into vaccine-associated adverse reactions and vaccine-preventable diseases.
- Because the needs are so great, the CPS also works with many other organizations to promote the health of children and youth.

ON THE INTERNET

www.cps.ca: This is the primary online home of the Canadian Paediatric Society. Visit this site to access position statements, written by Canada's paediatricians on a range of child and youth health topics, and learn more about the organization. You can also find a series of resources and links to complement the material in this book.

www.caringforkids.cps.ca: Caring for Kids is the CPS website for parents and caregivers, with more than 150 documents with practical, easy-to-use information on everything from pregnancy and babies to behaviour and development. To access the French version of the site, *Soins de nos enfants*, visit www.soinsdenosenfants.cps.ca.

Acknowledgements

Children with School Problems reflects the efforts and wisdom of some of Canada's most respected paediatricians. Led by Dr. Debra Andrews and Dr. William Mahoney, the authoring team brings insight and expertise from years of caring for Canadian children and working with families. The Canadian Paediatric Society is tremendously grateful to them for sharing their wealth of knowledge.

We must also recognize the authors of the first edition of this book. Published in 1998 under the guidance of editors Dr. Mervyn Fox and Dr. William Mahoney, the book included contributions from Dr. Debra Andrews, Dr. Mark Handley-Derry, Dr. Helena Ho, Dr. Wendy Roberts, and Dr. Jay Rosenfield.

EDITORS

Dr. Debra Andrews is one of the original contributing authors to *Children with School Problems: A Physician's Manual,* and is currently associate professor of pediatrics and divisional director for developmental pediatrics at the University of Alberta. She is medical director of two tertiary interdisciplinary programs at the Glenrose Rehabilitation Hospital that provide assessment and intervention for children with complex learning and behavioural problems. Dr. Andrews divides her time between providing clinical care to this population and teaching medical students, residents, fellows, and practising physicians how to assess and care for children with developmental disorders.

Dr. William Mahoney is one of the co-editors of the first edition (1998) of *Children with School Problems: A Physician's Manual* and a contributing author. He is a clinical associate professor of Pediatrics, Faculty of Health Sciences, McMaster University, and former medical director of the Developmental Pediatric, Rehabilitation, and Autism Programs of McMaster Children's Hospital. He teaches about developmental problems to all levels of trainees, and participates in research in acquired brain injury in children and the genetics of autism spectrum disorders. He provides clinical care for children with developmental problems, including children with learning disabilities and attention deficit hyperactivity disorder.

AUTHORS

Dr. Brenda Clark is an associate professor at the University of Alberta's Department of Pediatrics, Division of Developmental Pediatrics. Her clinical and research areas of interest are related to the diagnosis and treatment of developmental disorders, including learning disabilities, attention deficit hyperactivity disorder, and autism, and the rehabilitation of brain injury.

Dr. Cara Dosman is a developmental-behavioural paediatrician at the Glenrose Rehabilitation Hospital in Edmonton, and is medical director of the 1–2–3 Go! Glenrose Child and Family Early Intervention Service. She has experience in the assessment and management of children with developmental disorders in both community-based and tertiary hospital-based clinics. Dr. Dosman is an assistant professor of pediatrics and rotation coordinator for the general paediatric residents' rotation in Developmental Pediatrics at the University of Alberta.

Dr. G. Tyna Doyle is a developmental paediatrician at the Janeway Children's Health and Rehabilitation Centre in St. John's, and an assistant professor at Memorial University of Newfoundland. She received her medical degree and completed her paediatrics residency at Memorial University, and then completed a subspecialty residency in Developmental Pediatrics at the University of Alberta in 2010. At the Janeway, Dr. Doyle divides her clinical time between the child development and rehabilitation teams. Her interests include ASD, ADHD, LD, and CP.

Dr. Barbara Fitzgerald is a developmental paediatrician and clinical associate professor in the Division of Developmental Pediatrics at the University of British Columbia. She runs a unique outreach program that provides developmental assessment to inner-city children in their schools. She teaches child development to medical students, emphasizing a social paediatrics approach to learning and behavioural disturbances, and is a passionate advocate for children living in poverty. Dr. Fitzgerald developed an initiative providing a longitudinal experience for medical students in the inner city and is president of a charity aimed at alleviating child poverty and improving developmental outcomes.

Dr. A. Mervyn Fox is professor emeritus in the Department of Paediatrics at the University of Western Ontario in London. He was one of the co-editors of the first edition (1998) of *Children with School Problems: A Physician's Manual*. Before accepting an invitation to work in Canada in 1975, Dr. Fox was a lecturer in developmental paediatrics at London University's Wolfson Centre, Institute of Child Health, where he had qualified in medicine in 1960. In England he worked as principal physician in the Inner London Educational Authority, then the world's largest organization of elementary and secondary schools. Dr. Fox is a past chair of the CPS Psychosocial Paediatrics Committee and a past president of the Developmental Paediatrics Section.

Dr. Ana Hanlon-Dearman is a developmental paediatrician at the Child Development Clinic in Winnipeg. She trained at the University of Manitoba and completed her paediatric residency and fellowship training in developmental pediatrics at the Children's Hospital in Winnipeg. She is certified with the American Board of Pediatrics in developmental behavioural paediatrics, and is certified in behavioural sleep medicine with the American Association of Sleep Medicine. Dr. Hanlon-Dearman is currently an associate professor of pediatrics and child health at the University of Manitoba.

Dr. Helena Ho is a developmental paediatrician and clinical professor emeritus at the University of British Columbia, specializing in caring for children with learning and behaviour problems. She received degrees from the University of Ottawa, Radcliffe College, and McGill University. Dr. Ho founded the Multicultural Committee at Sunny Hill Health Centre for Children, and headed the autism team and child development diagnostic program there for many years.

Dr. Janet Kawchuk is a developmental paediatrician, autism team member, and residency program director for developmental pediatrics at the IWK Health Centre and assistant professor at Dalhousie University in Halifax. Dr. Kawchuk received her MD from the University of Alberta, completed her paediatric residency at the IWK, and worked as a community consultant paediatrician. She is an executive member of the Canadian Paediatric Society's Developmental Paediatrics Section, and a member of the section's curriculum committee.

Dr. Elizabeth Mickelson is a clinical associate professor, Division of Developmental Pediatrics,

Department of Pediatrics, at the University of British Columbia. She initially trained as a physiotherapist and has had a long-standing interest in neurologically based conditions affecting development as well as the behavioural phenotypes of children with underlying genetic conditions/syndromes. In addition to clinical evaluation, Dr. Mickelson participates in academic teaching and clinical research activities related to this population.

Dr. Ruth Neufeld is a developmental paediatrician at the Alvin Buckwold Child Development Program and assistant professor of pediatrics at the University of Saskatchewan in Saskatoon. She completed medical school and paediatric residency at the University of Saskatchewan, followed by subspecialty training in developmental pediatrics through the University of Alberta at the Glenrose Rehabilitation Hospital in Edmonton. Before entering medical school, Dr. Neufeld worked as an itinerant speech-language pathologist, serving rural school divisions in Saskatchewan.

Dr. S. Wendy Roberts is a developmental paediatrician at Holland Bloorview Kids Rehabilitation Hospital and co-director of the Autism Research Unit at the Hospital for Sick Children. She is a professor in the Department of Paediatrics at the University of Toronto and adjunct scientist at the Bloorview Research Institute. She has led the first Canadian site of the Autism Treatment Network in Toronto, with the goal of improving the quality of evidence-based medical care offered to all individuals with autism and their families.

Dr. Sarah Shea has been director and division head at the Developmental Pediatrics Clinic of the IWK Health Centre for more than twenty-five years, and is an associate professor in the Faculty of Medicine at Dalhousie University.

REVIEWERS

Thanks to all the reviewers who provided thoughtful comments on portions of this book: Ms. Michelle Bischoff; Dr. Susan Bobbitt; Dr. Heidi Carlson-Reid; Dr. Umberto Cellupica; Sharan de Waal, MScOT; Dr. Michael Dickinson; Dr. Mark Feldman; Dr. Charlotte Foulston; Dr. Frank Friesen; Dr. Sarah Gander; Dr. Anne Gillies; Dr. Fabian Gorodzinsky; Dr. Mark Handley-Derry; Dr. John Holland; Dr. Angie Ip; Dr. Elizabeth Jimenez; Dr. Kassia Johnson; Dr. Huma Kazmie; Connie Lillas, PhD, MFT, RN; Dr. Sally Longstaffe; Dr. Peter MacPherson; Dr. Marilyn Marbell; Dr. Susanna Martin; Dr. Rob Meeder; Dr. Oliva Ortiz-Alvarez; Dr. Wendy Roberts; Dr. R. Garth Smith; Dr. Joseph Telch; Dr. Sunita Vohra; Dr. Tannis Wiebe; and Dr. Sandra Woods.

OTHER ACKNOWLEDGEMENTS

Our thanks to the children who provided the original artwork for Chapter 10: Noah Hewett, Eliza Nadon, Meara Nadon, and Sydney Szijarto.

Finally, the editors and authors would like to acknowledge the hard-working CPS administrative team: Jennie Strickland, who helped with research and permissions; Lindsay Conboy, who patiently juggled schedules to set up our many teleconference meetings; and our team lead, Elizabeth Moreau, without whose excellent assistance and daily attention to this work over the past year this book would not have been possible.

INTRODUCTION

Debra Andrews and William Mahoney

It has been forty years since the Canadian Paediatric Society published *Learning Disabilities: A Practical Office Manual.* It was recognized that physicians needed information to help children who presented to their offices with the concern of having trouble in school. This initial volume, written by child neurologists John Crichton and Henry Dunn, provided physicians with both a framework and some tools to develop formulations and recommendations that could lead to improvements for their patients. The volume was revised in 1981 and was actually supplied by the CPS to new graduates in paediatrics.

At the time there were no Canadian training programs in developmental paediatrics, and child development issues were just being identified as core knowledge and skills for practicing paediatricians. By the mid-1990s, children with school problems had become a significant component of the practice of general, community-based paediatricians. The scientific basis of this practice had improved. It was this body of knowledge that led to the recognition of developmental paediatrics as a subspecialty by the Royal College of Physicians and Surgeons of Canada. *Children with School Problems: A Physician's Manual,* published by the Canadian Paediatric Society in 1998, was written and edited by a group of developmental paediatricians and aimed at community-based paediatricians to give them more precise information and tools to assist their assessment and management of children with learning disabilities, primarily. As the field has advanced over the past decade, it was felt that an updated, revised edition was in order.

We know that children don't appear in the physician's office with the diagnosis already made, and not all school problems are the result of a specific learning disability. The emphasis of the book has changed to become truer to its title of *Children with School Problems.* This revised edition provides information about a wider group of children, including those with intellectual disabilities. It also covers specific entities that affect a child both in school and in the community, such as developmental coordination disorder, recognizing that a community physician can make this diagnosis. We have also tried to make the information relevant to primary care physicians who see children with school problems.

HOW TO USE THIS BOOK

As in the previous volume, the book is organized into sections:

- Foundations
- Diagnostics
- Management
- Trajectories
- Resources

The components of each section were chosen to be useful to physicians in their clinical work with children with learning problems. Certain domains were not included, as this is not intended to be a textbook of developmental paediatrics or of child development.

The first section, **Foundations,** presents pertinent background information for physicians seeing children with learning problems in their offices and can be used as an introduction for medical students and residents. It begins with an overview of learning problems in children and general information about the education system, followed by discussions of the neurological underpinnings of children's development and how these and other factors influence child development leading to school entry. In Canada, children begin their formal education at four or five years of age. The section concludes with a summary of relevant educational processes in each province regarding children with special needs and key contacts that can help physicians and families access resources and supports. Assessing children with learning problems requires consideration of multiple dimensions and sources of information.

The second section, **Diagnostics,** provides tools and approaches to obtain the necessary information, to develop a diagnostic formulation and to begin to synthesize a plan. This section reviews history, use of questionnaires, physical exam, medical investigations, and developmental sampling and screening. If you are a primary care provider, you can use the questionnaires and other tools to assist you in triaging the less complex cases that you can manage in your practice from those that need a referral to a specialist. If you are a consulting general paediatrician or other specialist, you may use some of the materials in your own assessments. The assessment tools are also useful for trainees to get some direct experience of children with learning problems. A number of materials can be copied and used in your office, including questionnaires for parents and teachers, and the graded reading passages from the previous version. There is a specific teacher's questionnaire for the pre-school age group. These materials can also be downloaded from the CPS website at www.cps.ca.

There are many choices for treatments and interventions, depending on the diagnostic formulation. The third section, **Management,** provides information about the educational, behavioural, and medical management of children's learning problems, including options for community programs. The information can assist physicians at all levels in understanding and recommending management strategies for children across the range of challenges that they and their families experience.

Because learning problems tend to be lifelong and affect adolescents and adults in their functioning and educational and career options, the **Trajectories** section will help with managing students through the teen years and understanding prognosis, an important part of counselling families about these conditions, both initially and over the longer term. We hope that this will be especially useful for the primary care physicians, who remain the ongoing medical contact for older adolescents and adults and can incorporate the context of the individual's learning problem(s) in the provision of care.

The **Resources** section includes a chapter on our best tips for encouraging children to read, and a resource sheet to help you assemble the information about the key contacts in your area that you will need to assess and manage children with learning problems. There is a set of four illustrative cases that you can use to see how the pieces of assessment come together in a clinical setting; these cases may also be used for teaching trainees. There is also a glossary of items selected from the entire book, using the most up-to-date terminology, to help you easily negotiate the changes in diagnostic labels that have resulted from our increased understanding of developmental conditions.

Numerous e-resources have been added to the book. We have incorporated both key references and the websites to helpful documents and organizations. This is recognizing that much changes quickly in this electronic age. You can also find these links at www.cps.ca.

Finally, throughout the book we have included the best wisdom of the authors, as well as the supporting evidence. The research supporting the field remains at an early level, and there are inconsistencies between sources. We hope that our observations are helpful in filling gaps where good evidence is not yet available.

CHAPTER 1

Part I: Foundations

Overview of Children with Learning Problems, Schools, and Approaches to Helping

William Mahoney

In most societies, educating children is a universal goal that takes between ten and twenty years. One's level of education has long-term economic, social, and personal implications; a child's failure or perceived failure in school has a significant impact, leading to a series of responses by families and educators intended to solve the problem or improve academic performance.

The field of learning problems continues to evolve as new information emerges and approaches change. This chapter provides an overview of the field of learning problems and the different entities that lead to problems in school.

PREVALENCE OF LEARNING PROBLEMS

Estimates of the prevalence of learning problems vary from 3% to 20%(1), but the current consensus is that 10% to 15% of school-aged children are experiencing difficulty at any point in time. This includes those with a number of different difficulties that require further definition for appropriate interventions.(2)(3)

For specific learning disabilities (LDs), the variability in prevalence is also a result of different cut-points or formulas used to define them. Depending on the range of intelligence quotient (IQ) chosen to determine average ability and the instrument used to measure academic achievement, different boundaries will lead to a different prevalence.(4) However, the figure of 10% remains the most consistent and supportable estimate.

Numerous attempts to define learning problems have been made as understanding has improved, and different models have been found useful. Many disciplines, including education, psychology, psychiatry,

neurology, and paediatrics, have looked at the issues. So it is not surprising that different aspects of the definitions have concerned investigators from different professional backgrounds. The most common reason for a child not acquiring academic skills is a learning disability. In 2002, the Learning Disabilities Association of Canada adopted a definition that is used by the national and provincial LD associations in Canada:(5)

> *Learning disabilities* refer to a number of disorders which may affect the acquisition, organization, retention, understanding or use of verbal or nonverbal information. These disorders affect learning in individuals who otherwise demonstrate at least average abilities essential for thinking and/or reasoning. As such, learning disabilities are distinct from global intellectual deficiency.

Learning disabilities result from impairments in one or more processes related to perceiving, thinking, remembering, or learning. These include, but are not limited to: language processing; phonological processing; visual-spatial processing; processing speed; memory and attention; and executive functions (e.g., planning and decision-making).

Learning disabilities range in severity and may interfere with the acquisition and use of one or more of the following:

- oral language (listening, speaking, understanding)
- reading (decoding, phonetic knowledge, word recognition, comprehension)
- written language (spelling and written expression)
- mathematics (computation, problem-solving)

Learning disabilities may also involve difficulties with organizational skills, social perception, social interaction, and perspective-taking.

Learning disabilities are lifelong. The way in which they are expressed may vary over an individual's lifetime, depending on the interaction between the demands of the environment and the individual's strengths and needs. Learning disabilities are suggested by unexpected academic under-achievement or achievement that is maintained only by unusually high levels of effort and support.

Learning disabilities are due to genetic and/or neurobiological factors or to injury that alters brain functioning in a manner which affects one or more processes related to learning. These disorders are not due primarily to hearing and/or vision problems, socio-economic factors, cultural or linguistic differences, lack of motivation or ineffective teaching, although these factors may further complicate the challenges faced by individuals with learning disabilities. Learning disabilities may co-exist with various conditions, including attentional, behavioural, and emotional disorders; sensory impairments; or other medical conditions.

To succeed, individuals with learning disabilities require early identification and timely specialized assessments and interventions involving home, school, community, and workplace settings. The interventions need to be appropriate for each individual's learning disability subtype and, at a minimum, include the provision of the following:

- specific skill instruction
- accommodations
- compensatory strategies
- self-advocacy skills

Some, but not all, provincial ministries of education in Canada use this definition of learning disabilities. Other countries also have been wrestling with these issues, coming up with different terminology and definitions. In the United States, there is a federal definition for purposes of identifying who qualifies for programs for children with special needs:(6)

A disorder in one or more of the basic psychological processes involved in understanding or in using language, spoken or written, that may manifest itself in an imperfect ability to listen, think, speak, read, write, spell, or do mathematical calculations, including conditions such as perceptual disabilities, brain injury, minimal brain dysfunction, dyslexia, and developmental aphasia.

These variations contribute to some of the confusion in the field, as these definitions may be different from the "medical" terminology.

Although the above definition describes the population, most assessment systems use a discrepancy formula to determine who is labelled as having an LD and who is labelled as having a cognitive delay, and therefore who is entitled to receive services and who is not. Medical assessment can define a child with *attention deficit hyperactivity disorder* (ADHD) (see the Glossary). Traditionally, the difference between a child's IQ (or cognitive potential) and the child's academic achievement is felt to quantify the presence and "severity" of an LD and to justify the level and type of service a child should receive.(7) This conceptual framework requires a full psychometric examination prior to diagnosis(8), which can lead to a block in service provision while waiting for the testing. However, the discrepancy formula may not be the most appropriate way to define the population of those with a reading LD, and an in-depth assessment may not be needed to provide interventions.(9)(10)(11)

Intellectual disability

The term *intellectual disability* (or ID; see the Glossary) is now used to describe children whose overall intellectual skills are significantly sub-average and have significant delays in their adaptive behaviour.(12) The specific level of intellectual disability will determine the educational program and prognosis. Chapters 11 and 17 discuss this further. Children with an intellectual disability will require support throughout their education.

Mild intellectual disability (MID)

School systems differentiate between children who have an average IQ and difficulties acquiring specific academic skills who have a diagnosis of an LD, and those with a below-average IQ who are felt to have a general delay in the acquisition of most academic skills, which is known as a *mild intellectual disability* (MID) (see the Glossary). The specific IQ that differentiates these two groups varies from province to province but most use this model. Depending on the criteria used, between 2% and 5% of children would be identified with an MID. The approach to education is often modified to a lower level, and slow but gradual progress is expected. Children on this path will often be referred to vocational programs as they enter high school and may not be considered able to qualify for post-secondary education. With the new terminology regarding intellectual disability, this may become a source of confusion, as many children with this educational classification will have intellectual skills above the range for a diagnosis of intellectual disability.

Attention deficit hyperactivity disorder (ADHD)

Over the past ten years, there have been significant advances in knowledge about the diagnosis and treatment of ADHD. The current criteria for the diagnosis are listed in DSM-IV-TR(13), which separates the criteria for inattention and hyperactivity/impulsivity. Three subtypes of ADHD—predominantly inattentive, predominantly hyperactive/impulsive, and combined—are the current accepted diagnoses in North America. The predominantly hyperactive/impulsive type is expected to be eliminated in the next DSM revision. The ICD-10 criteria (14), used in Europe, are more stringent. A number of evidence-based guidelines and algorithms have been developed to support the evaluation of a child with possible ADHD. They include those published by the American Academy of Pediatrics, the American Academy of Child and Adolescent Psychiatry, and the *National Institute for Health and Clinical Excellence (NICE)* (see the Glossary) in Europe. The Texas Algorithm gives an approach to the medical treatment of ADHD.(15) Medical management is discussed in detail in Chapter 15.

ADHD is a common problem. Estimates of prevalence vary from 1% to 14%, with good evidence that at any point in time 9% of boys and 3.3% of girls will meet criteria for the diagnosis.(16) About half continue to show evidence of ADHD over time. (See Chapter 18.) One of the core weaknesses currently felt to explain the challenges children with ADHD experience is with "executive functioning."

Executive functioning describes the skills necessary to be successful in school in the higher grades and, ultimately, in one's vocation. *Executive functions* (see the Glossary) are skills involved in planning, organizing, strategizing, paying attention to and remembering details, and managing time and space. Understanding of the neurological basis of these functions and their measurement is evolving, and much of this literature comes from evaluating adults with acquired brain injuries. Measuring and tracking the development of these functions is an area of current investigation. Executive functioning is a theoretical framework, with different models advocated by different experts. A common application to ADHD is by Thomas Brown.(17) (See Figure 1–1.)

Executive functions affect skills necessary for social interaction and behaviour as well as academic functioning. Working memory, for example, describes the ability to keep information in active memory in order to manipulate and apply it. This is necessary for efficient performance in school, and children with different types of learning disabilities as well as children with ADHD are felt to have weaknesses in this particular function, compared to their peers.

Poor school performance is often attributed to attention difficulties, which include inattention to a teacher's instruction and to quality of academic performance. But children with ADHD can show variable academic performance, including some marks above average.(18) Because medications are commonly used to treat attention problems, children are referred to a physician when they are not doing well in school, as caregivers and teachers wonder if ADHD is the explanation and if medical therapy will lead to significant improvement. Meeting such children's needs is a driving force for the development of manuals such as this one. The relationship between problems with academic performance and attention difficulties is a source of ongoing study and clinical debate. A critical

Figure 1–1 Executive Functions Impaired in ADHD

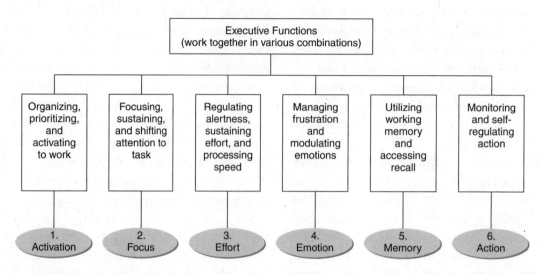

Source: Brown. Attention Deficit Disorder: The Unfocused Mind in Children and Adults. New Haven CT: Yale University Press, 2005. Used by permission of the author.

difference between the two is that the diagnosis of a specific or general learning difficulty implies some measurement of a child's skills and aspects of functioning, while the diagnosis of ADHD is based on behavioural criteria and, usually, involves multiple observers.

There is evidence that both the structure and functioning of the central nervous system is different in children with ADHD, but the measurement of these factors remains experimental. There are also significant differences in the treatment of the two conditions. (See Part III.) There is a high incidence of co-morbidity with ADHD—including language disorders, LDs, anxiety, family problems, and other behaviour challenges(19)—leading to recommendations for multi-faceted support in clinics that deal with moderate to severe ADHD.

The critical issue is that the learning component of a child's problem is identified and dealt with as part of the overall treatment plan, and the physician can be a critical resource in ensuring that this factor is addressed.

TYPES OF LEARNING DISABILITIES

Since LDs clearly form a heterogeneous group, it should be possible to generate descriptions of

discrete types meeting the general definition. The first step in classification is to examine the skills and academic functions expected in school. These include language skills, reading, spelling, writing, and mathematics. Any or all domains may be affected individually or together, and within each function there appear to be a number of subtypes. Specific problems are labelled as dyslexia for problems reading, dyscalculia for problems with mathematics calculations, and dysgraphia for problems writing.

Even within one domain, there are different subtypes. For example, within the mathematics domain, one subtype might be represented by developmental Gerstmann syndrome, a primary difficulty remembering mathematical facts, itself overlapping with developmental dyscalculia.(20) Another is a so-called "nonverbal learning disability," applicable to children who demonstrate, initially, good skills in reading and spelling but weaknesses in mechanical mathematics. They often have good automatic language skills. As they get older, they demonstrate increasingly severe problems dealing with new and complex material, concepts, and situations. They appear to be at high risk for the development of internalized emotional dysfunctions.

Reading difficulties may reflect specific developmental delays at different levels of complexity, such as phonemic analysis or word recognition, word analysis, oral or silent reading, or comprehension of written language, or they may specifically involve apparently discrete aspects of written language such as reading (receptive language), spelling, handwriting (graphomotor problems), or composition skills (written expressive language). The most common and certainly the most obvious manifestation in the early grades is difficulty in word recognition.

With the greater understanding of other processes that contribute to effective academic performance, there is also an attempt to identify underlying disorders such as *developmental coordination disorder* (DCD) (see the Glossary), which may cause significant difficulties with producing written work or participating in gym. This also helps identify that children often have trouble with their function outside school, in this example, with skills requiring motor coordination such as team sports.

While theoretical models are intriguing, there is no consensus on the classification of subtypes of LDs. Progress is being made with greater numbers of longitudinal studies. Regardless of uncertainty as to the existence of discrete subtypes, when a child is experiencing difficulty in school all of the various academic functions must be reviewed, as well as challenges in participation in activities outside the school environment.

RESPONSE TO INTERVENTION

The response to intervention (RTI) approach identifies children who are having trouble with academic development at an early age—around age six—and provides direct interventions to improve the skills without first undergoing any definitive diagnostic process. This is mandated as an approach in the United States and is used in some parts of Canada. Children are screened in school for difficulty, and those identified receive a structured systematic intervention and the results are measured. This has been most studied in the area of reading, and there is good evidence that a significant proportion of children experiencing difficulty improve to the point where their skills are the same as their peers. There also

has been demonstrated normalization of the brain functions needed for reading associated with the intervention. Children who make slower progress receive a more intensive program, and if difficulties continue, then more formal assessment and classification occur. This is different from the "waiting to fail" approach, as many children do respond to the intervention program. A description of the process, tools, and interventions can be found at www.rti4success.org.

ETIOLOGY/MECHANISMS OF LDs

No single etiology accounts for all LDs. Inherited forms have been identified; some cases may reflect disruption of neuronal migration in early gestation; some may reflect discrete injury; and some may be secondary to other neurological disorders. A number of faulty mechanisms involved in the processing of information through auditory or visual channels, alone or in combination, can be recognized in clinical, neuropsychological, or neurophysiological examinations. In the absence of a totally acceptable classification system, the relationship between pathology and dysfunction often remains obscure.

The understanding of the underlying mechanisms for LD has evolved through the analysis of the performance of certain tasks by persons with known brain lesions, usually adults. For example, it is known that people with a lesion in Broca's area of the left frontal lobe have difficulty with an expressive aphasia. It was recognized early in this century that children with brain damage had significant problems with traditional academic learning, and such findings suggested that children with LDs similarly had some kind of neurological lesion affecting the areas responsible for the dependant function.

Explanatory models such as minimal brain damage or minimal brain dysfunction (MBD) grew from these associations, leading to searches for signs of "organicity" and recommendations for increasingly more elaborate neurological evaluations. There is evidence that routinely including electroencephalograms (EEGs) or neuroimaging in investigations of LD is unrewarding.(21) Newer technological advances, such as computerized EEG analysis, positron emission tomography (PET) scans, magnetic resonance and functional magnetic resonance imaging (MRI and fMRI), are proving to be more helpful and are leading to clearer understanding of the mechanisms of learning problems and their response to intervention, although these remain largely research tools and are not used clinically at this time.

As noted, LDs can lead to difficulties in performing a number of different functions and tasks, depending on an individual's profile of strengths and weaknesses. Most of the research on LDs has focused on reading, but recent information is beginning to define more precisely the normal processes involved, as well as possible mechanisms responsible for the different types of LDs.

Traditionally, it was thought that the process of reading involved a pathway encompassing numerous areas of the brain sequentially. Information relay from visual to language to speech to motor centres in the occipital, parietal, temporal, and frontal areas were assumed to be anatomic and functional substrates of the reading process.

Recent studies suggest involvement of two mechanisms that are somewhat independent. Neurophysiological experiments with skilled adult readers provide some evidence for an area in the visual cortex, near the occipital-temporal junction, that recognizes familiar words without involvement of the temporal lobe. Frontal areas are involved in giving meaning (semantic processing) to the words on the printed page.

Reading unfamiliar words includes the process of sounding them out (phonological processing). It is known that the left temporal-parietal area, specifically the angular and supramarginal gyri of the inferior temporal lobe, is involved in this activity. Until recently, it was thought that reading always involved some phonological processing; however, current findings suggest that skilled readers bypass the left temporal lobe.

Studies of known poor readers or so-called "dyslexics" have demonstrated some differences in the relative size of bilateral brain structures, such as the planum temporale, which is usually larger on the left side. Studies have shown a reversed asymmetry (planum temporale larger on the right) or a symmetrical planum in some persons with problems reading.(22)

Recent fMRI studies have confirmed that this area is underactive in some patients with dyslexia.

Neuropathological studies of persons with known LDs who died from other causes(23) have shown specific patterns of abnormality on microscopic examination. Numerous areas of architectonic dysplasias and neuronal ectopias have been found, with all individuals having involvement of the left inferior frontal and superior temporal regions. Such dysplasias are found in approximately 20% of autopsies of persons with LDs. In persons without known LDs, such findings are not found in the same numbers or concentrated in these areas. These lesions are felt to arise in the middle trimester, associated with microscopic brain maldevelopment, when neuronal migration is occurring. Researchers have suggested an autoimmune process, but there are no definitive explanations for the finding. The planum temporale was symmetrical in all subjects with LDs in one study, which is consistent with other data. Neuropathological studies, some of which are contradictory, have not produced complete explanations for the clinical phenomenon of LDs.

Clinicians involved with children with LDs are often struck by the apparent family history of similar problems, and there is some evidence of familial aggregation of LD in both chromosomal and family history studies. Although some genetic disorders, such as fragile X syndrome, may be manifested as LD(24), the search for genetic markers in most families has been elusive. With newer technology, a number of genetic markers are being discovered.(25) It is also difficult to prove the same type of LDs in adults and children because test profiles and performance may change with the passage of time. The linkage of the genetic and neurological data is assisting in the delineation of the pathophysiology in some individuals.

Groups of persons with LDs have been shown to have problems with a number of neuropsychological functions, including visual and auditory memory, integration of visual and auditory information, left-right confusion, auditory synthesis, temporal order judgment, spatial orientation, and phonological processing. Few persons with LDs have all of these problems, but most persons with LDs have some of these problems. Improved neurophysiological imaging techniques should provide greater understanding of these brain-behaviour relationships.

Pregnancy and birth complications have sometimes been considered as probable, common, and significant contributors to learning problems. Prospective longitudinal studies, however, have questioned the validity of many perinatal influences as having a causal role for school dysfunction.(26) A prospective study of infants with very low birth weight found no increased incidence of reading problems at age eight(27), when allowances were made for social class and confounding attentional or behavioural problems. Very low birth weight does, however, appear to be associated with an increased incidence of both attention and fine-motor problems.

There is current interest in the role of environmental or dietary factors, such as exposure to toxins during the pregnancy, subtle lead intoxication, or iron deficiency.(28) From the perspective of the child in school, the determination of causation may have little practical value unless there is a correctable factor such as iron deficiency. If a thorough initial history and physical exam does not suggest further investigations, an extensive search is unlikely to be profitable and is not recommended.

Emotional disturbance or an adverse environment are specific exclusionary criteria for the diagnosis of LD, but are felt to contribute to other learning problems. The issues are complex. For example, it should be noted that:

- Family influence and dynamics are extremely important to persons with learning problems, perhaps even more than to other families, because these are chronic, disabling conditions.
- Children with chronic conditions are at significantly increased risk for mental health problems as a result of their disability.(29)
- The incidence of learning problems, including LDs, is greater in lower socio-economic groups.(30)

It remains difficult to sort out all the different mechanisms that may be contributing to an individual child's school performance, so that the physician's best efforts may culminate in a descriptive formulation rather than a single, simple diagnosis. The high prevalence of learning problems such as ADHD and specific learning disabilities suggests that it is important to consider them whenever a child's academic achievement lags behind peers. In a multifactorial situation, learning problems may prevent the child from enlisting existing coping mechanisms. The physician needs to search for factors—at home or in school—that interfere with the individual's ability to adapt, as so many do, to their unique profile of strengths and weaknesses. Then the physician must identify the individual, family, and community resources that may be deployed to facilitate the child's adaptation.

NATURAL HISTORY

Some have claimed that infantile colic or fussiness may be an early warning sign of a variety of neuro-developmental disturbances, but there are no sound longitudinal studies to determine the degree of risk associated with these early symptoms. Good evidence indicates that children with language delays—whether expressive, receptive, or mixed—are at high risk for having difficulty acquiring reading skills.(31)

Although there has been concern about preschool children with isolated perceptual-motor problems, this group seems to represent a relatively small proportion of the population with LDs. Preschoolers with *developmental coordination disorder* (DCD) (see the Glossary), however, are at higher risk of later LDs. Kindergarten teachers are able to reliably identify many children who will have problems in the primary grades. The response to intervention initiative has used universal screening of five- and six-year-olds to identify those needing intervention. Unfortunately, however, many educational authorities still do not provide assessment or programming for such children until after Grades 1 or 2, despite the evidence of the effectiveness of early intervention programs (EIPs).

Recurrent otitis media (ROM) has been another identified risk factor. Hearing losses and distortions associated with persistent or intermittent middle ear effusion have been alleged to affect phonemic analysis skills, language development, and subsequent reading skills, but prospective studies have questioned this association despite a possible influence on attentional behaviour.(32) Evaluation of hearing and visual acuity is part of the basic assessment of children experiencing difficulty in school, and any findings require pursuit and correction if possible.

Once a child's difficulty is established, teachers and parents often express a desire for assessment, but the amount of assessment needed for diagnosis and a remedial program is controversial.(33) Attention problems may lead to requests for medical evaluation and treatment. Many school systems request a medical assessment of children being considered for special education, but expectations vary widely as to its scope or usefulness. (The issue of assessment is further discussed in Part II.)

When the diagnosis has been established and accepted as the basis for educational planning, the child may receive different types of help designed to improve the areas of difficulty, often with the goal of the child returning to a regular program if he or she has a specific LD. Special services may be needed for a short time or for many years. As children get older, the skills needed to achieve in school also change. Youngsters with learning problems often grow into their problems despite early optimism that they will grow out of them with maturity. Children with known learning problems may find new expectations difficult to meet just when they are beginning to overcome some of their previous weaknesses. For example, many children will find spelling difficult despite having developed good reading skills. Another group of children, with problems in such areas as reading comprehension, may have had acceptable achievement up until Grade 4 or 5, but be unable to cope with the demands of senior grades without assistance. Children with writing problems frequently experience increasing difficulty as demands are made for ever-greater output.(34)

In junior high school, the organization of many schools changes: the child no longer has only a homeroom or single teacher. Young adolescents experience greater social pressures. Some school systems de-emphasize remedial assistance at this stage and begin helping with organizational and planning strategies. While very appropriate for some, these interventions may be very difficult for youth lacking the basic literacy skills for the core subjects. When there are many teachers, it may be very difficult to implement recommendations consistently, such as for classroom interactional styles, modified expectations, or individualized curricula.

As high school approaches, vocational or "basic" programs will often be recommended. There are excellent vocational courses and specialized secondary schools with good retention records, whose graduates consistently acquire useful technical and social skills. For students with specific LDs, however, this emphasis often reinforces the belief that they have insufficient skills and/or abilities to cope with an academic high school program. Unfortunately, some vocational or basic programs have high dropout rates (up to 65%), and graduates may not be eligible for post-secondary education. Even a very slow progress through regular high school courses may be a positive experience and leave the eventual graduate better equipped for ongoing learning. Continued instruction and accommodation may allow students with LDs to accomplish this goal.

It is also important to remember that some students with LDs proceed through high school to post-secondary programs, including university. Most will require some accommodations to be successful at the post-secondary level, particularly if they had help in high school. Many post-secondary institutions have modified entry requirements and/or provide resources to aid students with all types of disabilities. Confirmation of diagnosis may be necessary to qualify for services. The physician may be called upon to assist a family in decision-making regarding a high school program, which is crucial for the child's future. Decisions must be made on an individual basis, weighing the strengths of the child and family and not just the child's difficulties and the rules for inclusion in a particular educational category.

Secondary or reactive problems such as poor self-esteem, depression, and maladaptive coping strategies, such as *learned helplessness* (see the Glossary) or "acting out," are a significant concern for families of children with LDs and for those who work with them professionally. Preventing chronic failure through appropriate educational experiences and strategies should help children learn to take advantage of their strengths to compensate for weaknesses. Higher self-esteem should lead to higher levels of motivation and work that students with learning problems need to achieve. High self-esteem is also felt to buffer students against adverse influences such as substance abuse and delinquent behaviour.

Those working in the field are often struck by the obvious suffering of children who are exposed to failing situations. One sees their anger, frustration, and sadness. Unfortunately, although many learning problems can be predicted from the developmental or family history or kindergarten experience, most systems require a record of established problems or failure before assessment or remedial services will be implemented: the "waiting to fail" approach. The fear of labelling and stigmatizing children inappropriately and creating a self-fulfilling prophecy leads some systems not to recognize the evidence of the cumulative files and the impressions of their own teachers. Yet children who fail will label themselves, often more destructively than the cruellest of peers or the most intrusive delivery of special educational support. This occurs long before their academic delay reaches the statistical requirements of certainty. For the physician, the question should be "Does this child need support?" rather than "What learning problem should be diagnosed?"

TREATMENT/MANAGEMENT

Many types of treatments are recommended and used for children with LDs. Some examples are mentioned briefly here and discussed in greater detail in subsequent chapters. Many disciplines both within and outside the educational system offer treatment or remediation. These interventions and their efficacy were usefully reviewed by Feldman.(35) Within the domain of education, these interventions can be classified as follows:

- direct remediation of skills (e.g., reading)
- use of cognitive strategies, such as mnemonics, to assist the retention of material or execution of processes
- deficit improvement directed, for example, to basic prerequisites, including memory or motor skills

- accommodation or modification of curriculum expectations
- bypass, circumvention, or substitution strategies, such as using computers and calculators to improve a function or to circumvent a disability

In addition to classroom teachers and remedial or special educators, educational psychologists may also be involved. Other disciplines, including speech-language pathology, occupational therapy, audiology, and social work, also can have a role in treating children with LDs. These disciplines are often accessed through health care systems and may be associated with multidisciplinary LD clinics. Research continues into the role of these added personnel and the efficacy of their treatments.

Physicians are often consulted about prescribing medication for children whose problems are associated with concentration difficulties or hyperactivity. There is considerable overlap between attentional and learning disorders, with many children having both problems. It is also true that children who are asked to do impossible tasks will have difficulty maintaining attention on them. It is not uncommon to encounter children whose needs for special educational help have never been addressed because medication has suppressed their behavioural difficulties. Prescribing medication for children in school should occur only after appropriate educational assessment and remediation plans have been implemented, or after it has been clearly established that there is only a problem with behaviour and attention. This issue is more fully discussed in Part III.

For students with *mild intellectual disability*, academic programming may be modified to a level lower than the expectations for other children of the same age. Direct teaching of skills occurs, but the content may be simplified, and slower progress is expected. There is emphasis on practical skills needed for life in the community.

SUMMARY

There are a variety of differing approaches to assist children who are slow to master the tasks of childhood required to acquire academic skills. With increasing knowledge of biological markers, brain-behaviour relationships, and genetics, it is clear that LDs reflect innate individual differences in neurological functioning.

Early identification, particularly in the preschool period and ideally by the end of the kindergarten year, should lead to early interventions and allow most children with LDs to participate in programs that improve academic functioning, prevent the development of maladaptive coping mechanisms and poor self-esteem, and thereby reduce the need for ongoing, expensive, educational and mental health interventions at a later age.

REFERENCES

1. Broman S, Bien E, Shaughnessy P. Low Achieving Children: The First Seven Years. Hillsdale: Erlbaum, 1985.
2. Shaywitz SE, Escobar MD, Shaywitz BA, et al. Evidence that dyslexia may represent the lower tail of a normal distribution of reading ability. N Engl J Med 1992; 326: 145–50.
3. Learning Disabilities: A Report to the U.S. Congress. Bethesda MD: National Institutes of Health, Interagency Committee on Learning Disabilities, 1987.
4. Op. cit., Reference 2 (Shaywitz).
5. Learning Disabilities Association of Canada (2002). Official Definition of Learning Disabilities. <www.ldac-acta.ca/en/learn-more/ld-defined.html>
6. Horowitz, Sheldon (2006). Checking Up on Learning Disabilities. National Centre for Learning Disabilities. <www.ncld.org/ld-basics/ld-explained/basic-facts/checking-up-on-learning-disabilities>
7. Learning Disabilities: A Report to the U.S. Congress. Bethesda MD: National Institutes of Health, Interagency Committee on Learning Disabilities, 1987: 107–18.
8. Taylor HG. Neuropsychological testing: Relevance for assessing children's learning disabilities. J Consult Clin Psychol 1988; 56: 795–800.
9. Siegel LS. IQ is irrelevant to the definition of learning disabilities. J Learn Disabil 1989; 22: 469–78.
10. Rispens J, van Yperen TA, van Duijn GA. The irrelevance of IQ to the definition of learning disabilities: Some empirical evidence. J Learn Disabil 1991; 24: 434–8.
11. Berniger V, Hart T, Abbott R, et al. Defining reading and writing disabilities with and without IQ: A flexible, developmental perspective. Learn Disabil Quart 1992; 15: 103–18.
12. American Association of Intellectual and Developmental Disabilities. Definition of Intellectual Disability. <www.aaidd.org/content_100.cfm?navID=21>
13. American Psychiatric Association. Diagnostic and Statistical Manual of Mental Disorders, 4th Edition. Washington: The Association, 2000.
14. World Health Organization (2010). International Statistical Classification of Diseases and Related Medical Conditions (10th Edition). <http://apps.who.int/classifications/icd10/browse/2010/en>
15. Pliszka SR, Crismon ML, Hughes CW, et al. Texas Consensus Conference Panel on Pharmacotherapy of Childhood Attention Deficit Hyperactivity Disorder. The Texas Children's Medication Algorithm Project: Revision of the algorithm for pharmacotherapy of attention-deficit/hyperactivity disorder. J Am Acad Child Adolesc Psychiatry 2006 Jun; 45(6): 642–57.
16. Szatmari P, Offord DR, Boyle MH. Ontario child health study: Prevalence of attention deficit disorder with hyperactivity. J Child Psychol Psychiatry 1989; 30: 219–30.
17. Brown, Thomas. Executive functions: Describing six aspects of a complex syndrome. <www.drthomasebrown.com/pdfs/Executive_Functions_by_Thomas_Brown.pdf>
18. Halperin JM, Gittleman R, Klein DF, et al. Reading-disabled hyperactive children: A distinct subgroup of attention deficit disorder with hyperactivity? J Abnormal Psychol 1984; 12: 1–14.
19. Silver LB. The relationship between learning disabilities, hyperactivity, distractibility, and behavioral problems: A clinical analysis. J Am Acad Child Psychiatry 1981; 20: 385–97.
20. Shalev RS, Gross-Tsur V. Developmental dyscalculia and medical assessment. J Learn Disabil 1993; 26: 134–7.
21. Hynd GW, Marshall R, Gonzalez J. Learning disabilities and presumed central nervous system dysfunction. Learn Disabil Quart 1991; 14: 283–96.
22. Posner MI, Petersen SE, Fox PT, et al. Localization of cognitive operations in the human brain. Science 1988; 240: 1627–31.
23. Op. cit., Reference 21 (Hynd).

24. Brown WT. The fragile X syndrome. Neurol Clin 1989; 7: 107–21.

25. Scerri TS, Schulte-Körne G. Genetics of developmental dyslexia. Eur Child Adolesc Psychiatry 2010 Mar; 19(3):179–97. Epub 2009 Nov 29.

26. Nelson KB, Ellenberg JH. Apgar scores as predictors of chronic neurologic disability. Pediatrics 1981; 68: 36–44.

27. Saigal S, Szatmari P, Rosenbaum P, et al. Cognitive abilities and school performance of extremely low birth weight children and matched term control children at age 8 years: A regional study. J Pediatr 1991; 118: 751–60.

28. Pollitt E, Hathirat P, Kotchabhakdi NJ, et al. Iron deficiency and educational achievement in Thailand. Am J Clin Nutr 1989; 50 Suppl 3: 687–97.

29. Cadman D, Boyle M, Szatmari P, et al. Chronic illness, disability, and mental and social well-being: Findings of the Ontario Child Health Study. Pediatrics 1987; 79: 805–13.

30. Melekian BA. Family characteristics of children with dyslexia. J Learn Disabil 1990; 23: 386–91.

31. Silva PA, Williams S, McGee R. A longitudinal study of children with developmental language delay at age three: Later intelligence, reading and behaviour problems. Dev Med Child Neurol 1987; 29: 630–40.

32. Lous J. Otitis media and reading achievement: A review. Int J Pediatr Otorhinolaryngol 1995 May; 32(2): 105–21.

33. Berniger V, Hart T, Abbott R, et al. Defining reading and writing disabilities with and without IQ: A flexible, developmental perspective. Learn Disabil Quart 1992; 15: 103–18.

34. Sandler AD, Watson TE, Footo M, et al. Neurodevelopmental study of writing disorders in middle childhood. J Dev Behav Pediatr 1992; 13: 17–23.

35. Feldman W. Learning Disabilities: A Review of Available Treatments. Springfield: Charles C Thomas, 1990.

2

Understanding and Working with Schools

William Mahoney

There are differing opinions about the most appropriate aims of education: preparing for an individual's future, learning how to learn, helping students to feel good about themselves, accumulating facts and techniques, conserving and conveying societal values, or equipping a nation for economic success. Each perspective has its proponents, and each belief system has particular implications and repercussions when applied to children with special needs.(1)(2)

Physicians working with children with school problems require some knowledge of the varied approaches and philosophies followed by educators and school systems. These approaches determine differences in classroom practice and expectations that affect all children and their families, and they have particular impact upon those with any type of neurological exceptionality. Physicians require, at the very least, an overview of educational philosophy and theory to be able to collaborate effectively with the education system. It is important to avoid value judgments and focus on understanding the effects of particular policies and processes upon a specific individual or group, leading to change that benefits them.

Education, like medicine, develops new approaches and philosophies over the years. As in medicine, some innovations have been implemented without full evaluation or consideration of the impact on the target population. Children with learning problems are particularly vulnerable to such innovations, since their abilities to adapt may not be as strong as those of other children.

In this chapter we present some of the background principles and basic vocabulary that are useful in collaborating with school personnel.

EDUCATIONAL LEGISLATION AND SCHOOL ORGANIZATION

In Canada, provincial governments provide general guidelines and minimum standards for educational programs through legislation, including details such as class size; specific policies and structures about implementing guidelines are the responsibility of each school board. The resulting differences in services from school to school, particularly those that are geographically close, may be confusing for both parents and physicians.

The role of schools in society and children's daily experience in the classroom and playground has changed radically in recent years. Schools are expected to socialize children as well as to teach them. They help shape attitudes on racism, sexuality, morals, and health promotion. They are called upon to help prevent child abuse, sexually transmitted diseases, and unwanted pregnancies. They are asked to individualize programs and to develop basic skills in all students.

School systems are governed by elected boards, and some provincial mandates provide two or more school boards for a single geographical area, based on language and/or religion. Faith-based school boards are a Canadian phenomenon that date back to issues that were important at the time of Confederation. The resources available to a particular board may reflect its tax base, so that the board serving the majority may offer programs not available elsewhere. However, one school board may purchase services from another.

From the child's perspective, the **teacher** is the most important person at school. The teacher instructs and evaluates the student, reports progress to the student's parents, identifies children with difficulties, and requests support. The teacher is the first point of contact when parents have a concern about their child. If an **educational assistant** is in the classroom to support the student, the assistant is accountable to the teacher, again making the teacher the main point of contact.

In each school, the **principal** is accountable for the implementation of policies on instruction and discipline, and for the organization and management of the school. Teachers are accountable to the principal. When a child is having significant problems, the principal is an important contact person for the physician when there are issues that cannot be resolved by the teacher. The principal is also aware of the board's policies about assessment and procedures for children experiencing difficulties and is involved in placement decisions.

A **superintendent** is responsible for a group of schools, and his or her portfolio may include the special education services for the school board. Such an administrator can be helpful when complex issues cannot be resolved at the school level.

Parents have open access to their representative on the **local school board**. School board members are elected, and they are accountable first to taxpayers and then to children and parents. In some cases of dispute, the school board may be parents' final appeal and their only chance of exerting influence within what can seem like an unresponsive system. In many jurisdictions, however, appeals against placement decisions can be made to the **minister** responsible for education. Some of the key policies of each province are discussed in Chapter 5. Physicians working with parents in a dispute with the school system should counsel them to go through appropriate channels—teacher, principal, superintendent—before choosing the political route. They should be familiar with the advocacy role of parent groups such as the Learning Disability Association, which are often familiar with policies and can help parents navigate the system.

Visits from physicians to schools are usually welcomed. Physicians may have much to contribute to formal conferences and have much to learn from informal classroom observation and participation in case conferences. However, a collaborative and consultative approach is essential. The principal has authority over educational matters, including placement and access to educational assistants. Ensure that the principal is aware of an upcoming school visit, as you may need his or her permission. Treating a visit as an opportunity to share information and collaborate with school staff in formulating an intervention plan is the most effective approach.

Most school systems have a special services department. In addition to special educators, the staff is likely to include psychologists, speech-language pathologists, and social workers. What other consultants are available may vary by school board. The special services department is responsible for assessing students with special educational needs, and often is also responsible for the development of special educational resources and policies. The assessment information is often used to classify a child's problem and to determine the types of services, including special classes, for which this child is eligible. The role of the special services department may be advisory, as the implementation of its recommendations remains the mandate of the school, under the supervision of the principal.

TERMS USED BY THE EDUCATION SYSTEM

The education system, like medicine, has its own unique language. To communicate effectively with the school system, it helps to have an understanding of common terms. Some are explained here, and others are in the Glossary at the back of this book. Note that terms may vary from province to province.

- *Regular classroom*, *resource room*, and *segregated or self-contained classroom* indicate choices of classroom placement for children with problems that require special education. A regular class is a class for all students, and the resource room is an area in a school where extra help is provided although most of the child's time is spent in a regular class. A segregated or self-contained class is a special class for students with special education needs, though not all schools will have this type of class.

- *Specific learning disability (SLD); general learning disability (GLD); mild intellectual disability (MID); moderate intellectual disability or developmental disability; communication or language disability; motor disability; social-adjustment or behaviour disordered; emotionally disabled or disturbed; autism spectrum disorder (ASD); and gifted* are some of the categorical labels that identify the children whose performance or problems have led to consideration of the need for special educational provisions. These labels may lead to special education programs for such children. As well, the labels are often the titles of the actual special education classrooms or programs into which children will be placed.

  Many people feel that such labels are inappropriate for children because of their stigmatizing effect, because of inadequate diagnostic criteria allowing reliable placement in one or another group, or because of failure to demonstrate program effectiveness. There is movement toward non-categorical identification of children with functional descriptors of their learning and developmental needs.

- *Individual program plan (IPP), individual educational plan (IEP),* and *personal program plan (PPP)* are terms that refer to a written document developed by the school that outlines a child's needs and how these will be addressed. This type of document can be used to communicate to teachers and parents the strategies for assisting students.

- *Ungraded curriculum* is an approach to the education of children, particularly in the early elementary years, that eliminates grades but allows progress based on individual successes in different academic domains.

- *Streaming* is a process by which students of the same age may be enrolled in different levels of a program that have different goals. In some provinces, students are asked to choose an academic program (or stream) at high-school entry. Choices include an academic stream (leading to university education), the general or applied stream (which leads to community college education), and the basic or locally developed stream (for developing skills for entry to the employment market).

- *Regular teacher, resource teacher, special educator, special education/learning resource teacher,* and *consultant* refer to teachers with differing responsibilities for helping children with special needs. The terms are often referred to by their acronyms; you may need to ask about the precise implications of the terms used in your area. The qualifications and experience of teachers fulfilling these roles vary considerably; some are specialists with significant post-graduate training, and others may have limited additional training in special education beyond basic teacher training.

- *School-team meeting* or *team staffing* refers to an opportunity to meet to exchange information, to solve problems, and to make plans for a child who is experiencing difficulties. Ideally parents will also attend. Acronyms include DART for "diagnostic and review team," IPRC for "identification placement and review committee," or IPP meeting. Physicians and other consultants may be invited. The physician must distinguish between informal problem-solving gatherings and meetings, like the IPRC in Ontario, that are statutory hearings held under specific legislation with specific rules and appeal procedures.

- *School records* or *cumulative files* are files that contain the records of each individual student, which most school legislation requires. Access to the file by the parent or student and the right to change or remove information depends upon the jurisdiction. Physicians should not assume that their communications with the school about a student will necessarily be entered or remain in the file. Physicians should also be aware of which staff members have access to these files and any confidential health or family information. These records may be available long after someone has left the school system. Like medical records, school records are considered confidential, but there may also be rules and procedures for obtaining access.

- *Mainstreaming, integration, least restrictive (most enabling, most appropriate) environment, normalization,* and *non-categorical education* refer to approaches to education for students with disabilities. (See the Glossary for more information.)

- *Whole language, whole word, phonics, visual-auditory-kinaesthetic-tactile (VAKT), and multisensory approach* are different ways of teaching reading. (See the Glossary for more information.)

CONTROVERSIES IN EDUCATION

The field of education and its approach to children experiencing difficulty has evolved and changed over time. Change is often based on evolving philosophical and moral beliefs. Whether these changes are progressive and improve performance and outcomes or lead to negative results is sometimes discovered after fairly long periods of time. Discussion of change can be passionate, polarizing, and based on the beliefs that are prominent at a given point in time. The following is a discussion of some of the current controversies in the field of education.

Inclusion/Integration

In many developed and developing nations, the second half of the twentieth century saw the acceptance, as a moral proposition and as a political reality, of the right of persons with disabilities to an educational system that, at the least, should not contribute to their handicap. At best, the system graduates them on equal terms with their "normal" or typically developing peers into a society free of prejudice. There is ongoing debate about the degree of inclusion (the presence of students with disabilities in the regular classroom), the means of its implementation, and the availability of staff and financial resources to make this approach an improvement on the past. Governments in Canada and all over the world have recognized the moral justice of inclusion, but sometimes without allocating the resources necessary to lead to success for the individual student.

It can be quite challenging if there is no provision for segregated services where this may be in the best interests of the child. Special education that responds to individual differences must consist of a spectrum of services(3), which can include the following:

- Regular experience—placement in the regular classroom with use of special equipment or assistance, with specific curriculum modifications.

- Lesser or greater periods of withdrawal from the regular classroom—for small group instruction, one-on-one instruction, therapy, special programs with more or less integration in areas of strength, or for socialization.
- Full-time placement in a special class or school.

Philosophical beliefs promoting the education of most, if not all, children within a regular classroom in their neighbourhood school originate from two sources. The field of intellectual disability gave birth to the normalization, inclusion, and community living movements, stressing societal integration of those with cognitive impairment as a human rights issue. The complementary belief that most children, particularly those with "mild" disabilities such as LDs, will learn more from good teaching in regular classes than in segregated settings originated within the field of education. This position promotes the view that many LD problems are the result of normal variation in learning style, poor teaching, or environmental stresses. It emphasizes a non-categorical approach in which the commonalities among children—rather than the differences imposed by impairments—are salient. There is experimental support for the non-categorical approach, but there is little research evidence to support one classroom setting over another for specific conditions. Children do imitate other children, and there is evidence that behaviour classes can lead to more, rather than less, deviant behaviour. Finally, most provinces in Canada have as a legislated principle that education will be provided in the least restrictive setting.

The learning process

Another source of conflicting views is the nature of the learning process. One view suggests that children must "learn how to learn" and that developing this cognitive process is the true objective of education. According to this view, the learning experience generates satisfaction and further motivation to learn. A variety of experience is intended to provide the child with opportunities to learn concepts and skills. The actual specific competence gained is of less concern than the enjoyment of the learning experience that leads to the desire to do and learn more. The contrary view is that children must learn specific skills that form the foundation for the development of knowledge and skills. To build this foundation requires specific instruction and practice of prerequisite skills, such as following a specific phonetic reading program. As noted in the response to intervention (see Chapter 1), children falling behind need and respond to a direct structured approach to reading instruction.

Coaching the regular teacher versus using special education staff

There is controversy over the role of the regular teacher compared with the special education teacher in assisting children with learning problems.(4)(5) In the educational literature, terms such as LD are often referred to as a "mild handicap or disability." Some believe that many children so identified are affected by other contributing factors—social, emotional, physical, and nutritional—that contribute significantly to their underachievement. This view holds that most of their educational needs can be handled within a regular classroom with regular programs. The opposing view is that children with learning problems have an inferred neurological difference or impairment that prevents them from being able to develop skills with the usual instructional techniques, and that they need an individualized assessment and program, often delivered in a special education environment by a special education teacher. Teachers and paraprofessionals can be trained in early intervention, and there is evidence that they can effectively deliver these interventions. There is emerging evaluation of using computer-based programs to build skills, which can reduce the costs of intervention and can extend to the home environment.

SUMMARY

By the time family members appear in a physician's office, they may be quite upset by their experiences interacting with school personnel and their attempts to get help for their child. They may be frustrated at the lack of resources and the length of time it takes to access available support while agreeing that there are quite reasonable issues that need to be addressed. Avoid taking sides. Start out by finding out as much as you can about the child's difficulties and the school's resources. Be aware that it can be just as difficult for a physician to effect change within the educational system as it is for families. You will need to build relationships with the child's education team for optimal outcomes and may serve a bridging role between family and school. The following observations may be useful in effective collaboration with educational systems:

- Respect the expertise of educators as professionals. When interacting with educators, it is most useful to start by asking the teacher's view of the problem. This assists you in understanding the issue from an educator's perspective. School staff will also let you know what resources are available so that the interventions suggested have a good chance of being implemented. There is no point in making recommendations that cannot be put in place, and such promises may create unreasonable expectations.

- When a child is experiencing difficulty, it is tempting to blame someone for the problem. The physician can be very helpful in shifting the focus from blame to a careful description of the child's difficulties and what may be done about them, leading to possible win-win solutions.

- Some may see the physician as an outsider to the educational system. Regular interaction with schools can help shift your role from outsider to an integral member of the special education team. An atmosphere of collaboration and mutual respect increases the probability that the medical perspective will be heard and recommendations attempted.

- Physicians (and parents) must remember that their goal is the best interests of an individual child, whereas both the classroom teacher and the principal have to consider the needs of groups of children with many different needs competing for the same pool of resources. Individual school personnel are not responsible for systems issues such as under-resourcing. Most principals and teachers truly want the best for each of their students, and are just as concerned as doctors (and parents) that they do not have the resources they need to teach all children. Understanding this is critical to school-physician collaboration.

Dealing with systems issues falls in the political realm and is best addressed by advocacy. Physician opinion and participation are valued, whether regarding an individual child or advising about educational policies at the local level.

Developing positive relationships with schools can lead to meaningful participation of physicians in special education planning, benefiting not only the individual child but also populations of children with similar difficulties and needs. The physician can be very helpful in supporting change by working with government policy personnel and/or advocacy groups such as local learning disability associations. Suggestions for specific resources for each province/territory are in Chapter 5.

REFERENCES

1. Vaughn S, Klingner JK. Students' perceptions of inclusion and resource room settings. J Spec Educ 1998; 32: 79–88.

2. Zigmond N. Where should students with disabilities receive special education? Is one place better than another? In: Cook B, Shermer B, eds. What Is Special about Special Education? Austin, TX: Pro-Ed, 2006: 27–136.

3. Walker DK, Palfrey JS, Handley-Derry M, et al. Mainstreaming children with handicaps: Implications for pediatricians. J Dev Behav Pediatr 1989; 10: 151–6.

4. Hocutt AM. Effectiveness of special education: Is placement the critical factor? Future Child 1996; 6(1): 77–102.

5. Trent S. Much to do about nothing: A clarification of issues on the regular education initiative. J Learn Disabil 1989; 22: 23–5.

3

Early Development of the Nervous System and School Performance

Janet Kawchuk and Sarah Shea

Brain development from conception until six years of age is a critical factor in the subsequent educational and social success of children. The typically developing infant, toddler, and preschooler have predictable patterns of skill acquisition, reflecting both genetic and environmental influences. In this chapter we will review what is known about the development of the brain and nervous system and factors that impact that developmental process that could subsequently affect school performance.

BRAIN DEVELOPMENT IN UTERO

Neurolation, the process of neural tube formation from the neural plate, occurs in early fetal development. Disruption of this process leads to neural tube defects. The neural tube closes by the twenty-sixth day post-conception.

At week five, the forebrain divides into the telencephalon and the diencephalon. Development of the cerebral cortex requires the following processes, which overlap in time with one another:

- **Cell proliferation:** The undifferentiated precursor cells of the telencephalon divide to form neuroblasts in the ventricular neuroepithelium and the subventricular zones. Proliferation abnormalities may result in microcephaly or megalencephaly.
- **Neuronal migration:** This peaks during weeks twelve to twenty-four. Neuroblasts from the periventricular neuroepithelium are guided to migrate outwards along radial glial fibres, forming the six layers of the neocortex from the inner to outer portions. The newer layers are therefore more superficial. This process is influenced by molecules that signal and guide migration, and

others that signal the neurons to stop migrating. Neurons are organized in many vertical columns extending through all six layers, with horizontal connections between columns. The neurons in the different layers within a column have similar properties. Although the right and left hemispheres are forming by week five, sulci don't develop until week twenty-four. Migration abnormalities include:

- Disorders of initiation of neuronal migration, which can result in periventricular heterotopia.
- Disorders of migration to form the six layers. One mechanism for the genetic control of neuronal migration has been linked to a gene REELIN (RELN). Those who lack REELIN protein develop *lissencephaly* (see the Glossary) and cerebellar hypoplasia.(1)(2)
- Disorders of cessation of migration, which can result in cobblestone lissencephaly.
- **Cortical organization:** This occurs once neurons reach their destination. An example of an abnormal cortical organization is polymicrogyria (small gyri, excessive in number, and with underdeveloped sulci). In addition to the development of dendrites, ongoing processes include maturation of neurons, synaptogenesis, pruning of synapses, and neuronal apoptosis. These processes continue postnatally, as discussed later in this chapter.

BRAIN DEVELOPMENT AND THE ORIGIN OF LEARNING DIFFICULTIES

Advances in neuroscience and genetics provide increasing evidence for underlying mechanisms resulting in learning difficulties in children. Genetic conditions can predispose children to both generalized and specific learning impairments. Neuroscience provides strong evidence that disruptions during critical periods of in utero development may alter central nervous system (CNS) development. Teratogens affect proliferating cells and will therefore affect those neurons actively proliferating at the time of the exposure. In addition, the learning and social environments to which a young child is exposed affect his or her behaviour, development, and interactions with others. Knowing the factors contributing to children's learning difficulties can assist with early identification of risk, demystification for families, optimization of intervention, and, in some cases, primary and secondary prevention.

Genetic factors and learning difficulties

Many genetic disorders are associated with intellectual disabilities or learning disabilities. Examples include Down syndrome, 22q11.2 deletion syndrome, Prader-Willi and Angelman syndromes, Williams syndrome, and Turner syndrome. In some cases there is quite a lot known about the neurobiologic impacts of the genetic condition. The brains of individuals with Down syndrome, for example, are known to demonstrate hypocellularity, fewer dendrites, and disproportionately small hippocampi, as well as early neuronal death and development of fibrillary tangles.

Fragile X syndrome is another genetic disorder for which the mechanism of brain dysfunction has been described. The methylation of the FMR1 gene blocks the production of FMR protein, which results in weak synaptic connections during brain development. Affected males most commonly have an intellectual disability, and may also have an autism spectrum disorder. Affected females may have an intellectual disability, but frequently show a specific learning disability profile. ADHD is also found in many people with fragile X syndrome.

The recent availability of array-based CGH (comparative genomic hybridization—see Glossary), which detects copy-number variants across the entire genome, is increasing the identification of microdeletions and/or duplications associated with learning problems. Current guidelines support using this as an initial investigation of patients with intellectual disability or autism spectrum disorder, instead of G-banded karyotype analysis. However, genetic investigation is not yet recommended for children with specific learning disabilities without phenotypic features suggesting a specific syndrome.

A child with a learning disability often has a similarly affected parent and/or sibling, and genetic linkage studies are starting to identify risk loci for heritable factors. But this work is at an early stage, and not yet clinically applicable.

Early identification of genetic disorders and genetic counselling may modify the risk for subsequent siblings of an affected child. Moreover, research into genetic disorders and how their effects are mediated is progressing at a rapid pace and increasingly contributes to our understanding of neurobiological processes. It is hoped that this will lead to the development of biologic interventions for some of the conditions affecting learning.

DISRUPTIONS IN CNS DEVELOPMENT— CRITICAL PERIODS IN UTERO

The following are examples of disruptions in CNS development:

- **Fetal alcohol spectrum disorders (FASD):** Alcohol is teratogenic throughout pregnancy. Exposure at any stage may result in the neurodevelopmental impairments of FASD even if the phenotypic features of fetal alcohol syndrome (FAS) are absent. CNS effects can include ADHD, intellectual disability, and learning disability. Maternal alcohol use in the first trimester can result in the phenotypic facial features of FAS. In the second trimester, in utero alcohol exposure affects neuronal migration, resulting in heterotopias. Third-trimester exposure affects neuronal growth and maturation. These risks can be eliminated with alcohol abstinence during pregnancy and modified by reduction of alcohol use and improved prenatal health.
- **Maternal cigarette smoking:** Smoking during pregnancy can result in intrauterine growth restriction (IUGR) and premature labour, with their associated risk of co-morbidities.

Smoking has also been linked in some studies to an increased risk of attention deficit hyperactivity disorder, although there are often other confounding factors.(3) Smoking cessation supports for the pregnant mother are important to modify these risks.

- **Maternal illicit substance use:** Limited studies on isolated cannabis use suggest an increased risk in offspring of ADHD and learning difficulties, especially impaired memory and possibly visual-spatial skills. Prenatal cocaine exposure is associated with an increased risk for deficits in working memory and visual-spatial skills. Exposed children adopted or placed in other stimulating care settings have better outcomes, indicating the significant mediating benefit of a nurturing environment.(4) Toluene embryopathy results from inhalant abuse in pregnancy. Affected children, often born prematurely with low birth weight, have microcephaly and craniofacial abnormalities. Deficits in speech, motor, and cognitive skills are reported.

- **Methylmercury:** Methylmercury has been shown in animal models to disrupt mitosis, which reduces neuron numbers. Neuronal migration is also affected. In utero exposure is more neurotoxic than exposure in childhood, and can result in impairment of cognition, memory, attention, language, and fine motor development. The most common source of methylmercury exposure at present is from fish consumption. Current recommendations are to limit maternal intake of fish during pregnancy, as well as fish intake in young children, especially for fish known to have higher mercury levels.

- **Pesticides:** In utero exposure to pesticides affects synaptogenesis.

- **Prescription teratogens:** Management of maternal disease may require medications found to be teratogenic. Maternal use of phenobarbital, hydantoin, retinoic acid, and valproic acid have effects on the CNS which may result in learning difficulties in the child. Genetics may play a role with some of these teratogenic effects. (More information on specific medications can be found on Health Canada's website at www.hc-sc.gc.ca or the Motherisk website at www.motherisk.org.)

- **Maternal disease:** Active lupus (SLE) with the presence of anti-Ro/La antibodies during pregnancy has been associated with an increased risk of learning disabilities in male offspring.(5) Uncontrolled maternal phenylkentonuria (PKU) during pregnancy can cause intellectual disability and microcephaly in the child. Low T4 levels in early pregnancy due to maternal hypothyroidism have been associated with an increased risk of cognitive impairment.

- **Neural tube defects:** The use of folate supplements has significantly reduced the number of new cases of neural tube defects, with their associated learning difficulties. The use of higher amounts of folate for the month prior to conception with continued use during the first trimester also significantly reduces the recurrence risk for subsequent pregnancies in families with an affected child.

- **Poor maternal nutrition:** In the second and third trimesters of pregnancy, this may result in fewer neurons with poor maturation. Postnatal malnutrition (for the first twenty-four months) affects myelination.

- **Congenital infections:** Many of these result in impaired neuronal cell growth and cell necrosis. Even in the absence of severe neurological sequelae, the affected child is at risk for developmental disorders. Learning difficulties can be exacerbated by hearing loss, which is associated with some of these infections:
  - Congenital rubella is infrequently seen in North America due to the effectiveness of vaccination. Affected children are at risk for hearing loss and developmental disorders.
  - Toxoplasmosis is associated with seizures, hydrocephalus, and developmental delay; therefore, pregnant women should avoid exposure to soiled kitty litter.
  - Primary cytomegalovirus (CMV) infection is associated with microcephaly, hearing impairment, and delayed development. Good hand washing, especially around young children, is important to prevent infection in previously unaffected pregnant women.

- HIV can present with spasticity, developmental delays, and subacute encephalopathy. Improved obstetrical care, including testing for HIV and management in the perinatal period, can help prevent mother-to-child transmission of HIV.

THE NEWBORN PERIOD

Most neuron production has taken place by birth, and very few neurons develop in the mature brain. Brain plasticity is most prominent in the developing brain. Postnatally, the cortex rapidly increases in size due to increasing dendritic growth and overproduction of synapses during the first two years after birth. Neurodevelopment is influenced by activity/use patterns and early sensory experiences, especially during specific sensitive periods. Apoptosis of excess neurons takes place, and synaptic pruning reduces unused synaptic connections. Myelination is an important ongoing process in the third and fourth years of life, and is not complete in the prefrontal cortex until the adolescent years. Below is a list of some of the conditions affecting newborns that may result in learning difficulties:

- Prematurity, intrauterine growth restriction, and their many complications (hypoxia, CNS infection, sepsis, shock, CNS bleeding, sensory deficits, iron deficiency anemia, etc.)
- Extremely low birth weight and very low birth weight
- Hypoxic-ischemic encephalopathy in term neonates (neonatal encephalopathy)
- Hypoglycemia

- Metabolic disorders: Neonatal screening has improved outcomes for many metabolic disorders. When PKU dietary recommendations are closely followed, affected children typically have normal IQ levels.
- Endocrine conditions: Congenital hypothyroidism is usually associated with normal cognitive abilities with early diagnosis via neonatal screening, early treatment, and good control for the first three years of life. A small percentage of affected children have academic challenges. High-risk groups include those with thyroid agenesis and more severe disease, especially those with very low T4 levels and delayed bone age at birth, as well those with delayed diagnosis and later onset of treatment.
- Neonatal bacterial meningitis: Approximately 25% have developmental delays. See the discussion to follow on viral CNS infections.

ACQUIRED BIOLOGIC CHILDHOOD FACTORS

Children without the previously mentioned risk factors (Table 3–1) may acquire brain dysfunction resulting in learning difficulties through a number of different mechanisms. These are discussed below, and are summarized in Table 3–2.

- Infectious:
  - **Viral meningitis:** Most childhood viral meningitis is not associated with an increased risk of learning disorders. Studies have been inconsistent regarding the long-term developmental sequelae for enterovirus meningitis in neonates and young infants.

Table 3–1 Early Risks for Learning Difficulties (Intellectual Disability, Specific Learning Disability, ADHD)

Genetic factors	In utero risks	Newborn complications
• positive family history of ADHD or specific learning disability • recognized genetic disorders	• teratogen exposure • maternal substance use • environmental exposures • maternal disease and disease treatment • poor maternal nutrition during pregnancy, or low folate intake • congenital infections	• complications of prematurity and low birth weight • neonatal encephalopathy • hypoglycemia • endocrine and metabolic disorders • bacterial and viral meningitis and viral encephalitis

- **Viral encephalitis:** Neurologic outcomes are worse for children less than five years old; those with seizures, focal signs, or coma at presentation; the need for ICU admission; and herpes simplex virus (HSV) encephalitis, especially in the neonate. In a study of ninety-three children treated for acute encephalitis in Sweden, the most common persisting conditions at discharge were cognitive difficulties, including concentration problems and memory loss in twelve patients.(6) Neonatal western equine encephalitis has significant long-term morbidity, with 50% of those affected having motor or cognitive disabilities.

- **Bacterial meningitis:** Intellectual disability has been reported in approximately 4% of children following bacterial meningitis. A systematic literature search published recently of 1,433 children who survived childhood bacterial meningitis reported that 49.2% had one or more long-term sequelae, and of these, 45% were behavioural and/or intellectual and academic disorders.(7) Sensorineural hearing loss is a complication of bacterial meningitis in 11% of children.

- **CNS tumour:** Educational outcomes for children with brain tumours are often good, with reports of some mild school difficulties. A nationwide register-based study in Finland assessed the educational outcome of 300 children with brain tumours compared to population controls. Only 6% of the children with brain tumour failed to finish their comprehensive school (Grade 9) at the usual age. The brain tumour group had lower averages overall for all academic subjects, and especially for foreign languages. In girls, this was independent of age of diagnosis and cranial irradiation, but boys with cranial radiation at school age had poorer outcomes.(8)

- **Childhood cancer survivors:** A multicentre Canadian study using parental reporting of 800 paediatric cancer survivors reported grade repetition in 21% of cancer survivors compared to 8.5% controls. In addition, 46% of the cancer survivors were reported to have academic difficulties compared to 23% in the control group. Those who received cranial radiation therapy alone or with intrathecal methotrexate had higher reports of academic difficulties than the cancer survivors who did not require these treatments.(9)

- **Hypoxia:** Severe hypoxic events in children (such as choking, strangulation, or near drowning) can result in long-term neurologic sequelae, including coma, seizures, neuro-motor symptoms, cognitive impairment, and behavioural disturbances, including ADHD.

- **Traumatic brain injury (TBI)—accidental and non-accidental:** In children less than two years of age, a common cause of TBI is child abuse. Preschoolers, older children, and youth more typically have accidental trauma as the cause, such as falls, sports injuries, and motor vehicle accidents. In one report, children with moderate to severe TBI acquired before six years of age demonstrated persistent academic impairment at an average of 5.7 years following the TBI, regardless of the cause. And 48% of the children failed a grade or required special education support, and they had an eighteen times greater risk of impaired academic performance compared to the control group. They did not demonstrate improvement over time in lessening the performance gap.(10) Other studies have demonstrated that, in addition to academic impairments, TBI in young children may have a long-term negative impact on executive function and social competence.(11)(12) Helmets reduce head injuries in many sports, including bicycle riding, football, hockey, skiing, and snowboarding. Compliance is more successful when helmet use is legislated.

- **Iron deficiency anemia:** Numerous studies have documented cognitive and behavioural impairment with iron deficiency anemia in early childhood, which persists even after the anemia is corrected. This is thought to be related to changes in neurotransmitters, organization and morphology of neuronal networks, and neurobiology of myelination.(13)(14) Iron deficiency in adolescent girls affects attention, learning, and verbal memory, with more impairment with more severe deficiency. These improve with iron replacement.(15)(16)

- **Environmental exposures (lead poisoning):** Young children, with their incomplete blood-brain barrier formation, are at increased risk for CNS damage due to elevated lead levels. Typically, lead toxicity results from ingestion; therefore, younger children with frequent mouthing behaviours or older children with pica are at risk. Inhalation is another potential source, often due to renovations of older homes containing lead paint, which can generate lead-containing dust. Lead poisoning may result in hearing loss in addition to learning and behaviour problems in children. Canfield et al. showed that blood lead concentrations below 0.483 micromol/L (=10 micrograms/dl, the suggested level for public health activation by the Centers for Disease Control and Prevention) are inversely associated with IQ scores at three and five years of age.(17) CNS dysfunctions often persist even when the lead levels return to normal. Removal of lead from gasoline and paint products, as well as improved public awareness, and public notification and recall of toys and other objects found to contain lead, have been effective in decreasing lead poisoning.
- **Mercury:** See the previous discussion for methylmercury (see page 21). Poisoning in older children and adolescents may result in impaired peripheral vision, and impairment of motor and speech coordination, as is seen in adults. Note: Thimerosol contains ethylmercury, a form which is broken down and excreted rapidly. There is no evidence of health problems arising from the small amount used in vaccines.

CHILDHOOD SOCIAL FACTORS

The social environment of a child plays an important role in their development, behaviour, and subsequent learning patterns. These influences start with infant/caregiver bonding and attachment, and respond to the stimulation from both their physical environment and from those who interact with them. Temperament is discussed in the next chapter.

Neglect and lack of stimulation

As noted above, neurodevelopment occurs under the influence of the environment and experiences to which the child is exposed. Extreme cases of neglect may result in marked delays in all aspects of development and even an autistic-like pattern of social withdrawal and self-stimulatory behaviour, as was seen in the past for children raised in severely suboptimal orphanages. Children who spend less time in the neglectful situation and are younger at the time of adoption have better outcomes. Behaviour and learning typically improve once a child is living in a stimulating, stable, and supportive home for two years, but cognitive impairment, attention difficulties, and learning disabilities are frequent ongoing problems. A more common condition resulting in lack of stimulation is maternal depression. This is associated with dysregulation of attention and arousal in the infant, and increases the risk for poorer cognitive function in children, particularly boys.(18)

Attachment

Attachment, as described by John Bowlby(19), is the relationship between the child and caregiver, which influences relationships, emotional security within the family, the development of friendships with peers, and the capacity to function within groups. It is dependent on maternal and infant factors. Attachment starts with early bonding during pregnancy and immediately after birth. It continues as infants elicit parental attention with vocalizations, eye contact, smiles, and laughter, or with distress signals by crying. When caregivers can correctly interpret these signals, the predictable source of support allows some control for the infant. This *secure attachment* promotes self-organization for the infant, and allows predictable expectations at times of stress. This eventually develops into self-regulation and coping skills, which are imprinted in the right hemisphere of the brain. Each separation increases the child's self-confidence and feeling of competence. Adverse experiences, however, such as repeated traumatic hospitalizations, family breakup, or parental death—perpetuate insecurity and separation anxiety.

Tolerance of separation also depends upon the availability of other attachment figures, the nature

Table 3–2 Childhood Risks for Learning Difficulties (Excluding Children with Major Malformations/ Dysmorphisms, or Major Neurologic or Sensory Disorders)

Acquired biologic childhood factors	Childhood social factors
• bacterial meningitis and viral encephalitis	• neglect and lack of stimulation
• CNS tumours and cancer survival	• attachment disorders
• hypoxic events	• low socio-economic status and low parental education levels
• traumatic brain injury	
• nutritional deficiency	
• environmental exposures	

and duration of the separation, and the presence of other stresses. The extent to which the child has been prepared for the separation and the child's temperament (see Chapter 4) also play important roles. In later childhood, those with secure attachment tend to form secure attachments with their peers and develop more cooperative peer interactions.

Some patterns of attachment behaviour are more likely to be associated with adverse developmental outcomes. If signals are ignored, misinterpreted, or result in unpredictable responses, the child develops mistrust. In the *ambivalent-resistant attachment* pattern, this may result in more demanding responses from the child, which in turn may create parental anxiety, stress, or even hostility (i.e., abuse). Often the timing is off, so that the contact depends more on parental factors than on the child's cues. This teaches the child that others are unreliable, and that he or she has little ability to influence events, which may undermine the child's emerging sense of competence and control.

Other children have *avoidant attachment*, and rarely cry. Often negative feelings are internalized, leading to a poor self-image and self-esteem. Neuroscience has shown that these latter two attachment patterns can result in right-brain dysfunction and are associated with more difficulty handling peer interactions in later years.

Disorganized/disoriented attachment describes children who may not make direct eye contact, and seem uncertain about the response they will receive, although they are happy when they are reunited with their parent. Hyper-vigilance and hyper-reactive arousal states have been described in which, in addition to dysregulation of the CNS, catecholamine

function may be impaired. This pattern has been identified with maternal depression or substance abuse, and is thought to relate to mixed messages from mother to child. Psychomotor Development Index and Mental Development Index scores on the Bayley Scales of Infant Development for a group of internationally adopted infants (adopted prior to their first birthday) were lower in those with a disorganized attachment pattern compared to those without this attachment pattern. This short-term assessment took place after adjustment to their adoptive home.(20) Longer-term studies indicate difficulty with social adaptation related to attachment issues rather than specific academic impairments.

SUMMARY

Multiple genetic and environmental factors have been identified as risk factors for learning dysfunction. Many can be detected long before school entry, while others will be diagnosed only when the child experiences academic difficulties. Children have higher risks if multiple factors are present. Some risks can be eliminated or modified, but others have no current preventive measures. In general, a supportive and stimulating home environment rich with language and literacy exposure, as well as higher socio-economic status and higher parental education levels, mitigate some of these risks.

School success is founded upon skills in many different domains, the early acquisition of which is discussed in Chapter 4. Early identification of the discussed risk factors and active surveillance of all children to identify developmental lags and/or atypical development are important to maximizing opportunities to intervene in the critical early years. Deviations from the expected skill acquisition rate or pattern are most reliably detected using developmental surveillance and/or screening tools, followed by developmental assessment when indicated. Identification of early developmental differences will allow for identification of risk factors and targeted intervention, and should lead to better outcomes.

RESOURCES

Canadian Paediatric Society, First Nations, Inuit, and Métis Health Committee. Fetal Alcohol Spectrum Disorder (Principal authors: Godel J, Schröter H). Paediatr Child Health 2002; 7(3): 161–74 (Addendum 2010). <www.cps.ca>

Canadian Paediatric Society, First Nations, Inuit and Métis Health Committee. Inhalant abuse (Principal author: Baydala L). Paediatr Child Health 2010; 15(7): 443–8. <www.cps.ca>

Canadian Paediatric Society, Infectious Diseases and Immunization Committee. Prevention of congenital rubella syndrome (Principal author: Robinson JL). Paediatr Child Health 2007; 12(9): 795–97. <www.cps.ca>

Canadian Paediatric Society, Infectious Diseases and Immunization Committee. Testing for HIV infection in pregnancy (Principal author: Robinson JL). Paediatr Child Health 2008; 13(3): 221–4.

Health Canada. Lead and human health. <www.hc-sc. gc.ca/hl-vs/iyh-vsv/environ/lead-plomb-eng.php> (Version current at April 4, 2012.)

Health Canada. Mercury in fish: Consumption advice; Making informed choices about fish. <www.hc-sc. gc.ca/fn-an/securit/chem-chim/environ/mercur/cons-adv-etud-eng.php> (Version current at April 4, 2012.)

REFERENCES

1. Gressens P. Pathogenesis of migration disorders. Curr Opin Neurol 2006; 19(2): 135–40.
2. Hong SE, et al. Autosomal recessive lissencephaly with cerebellar hypoplasia is associated with human RELN mutations. Nat Genet 2000; 26(1): 93–6.
3. Linnet KM, et al. Maternal lifestyle factors in pregnancy risk of attention deficit hyperactivity disorder and associated behaviors: Review of the current evidence. Am J Psychiatry 2003; 160(6): 1028–40.
4. Singer LT, et al. Cognitive outcomes of preschool children with prenatal cocaine exposure. JAMA 2004; 291(20): 2448–56.
5. Ross G, et al. Effects of mothers' autoimmune disease during pregnancy on learning disabilities and hand preference in their children. Arch Pediatr Adolesc Med 2003; 157(4): 397–402.
6. Fowler A, Stödberg T, Eriksson M, Wickström R. Childhood encephalitis in Sweden: Etiology, clinical presentation and outcome. Eur J Paediatr Neurol 2008; 12(6): 484–90.
7. Chandran A, Herbert H, Misurski D, Santosham M. Long-term sequelae of childhood bacterial meningitis: An underappreciated problem. Pediatr Infect Dis J 2011; 30(1): 3–6.
8. Lähteenmäki PM, Harila-Saari A, Pukkala EI, Kyyrönen P, Salmi TT, Sankila R. Scholastic achievements of children with brain tumors at the end of compressive education: A nationwide, register-based study. Neurology 2007; 69(3): 296–305.
9. Barrera M, Shaw AK, Speechley KN, Maunsell E, Pogany L. Educational and social late effects of childhood cancer and related clinical, personal, and familial characteristics. Cancer 2005; 104(8): 1751–60.
10. Ewing-Cobbs L, et al. Late intellectual and academic outcomes following traumatic brain injury sustained during early childhood. J Neurosurg 2006; 105(4 Suppl): 287–96.
11. Ganesalingam K, Yeates KO, Taylor HG, Walz NC, Stancin T, Wade S. Executive functions and social competence in young children 6 months following traumatic brain injury. Neuropsychology 2011; 25(4): 466–76.
12. Yeates KO, et al. Social outcomes in childhood brain disorder: A heuristic integration of social neuroscience and developmental psychology. Psychol Bull 2007; 133(3): 535–56.
13. Beard J. Iron deficiency alters brain development and functioning. J Nutr 2003; 133 (5 Suppl 1): 1468S–72S.
14. Grantham-McGregor S, Ani C. A review of studies on the effect of iron deficiency on cognitive development in children. J Nutr 2001; 131(2S-2): 649S–68S.
15. Bruner AB, Joffe A, Duggan AK, Casella JF, Brandt J. Randomised study of cognitive effects of iron supplementation in non-anaemic iron-deficient adolescent girls. Lancet 1996; 384(9033): 992–6.

16. Murray-Kolb LE, Beard JL. Iron treatment normalizes cognitive functioning in young women. Am J Clin Nutr 2007; 85(3): 778–87.

17. Canfield RL, Henderson CR Jr, Cory-Slechta DA, Cox C, Jusko TA, Lanphear BP. Intellectual impairment in children with blood lead concentrations below 10 microg per deciliter. New Engl J Med 2003; 348(16): 1517–26.

18. Canadian Paediatric Society, Psychosocial Paediatrics Committee. Maternal depression and child development (Principal author: Bernard-Bonnin AC). Paediatr Child Health 2004; 9(8): 575–83. <www.cps.ca>

19. Bowlby J. Attachment and Loss. London: The Hogarth Press and Institute of Psycho-analysis, 1940; Vol 1.

20. van Londen WM, Juffer F, van Ijzendoorn MH. Attachment, cognitive, and motor development in adopted children: Short-term outcomes after international adoption. J Pediatr Psychol 2007; 32(10): 1249–58.

4

Development and School Entry

Sarah Shea and Janet Kawchuk

Knowledge of typical early development, along with familiarity with the expectations for learning in the first year of school and predictors of success, can be helpful in assessing children's school performance difficulties. In this chapter we review the concept of readiness for school entry and the important developmental attainments that are needed to support a successful transition to formal education.

SCHOOL READINESS

The construct of school readiness is used by educators, policy makers, parents, and professionals who work with children. At the time of school entry, a *readiness framework* (i.e., examining whether cognitive, physical, social, emotional, behavioural, and experiential development matches that associated with good school performance) can be used to assess the profile of an individual child, or groups of children. In the past, school entry screening tests were designed to identify individuals who were not "ready" for traditional school enrolment and therefore in need of special developmental programs. That practice has been largely abandoned, and the concept of school readiness has adjusted to place the emphasis on the readying. Knowledge of the skills and attributes known to contribute to success in school can be used to guide efforts to optimize children's early experiences. It is not just children who need to be readied; families and communities need to be readied for their children to succeed, and schools themselves need to be ready to meet the needs of children.

Reflecting on school readiness at the individual level by comparing a child's developmental profile to the typical expectations for school entry can assist in preparing the child, family, and receiving school. It may also identify factors that contribute to a child's difficulty in the first year of school. In some cases, consideration of the child's developmental "readiness" may be helpful in making decisions about school entry versus opting for an alternate educational setting, with or without deferral.

AGE OF ENTRY

The age of eligibility for school entry is generally determined provincially, although some school boards and independent schools have their own rules. Each province also decides whether junior kindergarten and/or kindergarten (or their equivalents) will be universal publicly funded programs. Some areas offer public preparatory programs only for higher-risk populations for the year prior to typical school entry. The most common cut-off birthdate for entry for the first year of "school" is December 31. There is uncertainty about the ideal age for entry, as is reflected in the fact that Canadian provinces have different age cut-off dates for entry. Most Canadian children start into a senior kindergarten (primary) program between the age of four years, six months and the age of five years, eight months.

The age of its students during the first year will logically influence a school's curriculum and expectations, and there should be flexibility in view of the wide age range of students within an early elementary classroom. Nonetheless, a child's age at the time of school entry is itself one of the many factors that may influence early school performance. Younger students as a group statistically lag somewhat behind their older peers on measures of academic achievement. The youngest students also have an increased risk of being identified as having school performance difficulty. Research looking at longer-term birthdate effects is somewhat limited and is mixed in its conclusions. Some studies have indicated that achievement differences in students who are born later versus those born earlier can still be identified in the junior high age range, whereas others have concluded that the birthdate effect on academic achievement disappears by the mid-elementary years.(1)(2)

Research on birthdate effects has been largely retrospective, and there are often many variables that make the results hard to interpret. More recently, for example, parents in affluent communities have been the ones more likely to defer school entry. Those children as a group would be predicted to have better school outcomes based on factors other than age.

There is also concern that late enrolment—or, for that matter, early enrolment for a child perceived as "ready" ahead of peers—may later be a disadvantage to some children socially and behaviourally when they are adolescents and out of sync with their peer group, especially with respect to pubertal development.(3) Educational research does not suggest that acceleration is socially harmful to gifted children, and it may, in fact, be associated with better academic and emotional outcomes.(4) Very little research has looked at the issue of age of enrolment for children identified as having developmental concerns or lack of "readiness" prior to school entry. There is certainly a strong argument in favour of getting the child from a suboptimal home or childcare setting into school rather than deferring and maintaining exposure to a disadvantaging environment. Children at risk can also improve their skills in a high-quality preschool program, and some children in a good preschool setting may thrive better in that environment than in formalized schooling. Funding issues may dictate a child's options. A child's readiness for school appears to be a stronger predictor of success than age among higher-risk children, which argues in favour of early intervention and good preparation prior to school entry.

TYPICAL PRESCHOOL LEARNING AND SKILLS PRESENT AT THE TIME OF SCHOOL ENTRY

Senior kindergarten (primary) is typically a blend of structured and unstructured activities with a progressive increase in the focus on early academic skill development over the school year, including reading, math, and printing. A review of senior kindergarten curricula from representative provinces reveals common expected outcomes for numeracy and literacy, as shown in the following lists:

Typical literacy skills developed during the kindergarten/primary year
- listening to stories
- discussing stories
- rhyming
- naming and printing letters
- recognizing some high-frequency words in print
- using letter-sound correspondence to sound out simple words
- printing some words

Typical numeracy skills developed during the kindergarten/primary year
- counting with one-to-one correspondence up to ten
- matching numbers to arrays
- recognizing and making patterns
- comparing objects on length, weight, or volume
- ordering and sorting

Development of visual perceptual and fine motor skills

Children develop an interest in pencil or crayon skills by fifteen to eighteen months, initially using a *fisted grasp*, and often without displaying a clear hand dominance. This matures into a *tripod* (thumb, index, and middle finger) grasp by thirty months, and by four years is a *dynamic tripod grasp* (using only the distal interphalangeal joints for maximal precision and economy of effort). The ability to imitate and later to copy drawing shapes develops in a predictable pattern, as laid out within the Gesell figures and human figure drawing tasks (see Chapter 10). Scissor skills develop at three years of age, and by four to five years, the child cuts out shapes and cuts along lines with accuracy. At this age, children have the dexterity to dress themselves, including fastening buttons, although some may still need help starting a zipper and tying shoelaces. (With the widespread availability of Velcro fastenings, some children may not have yet needed to learn to tie, and the lack of this skill should not be considered a delay unless there has been exposure.) Hand dominance is usually well established by age five.

Typical school-entry fine motor skills
- using scissors well
- employing a dynamic tripod grasp
- doing almost all self-dressing

Development of gross motor skills

Children will usually walk up and down steps while alternating feet by three years of age, which is when they successfully pedal a tricycle. Hopping on one foot emerges at four years of age, and by five to six years of age, children have a reasonable forward tandem gait and can ride a bicycle without training wheels. As with tying shoes, learning to ride a bike requires opportunity to master the skill.

Typical school-entry gross-motor skills
- running
- skipping
- kicking a ball
- playing catch
- balancing
- climbing a slide ladder

Development of language skills

There is considerable variation in the emergence of expressive language skills. Most children have ten or more clear words by eighteen months of age, and are combining words at two years. By thirty months of age, children identify a specific object from a group of objects when they are described by function. An example is choosing scissors when asked, "Which one do we cut with?" Three-year-old children use pronouns, plurals, adjectives, and past tenses. (Note: Late talkers with subsequently normal language skills have normal receptive language skills, and often communicate well with gestures and facial expressions. There is often a family history of other late talkers.)

As a child's language skills continue to increase at a rapid rate, some *dysfluency* (stuttering) may emerge, which is usually temporary. Self-talk or word and phrase repetition are rehearsal strategies used by many children as they develop language. The clarity of a child's speech is typically 25% comprehensible to strangers at two years of age, 50% by three years, and fully by four to five years, although minor developmental articulation errors may still be present.

Typical school-entry language skills:
- speaking 100% intelligibly (with possible sound substitutions)
- communicating in complex, grammatically and syntactically correct sentences
- engaging in appropriately reciprocal conversation
- understanding multipart directions
- defining words by use
- retelling an experience in sequence

Development of cognitive skills

Infants at three months of age use recognition memory to detect familiar stimuli, and they start to pay attention to objects around them. Object permanence develops, which leads to stranger anxiety and separation anxiety in later infancy. Symbolic and imaginative play develops by eighteen months of age, and imitation skills are well developed. Toddlers are egocentric and see things from their own point of view. They recognize sequences and routines, but have no concept of time. By four years of age, children increasingly appreciate the point of view of others. They are able to focus on more than one property of an object, and are therefore able to sort objects by shape and colour, for example. As children progress in school, they may demonstrate learning style preferences and/or strengths. A variety of cognitive styles have been described, including verbal versus nonverbal learners, auditory versus visual versus kinesthetic learners, reflective versus impulsive learners, and convergent or rigid versus divergent or creative learners.

Typical school-entry cognitive skills
- identifying, naming, and sorting by size, shape, and colour
- counting with one-to-one correspondence
- reciting the alphabet
- recognizing some letters and logos
- rhyming

Development of attention skills

Attention skills change over time, but can be observed from birth onward. During their first year, babies attend most to new objects and events, and early on they may have trouble disengaging attention from highly interesting stimuli. Over time they become more able to disengage and transition attention under executive control, and to sustain their attention for longer periods. At around eighteen to twenty-four months, children increase their visual attention and can focus on complex visual displays. Toddlers develop the ability to multi-task with their attention and, for example, can play with multiple toys at once. During the preschool years a higher-level control of attention gives the child the ability to plan ahead, engage in complex activity, and sustain attention when needed, even for less interesting stimuli.(5) These skills develop significantly between the ages of four and six years.

Typical school-entry attention skills
- following directions delivered to the group
- changing tasks as requested
- listening to a speaker
- completing an assigned task in a sustained manner (up to approximately fifteen minutes)

Emotional development and social skills

Social skills develop initially with family and caregivers. In the toddler years, children increasingly develop independent control, often challenging parents with eating, toileting, sleeping, and attention-demanding issues. As preschoolers, they develop self-confidence in these skills, and start to explore and expand relationships beyond the family unit. Two-year-old children engage in parallel play, but as they mature their play becomes more interactive and collaborative, and the preschooler develops the social competence to interact with peers. Cooperative play, sharing, and taking turns are usually present at age three years.

The framework of *temperament*, or innate behavioural style, is helpful in understanding children's emotional development. Each child has an intrinsic set of traits that influence activity level, biological regularity (patterns of sleep, eating, and bowel movements), adaptability, initial approach, emotional intensity, quality of mood, persistence, and distractibility. Children's temperament may affect their initial or longer-term adaptation to people, events, and experiences, including attending school. Children who are "slow to warm up" may, for example, require more active transition support or simply take longer to demonstrate their skills with confidence. "Difficult" children may also need more support as they learn to regulate their tendency to be reactive or negative.

Typical school-entry social skills
- separating comfortably from family for hours at a time
- cooperating and taking turns when playing with peers
- expressing emotions in acceptable ways
- displaying curiosity and enthusiasm about learning

OTHER PREDICTORS OF SUCCESS AT THE TIME OF SCHOOL ENTRY

Beyond looking for the factors that may affect neurobiological development outlined in Chapter 3 and the developmental skill expectations discussed above, one can assess other aspects of a child's profile at the time of school entry to identify elevated risk for subsequent poor school performance.

One study of almost 10,000 schoolchildren used early grade retention as a general proxy for school problems. It reported each of the following factors to be associated with an increased risk of retention:

- poverty
- male gender
- low maternal education
- speech defects

- low birth weight
- enuresis
- exposure to household smoking

These factors were associated with decreased risk of retention:

- high maternal education
- residence with both biologic parents at the age of six years(6)

Also demonstrated to decrease the risk of poor school performance is participation in high-quality early childhood development programs, as noted above.(7)(8)

Literacy development is another predictor of early success in school. Children whose parents read to them, and who begin school with stronger early literacy skills, are more likely to succeed even after controlling for social risk factors. (See Chapter 19 about encouraging reading.) This difference may be lessened by early school programming focused on developing reading.(9)

Finally, it is important to note that this chapter does not address issues of physical health nor of sensory dysfunction and other disabilities, all of which may affect development, expectations, and early school performance.

SUMMARY

Children do not enter school with identical ages, backgrounds, strengths, or needs. Knowing the skills expected at entry and during the first year of formal schooling allows physicians to better advise families and schools and, most importantly, to assist children in accessing intervention early. Physicians can provide critical support through developmental surveillance and by working with families and communities to build a strong foundation for early learning for all children.

REFERENCES

1. Kern M, Friedman HS. Early educational milestones as predictors of lifelong academic achievement, midlife adjustment, and longevity. J Appl Dev Psychology 2008; 30(40): 419–430.
2. Crosser S. He has a summer birthday: The kindergarten entrance age dilemma. ERIC Digest. ED423079 1998-09-00. <www.eric.ed.gov>
3. Byrd RS, Weitzman M, Auinger P. Increased behavior problems associated with delayed school entry and delayed school progress. Pediatrics 1997; 100: 654.
4. Diezmann CM, Watters J, Fox K. Early entry to school in Australia: Rhetoric, research and reality. Australasian Journal for Gifted Education 2001; 10(2): 5–18.
5. van de Weijer-Bergsma E, Wijnroks L, Jongmans MJ. Attention development in infants and preschool children born preterm: A review. Infant Behavior & Development 2008; 31: 333–51.
6. Byrd RS, Weitzman ML. Predictors of early grade retention among children in the United States. Pediatrics 1994; 93: 481.
7. Anderson LM, Shinn C, Fullilove MT, et al. The effectiveness of early childhood development programs: A systematic review. Am J Prev Med 2003; 24: 32.
8. Reynolds AJ. Resilience among black urban youth: Prevalence, intervention effects, and mechanisms of influence. Am J Orthopsychiatry 1998; 68: 84.
9. Kern ML, Friedman HS. Early educational milestones as predictors of lifelong academic achievement, midlife adjustment, and longevity. J Appl Dev Psychol 2008; 30(4): 419–30.

5

Provincial/Territorial Special Education Legislation

William Mahoney and Debra Andrews

Every province and territory in Canada mandates educational programming and services for children with intensive learning needs. Physicians involved with children who experience problems in school need to become familiar with legislation, guidelines, and resources for their jurisdiction. Being able to share even basic information about which school authorities to approach or about accessing local supports can be hugely empowering to families with a child having trouble in school.

The most consistent theme in current legislation in Canada is the emphasis on *inclusion*: keeping students with intensive needs with their peers in a regular classroom whenever possible, while providing appropriate levels of assistance, accommodation, or support.

There are considerable differences among educational systems in terms of who initiates, who is responsible for, and who is involved in identifying, assessing, or placing a student with intensive learning needs. The processes for developing learning plans, along with their evaluation, review, or appeal, vary as well.

To best help child patients in their own educational setting, it may be important to distinguish between services, placement, and programming. *Services* can mean an assistive technology, behavioural counselling, speech therapy, a professional referral, individualized program development, and/ or some other kind of intervention. *Placement* refers to the environment in which a learning program is delivered. The *program* refers to what is done to help the student: usually the collaborative development of an individual learning plan, with strategies and outcomes, by a school-based team, parents, and appropriate professionals as needed.

An important concept to keep in mind is the issue of accountability: Once a plan is in place, how is the outcome evaluated? What happens if there are perceptions that a plan is not working? Parents often come to appointments with questions about their rights and those of their child. Become familiar with the special education processes for your jurisdiction, e.g., know the government and school board websites that contain the information parents need and have a working knowledge of the contents. The provincial- and territorial-specific resources that follow in this chapter should help; websites are usually the most regularly updated sources for this kind of information. Some jurisdictions have defined bylaw issues such as parents' rights of consultation, review, and approval of their child's program plan. In others, their involvement may be incorporated in school board policies.

Descriptions of an appeal process indicate what is done when there is a disagreement between schools and parents or students. While parental involvement in developing and review of a child's learning programs is always provided for, parents' signed consent is not always required for assessment, placement, and programming decisions. Procedures to review and evaluate the success of students' programs can also vary widely.

Programs require resources for their development and implementation, and it does cost more per child to provide special education services than a regular education program. All provinces and territories have legislation allocating money for "special education" programs; however, the amounts of funds specified, the types of conditions considered eligible, and whether this funding is assigned to be used for a particular student or added to a school-based general special education budget also vary. Being familiar with the way things are done in your jurisdiction will help parents understand what interventions can (or cannot) be reasonably expected if their child meets special education eligibility guidelines. It is also important to know how schools in your district will handle the large group of children who have conditions perceived to be "less severe." For example, can a parent ask for a program plan? Will teachers access a special education facilitator and implement strategies? Can ADHD behavioural strategies be incorporated into classroom routines? Physicians are often in the position of advocating for this population.

The following overviews, drawn from the wealth of information available on government websites, identify a few key issues for each province and territory. Legislation refers to the statutes that provide for inclusive services and policies. The general process is indicated—the *what* and the *where* for parents and supporting professionals—concerning policies that define what schools and school boards do to help children with intensive needs. While education ministries define and steer inclusive education policy, school districts often shape and oversee placement and special learning processes, while individual school-based teams largely determine the character, strategies, and outcomes of specific programs for specific children.

In summary:
- Children with learning problems are receiving excellent and successful educational services across Canada. Sometimes, however, parents become concerned that their child's program is not appropriate or working. This is often the point when physicians are consulted for an assessment, advice, and/or support. In some cases it is the severity of the child's learning problem that has led to slow progress, and the physician may need to help parents to have appropriate expectations for their child and support the school's programming choices.
- Physicians need to know that much of the legislation in place to resolve disagreements remains permissive: the schools or ministries of education *may* allocate further services to resolve an issue but, ultimately, in most jurisdictions, the final say rests with school district or government decision-makers.
- Being familiar with community and provincial/territorial terminology and procedures facilitates communication both with families and local educational authorities.

BRITISH COLUMBIA

Legislation
- B.C. School Act
  <www.bclaws.ca/EPLibraries/bclaws_new/document/ID/freeside/96412_00>
- B.C. Ministry of Education
  <www2.gov.bc.ca/en/themes/education/special_education/index.page?WT.svl=Footer>
- B.C. Ministry of Education policy framework on special education, 2006
  <www.bced.gov.bc.ca/policy/policies/special_ed.htm>
- Ministerial order on IEPs (individual education plans)
  <www.bced.gov.bc.ca/legislation/schoollaw/e/m638–95.pdf>
- Special education services manual of policies, procedures, and guidelines (2011) covers roles and responsibilities, categories, and assessment of special needs, condition-specific approaches, IEPs, provincial resource programs, and Internet resources
  <www.bced.gov.bc.ca/specialed/ppandg.htm>

Key points
- School districts establish assessment, programming, placement, reporting, and evaluation procedures.
- Other service providers are often involved in identification, assessment, and planning to support a student.
- Parents are consulted about placement and the development of their child's IEP, and also have the right to examine all records kept by the board pertaining to their child.
- Each board of education must establish an appeals procedure, with further appeals going to the ministry.

Contacts and resourses

- B.C. Ministry of Education
  <www.bced.gov.bc.ca>
- Student support services by district
  <www.bced.gov.bc.ca/apps/imcl/imclWeb/
  SN.do>
- Learning Disabilities Association of B.C.,
  with chapters in Victoria, Vancouver, Surrey,
  Coquitlam, Vernon, Williams Lake, and Fraser
  Lake Northwest
  <www.ldabc.ca>
- Special Education Technology B.C., helping
  school districts provide assistive technologies
  to students with special needs
  <www.setbc.org>
- B.C. Council of Administrators of Special
  Education, a professional educational organization affiliated with the Council for Exceptional
  Children
  <www.bc-case.org>

ALBERTA

Legislation

- Educational placement of students with
  special needs policy under the School Act,
  and Alberta Education's Special Education
  Policy, 2003
  <http://education.alberta.ca/admin/special/
  legislation/special.aspx>
- For standards in special education, see
  Ministerial order in 015/2004
  <http://education.alberta.ca/department/policy/
  standards/sestandards.aspx>
- Alberta Education sets policy on inclusive education programming. The Inclusive Education
  Planning Tool is a digital resource incorporat-
  ing many elements of the individual program
  plan (IPP), including parental involvement. It is
  being piloted in Grades 1 to 9 in the 2011–2012
  school year, and replaces individual goals with
  supports and strategies matched to a child's individualized strengths and needs
  <http://education.alberta.ca/department/ipr/
  inclusion/capacity/planning.aspx>

Key points

- Boards provide programming, assessment,
  reporting, placement, and curriculum modifications, and assign support services.
- If a board cannot provide appropriate programming, it refers to a special needs tribunal,
  which may establish a plan (to be reviewed
  every three years).
- Schools consult with parents about special education programs. Parental involvement in the
  screening and identification processes, as well as
  their written, informed consent for specialized
  assessments and referrals, are required. Parents
  have right of access to information contained
  in their child's files as per the Student Record
  Regulation.
- Boards establish appeals procedures. Parents
  (or a student) may appeal the decision to the
  minister of education for review. Review is at
  the discretion of the minister.

Contacts

- Alberta Education, Authorities and Schools
  Directory
  <http://education.alberta.ca/apps/schoolsdir/>
- Learning Disabilities Association of Alberta,
  with chapters in Calgary, Edmonton, and Red
  Deer
  <www.ldaa.ca/aboutus/calgary.aspx>

Resources

- Special education resources include free, downloadable guides for different types of learners,
  including those with LDs, ADHD, FASD,
  and who are deaf/hard of hearing or visually
  impaired
  <http://education.alberta.ca/admin/special/
  resources.aspx>
- Handbook for Aboriginal Parents of Children
  with Special Needs, 2000
  <http://education.alberta.ca/media/448720/
  aboriginalparenthandbook.pdf>
- The Learning Team: A handbook for parents
  of children with special needs, 2003, provides

information and strategies for involving families in a child's special education program <http://education.alberta.ca/media/352698/learning.pdf>

- The Parent Advantage: Helping children become more successful learners at home and school, 1998, was produced in collaboration with the Learning Disabilities Association of Alberta, and is also available in French <www.lrc.education.gov.ab.ca/pro/resources/item.htm?item-no=361501>

SASKATCHEWAN

Legislation

- The Education Act, 1995 (especially Part IV, Sections 146 and 178), and accompanying Education Regulations, 1986, are applicable <www.qp.gov.sk.ca/documents/English/Statutes/Statutes/E0–2.pdf>
- Guidelines include an annual Student Support Services Review Process (revised January 2012) that school divisions engage in <www.education.gov.sk.ca/sss/review-process>
- The Ministry of Education's Student Support Services (Intensive Supports), within the (former) Supports for Learning Unit, helps school divisions and educational partners to meet special needs <www.education.gov.sk.ca/IntensiveSupports>
- The Student Achievement and Supports Branch guides and supports school divisions. It receives learning block funding, provides appropriate services/supports for its students, and responds to local needs <www.education.gov.sk.ca/Actualizing-a-Needs-Based-Model-to-Support-Student-Achievement>

Key points

- Each school division provides appropriate supports and services to accommodate students with intensive needs in the regular program of instruction.
- There is parental right of appeal to the school principal and, if an issue is unresolved, appeal to the Ministry of Education. The appeal is done

by an objective third party agreed upon by all, whose decision is final.

- School divisions provide qualified professionals to support students with intensive needs.
- A Personal Program Plan (PPP)/Inclusion and Intervention Plan (IIP) is a collaborative document that develops, implements, and monitors a student's priority outcomes during the school year. Students can access supports and services ranged in tiers of intervention, from universal to targeted for groups, intensive for individuals. See www.education.gov.sk.ca/PPP.
- Annual review and documentation of individual student progress is required.

Contacts

- The Learning Disabilities Association of Saskatchewan, with branches in Saskatoon, Regina, and Prince Albert <www.ldas.org/default.aspx>
- Council for Exceptional Children Saskatchewan <http://saskcec.ca>
- Regional superintendents of student support services <www.education.gov.sk.ca/Default.aspx?DN=bb70b589–9b8c-49a4-bb62–306e24b195a9>

Resources

- Sample PPPs/IIPs for a range of ages/grades and other instructional information <www.education.gov.sk.ca/PPP>
- Teaching Students with Reading Difficulties and Disabilities: A Guide for Educators, 2004 <www.education.gov.sk.ca/Reading-Difficulties-Disabilities>
- Policy and Procedures for Locally Modified Courses of Study, 2007 <www.education.gov.sk.ca/LMC>
- Policy, Guidelines, and Procedures for Functional Integrated Programs, 2006 <http://education.gov.sk.ca/FIP>
- Policy, Guidelines, and Procedures for Alternative Education Programs: Alternative Grade 10, 11, and 12, 2006 <www.education.gov.sk.ca/AEP>

MANITOBA

Legislation

- Rights and responsibilities are defined in the Public Schools Act, the Education Administration Act, and the Public Schools Amendment Act (Appropriate Educational Programming), S.M. 2004, c.9 (2005)
  <http://web2.gov.mb.ca/bills/38–2/b013e.php>
- Manitoba Education, Program and Student Services is responsible for special education <www.edu.gov.mb.ca/k12/specedu/index.html>. Requirements are set down in:
  - Appropriate educational programming in Manitoba: Standards for student services, 2006 <www.edu.gov.mb.ca/k12/specedu/aep/pdf/Standards_for_Student_Services.pdf>
  - Appropriate educational programming in Manitoba: A formal dispute resolution process, 2006
    <www.edu.gov.mb.ca/k12/specedu/aep/dr.html>

Key points

- School divisions develop policies and procedures, keep them current, ensure implementation in schools, and direct placement if a catchment school cannot meet a student's individual needs (as determined in consultation with the parents and the school team).
- School-based teams identify students with exceptional learning needs. Their IEP is developed and specialized assessments may be conducted to identify which academic, social, emotional, or behavioural outcomes are required to support in-class learning. Parents (and the student, when appropriate) are involved in IEP development.
- The school principal ensures that IEPs are monitored and evaluated, that professionals become involved when needed, and that parents have the opportunity to be involved in developing their child's IEP.
- Parents, or an older student with an IEP, can appeal issues of programming or placement. School divisions have their own appeal process, and parents can only request formal dispute resolution through the Ministry of Education once all local avenues have failed.
- Placement decisions are reviewed annually or as needed, and IEPs are evaluated at least annually.

Contacts

- Manitoba Education, Student Services <www.edu.gov.mb.ca/k12/specedu/index.html>
- The Learning Disabilities Association of Manitoba, with chapters in Brandon, Portage la Prairie, and Winnipeg <www.ldamanitoba.org/index.htm>
- Community Living Manitoba <www.aclmb.ca>
- Manitoba First Nations Education Resource Centre (Special Education Unit) <www.mfnerc.org>

Resources

- Manitoba Education, Student Services documents <www.edu.gov.mb.ca/k12/specedu/documents.html>. These include:
  - Manitoba Pupil File Guidelines, January 2012
  - Towards Inclusion: Supporting Positive Behaviour in Manitoba Classrooms, 2011
  - Student-specific Planning: A handbook for developing and implementing individual education plans (IEPs), 2010
  - Working Together: A Handbook for Parents of Children with Special Needs in School, 2004
  - The Manitoba Speech-Language Pathology Outcomes Measure evaluates change in an individual's performance as a result of speech-language pathology intervention <www.edu.gov.mb.ca/k12/specedu/slp/index.html>

ONTARIO

Legislation

- The Education Act on Special Education, and accompanying regulations. An Advisory Council on Special Education reports directly to the minister.

- Highlights of Regulation 181/98, Identification and Placement of Exceptional Pupils, provides a summary of the key provisions <www.edu.gov.on.ca/eng/general/elemsec/speced/hilites.html>

Key points

- Boards are required to provide special education programs and services to students who have been identified as exceptional by an identification, placement, and review committee (IPRC).
- Upon receiving a written request from a parent, the school principal refers the student to an IPRC. Once a parent has agreed with the IPRC identification and placement decisions, the board notifies the principal of the need to develop an individual education plan (IEP).
- If parents disagree with the IPRC decision, they may file a notice of appeal to the secretary of the board within thirty days. Parents who disagree with subsequent IPRC/appeal board decisions on identification or placement can appeal to a hearing by the Social Justice Cluster.
- An IPRC review meeting is held each school year unless parents notify the principal in writing that it can be waived.
- Schools can prepare an IEP for a student who has not been formally identified as exceptional. The IEP is a written, working document describing a pupil's strengths and needs, the special education program and/or services established to meet these needs, delivery methods, and the student's progress.

Contacts

- Most information on special education in Ontario is online <www.edu.gov.on.ca/eng/parents/speced.html>
- The Special Education Advisory Committees (SEACs) Information Program helps members to undertake the roles and responsibilities ascribed by legislation <http://seac-learning.ca>

- The Learning Disabilities Association of Ontario, with chapters in Chatham-Kent, Durham, Halton, Kingston, Kitchener-Waterloo, Lamton County, London Region, Mississauga, Niagara, North Peel, Ottawa-Carleton, Peterborough, Simcoe County, Sudbury, Toronto District, Wellington County, Windsor, and York Region <www.ldao.ca>

Resources

- Guidelines on developing and maintaining an IEP <www.edu.gov.on.ca/eng/general/elemsec/speced/iep/iep.html>. These include:
  - The Individual Education Plan: A resource guide, 2004 (provides advice to school boards on the process, format, and content for developing IEPs).
  - Individual Education Plans: Standards for development, program planning, and implementation, 2000
  - Standards for School Boards' Special Education Plans, 2000
- Learning for All: A guide to effective assessment and instruction for all students, Kindergarten to Grade 12 (draft, 2011)
- Ontario Curriculum Unit Planner, Special Education Companion, 2002 <www.ocup.org/resources/documents/companions/speced2002.pdf>
- Learning Disabilities Association of Ontario: A parent's guide to special education in Ontario, 2003 <www.ldao.ca/wp-content/uploads/A-Parents-Guide-to-Special-Education.pdf>
- Caring and Safe Schools in Ontario: Supporting students with special education needs through progressive discipline, Kindergarten to Grade 12, 2010 <www.edu.gov.on.ca/eng/general/elemsec/speced/Caring_Safe_School.pdf>
- Education for All: The report of the expert panel on literacy and numeracy instruction for students with special educational needs, Kindergarten to Grade 6, 2005 <www.edu.gov.on.ca/eng/document/reports/speced/panel/speced.pdf>

QUEBEC

Legislation

- The first paragraph of section 224 of Quebec's Education Act (R.S.Q, c.I-13.3) <www.canlii.org/en/qc/laws/stat/rsq-c-i-13.3/latest/rsq-c-i-13.3.html>
- Guidelines published by the Ministry of Education, Leisure and Sport <www.mels.gouv.qc.ca/gr-pub/m_englis.htm>. Includes:
    - Organization of educational services for at-risk students and students with handicaps, social maladjustments, or learning difficulties, 2007 <http://www.learnquebec.ca/export/sites/learn/en/content/pedagogy/insight/aldi/Resources/DASSC.pdf>
    - Methods for organizing and managing regional support and expertise services in special education, 2006 <http://collections.banq.qc.ca/ark:/52327/bs57214>

Key points

- School boards establish student services programs for supportive services, school activities, counselling, and promotional/prevention services for students with special needs. They ensure that special needs are being met by schools.
- Schools can implement a wide array of supportive, remedial services. The principal is responsible for developing and evaluating IEPs with the involvement of parents, staff, and (when appropriate) the student, and with periodic oversight by a regional governing board.
- An appeal process is established in each board, as well as a provincial mechanism for resolving issues that cannot be resolved at the school or board levels.
- Consultation with parents is required.
- Each board develops the process for evaluation and review.

Contacts and resources

- Regional education contacts <www.mels.gouv.qc.ca/ministere/nousJoindre/index.asp?page=education>
- The Inclusive Education Service is a provincial service offering support and expertise to the English sector for the organization of programs and adapted teaching to students with special learning needs in an inclusive setting <www.etsb.qc.ca/en/centre_of_excellence/aboutus.html>
- The Learning Disability Association of Quebec <http://aqeta.qc.ca>

PRINCE EDWARD ISLAND

Legislation

- The School Act (revised 2010) <www.gov.pe.ca/law/statutes/pdf/s-02_1.pdf>
- The minister's directive 2001–08 on special education outlines imperatives: providing a continuum of support, a process for assessment and intervention, and an accountability framework <www.gov.pe.ca/eecd/index.php3?number=1027961>
- A standing committee on special education and student services is an advisory body on the delivery of services and makes policy recommendations <www.gov.pe.ca/eecd/index.php3?number=1038312&lang=E>
- Department of Education and Early Childhood Development www.gov.pe.ca/eecd Support services include:
    - Assistive technology <www.gov.pe.ca/eecd/index.php3?number=1028702&lang=E>
    - Autism services <www.gov.pe.ca/eecd/autismservices>
    - Individual education planning <www.gov.pe.ca/eecd/index.php3?number=1027859&lang=E>
    - Individual education planning for students <www.gov.pe.ca/eecd/index.php3?number=1027859&lang=E>

- Transition planning
  <www.gov.pe.ca/eecd/index.php3?number=1027875&lang=E>

Key points

- The Department of Education approves programming, supplementary, and/or specialized instructional resources, and services in schools.
- The school board is responsible for assessment and placement, and for ensuring that support services, student services teams, IEPs, and transition planning are established.
- The school, led by the principal, initiates referrals, identifies and implements interventions, develops IEPs and transition plans collaboratively with parents, and shares this information as appropriate with the student, parents, staff, and board or department personnel.
- Informed parental consent for a student's IEP is required.
- No appeal process is provided, but parents are very involved in the process and can arrange for mediation at the school board level or higher.
- An IEP is reviewed at least once a year or as needed.

Contacts

- The Atlantic Provinces Special Education Authority is a cooperative agency of the provincial departments of education for New Brunswick, Nova Scotia, Newfoundland and Labrador, and Prince Edward Island, serving children and youth who are deaf, hard of hearing, deaf/blind, blind, or visually impaired
  <www.apsea.ca>
- The Learning Disability Association of Prince Edward Island
- Ministry contacts
  <www.gov.pe.ca/education/laecd-info/dg.inc.php3>

Resources

- Student Support Resource Guide, 2010–2011
  <www.gov.pe.ca/photos/original/eecd_StudentSup.pdf>

- Record of Course Adaptation (template)
  <www.gov.pe.ca/forms/pdf/1517.pdf>
- Provincial Joint Committee on Class Composition: Summary report, 2011
  <www.gov.pe.ca/photos/original/eecd_clascomp11.pdf>
- Individualized Educational Planning (IEP): Standards and guidelines: A handbook for educators, 2005
  <www.gov.pe.ca/photos/original/ed_ieplanning.pdf>
- Teachers and Support Staff Working Together: Standards and guidelines: A handbook for teachers and support staff, 2005
  <www.gov.pe.ca/photos/original/ed_tssworktog.pdf>
- Student Assessment Process: Standards and guidelines, 2004
  <www.gov.pe.ca/photos/original/ed_StAsPrStanGu.pdf>

NOVA SCOTIA

Legislation

- The Education Act
  <http://nslegislature.ca/legc/statutes/eductn.htm>
  - Sections 24–26, 38, and 64(2)(D), Regulations under the Education Act
    <http://gov.ns.ca/JUST/regulations/regs/edmin.htm>
  - Special Education Policy (updated 2008)
    <http://studentservices.ednet.ns.ca/sites/default/files/speceng.pdf>
- The Department of Education's Student Services Division provides policies, guidelines, and support documents
  www.studentservices.ednet.ns.ca

Key points

- A school-based program planning team, including parents, follow a staged, collaborative process for identifying, assessing, and developing individual program plans (IPPs) for students with special needs, and for evaluation.

This process can be initiated by a teacher or parent, with the school principal.

- The program planning team includes the principal or vice-principal, the child's teachers and parents, with additional members depending on pupil needs and school board/community resources.
- The principal is responsible for ensuring that appropriate IPPs are developed, implemented, monitored, and evaluated for students with special needs.
- Parents or a school board may appeal an IPP or placement. If issues cannot be resolved at the school board level, either can request the minister to establish a board of appeal whose decision is final and binding.
- Obligation exists for involving/informing parents at every stage.
- The program planning team reviews student progress and meets to discuss changes to the IPP as necessary.

Contacts

- Student Services Division, N.S. Department of Education
<http://studentservices.ednet.ns.ca/content/contact>
- Atlantic Provinces Special Education Authority
<www.apsea.ca>
- The Learning Disabilities Association of Nova Scotia
<www.ldans.ca>
- The Mi'kmaq Liaison Office is a mandated conduit between the Department of Education and Aboriginal communities in matters of education
<http://mikmaq.ednet.ns.ca/contact.shtml>

Resources

- The Department of Education's Student Services Division also provides contact information, special reports, an educators' area, and "continuum of services" resources
<http://studentservices.ednet.ns.ca/>
- Assistive Technology: Supporting student success, 2006
<http://studentservices.ednet.ns.ca/sites/default/files/assistive_technology.pdf>
- Increasing the Effectiveness of Service Delivery to Mi'kmaw Learners, 2008
<www.ednet.ns.ca/pdfdocs/mikmaq-resources/MinistersResponse-MikmawLearners.pdf>
- Mi'kmaw Kina'matnewey Special Education Policy Manual, 2005
<www.kinu.ns.ca/downloads/MK_Spec_Ed_Policy.doc>
- The Program Planning Process: A guide for parents, 2006
<http://studentservices.ednet.ns.ca/sites/default/files/program-planning-process.pdf>
- Program Planning: A team approach (fact sheet)
<http://studentservices.ednet.ns.ca/sites/default/files/program_planning.pdf>

NEW BRUNSWICK

Legislation

- Section 12 of the Education Act (1997)
<www.gnb.ca/0062/acts/acts/e-01–12.htm>
- The Department of Education and Early Childhood Development, Education Support Services is responsible for developing, implementing, and coordinating special education programs, including all areas of learning difficulty and learning disability. This unit provides consultative support to schools, school districts, and other government departments
<www.gnb.ca/0000/anglophone-e.asp#ss>

Key points

- District superintendents, and their student services supervisors and team members, are responsible for regular contact with schools and for programs and services.
- The school principal ensures proper special education planning and documentation, along with a school-based student services team. The child's teacher leads personal learning plan (PLP) development, monitoring, assessment, co-teaching, tracking, and information storage.

- Parents must be consulted during assessment and while developing individualized special education programs, E-PLPs, and services.
- Ultimate decisions about placement, programming, and services rest with educators, but parents can request an appeal.
- Programming is based on continuous assessment and evaluation.

Contacts

- Atlantic Provinces Special Education Authority <www.apsea.ca>
- The Department of Education and Early Childhood Development, Education Support Services (Branch) <www2.gnb.ca/content/gnb/en/contacts/dept_renderer.151.2471.20024.html#employees>
- School districts and sub-districts <www.gnb.ca/0000/schdist/district/subdist.asp>
- The Learning Disabilities Association of New Brunswick <www.nald.ca/ldanb/english/home.htm>

Resources

- Guidelines and Standards: Educational planning for students with exceptionalities, 2002 <www.gnb.ca/0000/publications/ss/sep.pdf>
- Learning Strategies Intervention Course, Grades 11–12, 2001 <www.gnb.ca/0000/publications/curric/LearningStrategiesCourse.pdf>

NEWFOUNDLAND AND LABRADOR

Legislation

- The Schools Act, 1997 <www.canlii.org/en/nl/laws/stat/snl-1997-c-s-12.2/latest/snl-1997-c-s-12.2.html>
- Department of Education, Student Support Services Division <www.ed.gov.nl.ca/edu/department/branches/pes/sss.html>
- Policies and protocols for teaching students with exceptionalities <www.ed.gov.nl.ca/edu/k12/studentsupportservices/exceptionalities.html>
- The Service Delivery Model for Students with Exceptionalities is a tool that describes programming options for K–12 students who are identified as needing extra support <www.cdli.ca/sdm/>
- The recent inclusive schools initiative features professional learning on inclusive practices, differentiated instruction, and co-teaching models <www.ed.gov.nl.ca/edu/k12/inclusion.html>

Key points

- The school's service delivery team oversees special education services, including deployment of resources, consultation with classroom teachers, and managing referrals for comprehensive assessment.
- A program planning team may be initiated for a student with one or more exceptionalities. This team manages a student's individual education plan (IEP) or record of accommodations. Parent or guardian involvement is critical, and the student participates as a team member when developmentally and emotionally appropriate.
- An IEP records and tracks the educational supports and services provided and is required for students in modified courses, or with alternate programs, courses, or curriculum. Accommodations are recorded in an IEP, but if only accommodations are required, an IEP is not necessary.
- A parent, as a program planning team member, is involved in the development, review, and signing of an IEP.
- An IEP records educational services only. Services provided by other government agencies are recorded, tracked, and coordinated on an individual support services plan (ISSP) (www.mcscy.nl.ca/issp.html). The ISSP process is currently under review by the government.
- Appeals by a parent or older student are provided for under the Schools Act, first to the school principal, then to the board, with the board's decision being final.

Contacts

- Atlantic Provinces Special Education Authority (APSEA)
  <www.apsea.ca>
- Eastern School District
- Nova Central School District
- Western School District
- Labrador School District
- Conseil Scolaire Francophone
  <www.csfp.nl.ca/conseil_scolaire.html>
- Learning Disabilities Association of Newfoundland and Labrador
  <www.ldanl.ca>
- List of K–12 schools
  <www.ed.gov.nl.ca/edu/faq/schooldatabase.html>

Resources

- Department of Education: Student Support Services
  <www.ed.gov.nl.ca/edu/k12/
  studentsupportservices/rts/index.html>

NORTHWEST TERRITORIES

Legislation

- The Education Act, 1996, especially:
  - Pt. 1 (Section 7) on "Inclusive Schooling"
    <www.justice.gov.nt.ca/Legislation/..%5C
    PDF%5CACTS%5CEducation.pdf>
  - Ministerial directive on inclusive schooling, 2006
    <www.ece.gov.nt.ca/PDF_File/Student
    Support/Ministerial Directive on Inclusive
    Schooling 2006.pdf>
- The Department of Education, Culture and Employment provides support to boards in implementing the inclusive schooling directive: www.ece.gov.nt.ca

Key points

- IEPs document the goals, objectives, instructional strategies, and evaluation methods for students on individual programs, and are reviewed twice a year.
- Parental involvement is sought and encouraged, and signed approval for IEPs is required.
- Parents have the right to appeal decisions reached during the IEP process.
- Student support plans (SSPs) document accommodations required by a student on a regular program and curricular outcomes for students on modified programs.

Contacts

- Education, Culture and Employment contacts: www.ece.gov.nt.ca

Resources

- NWT Student Support Services
  <www.ece.gov.nt.ca/divisions/kindergarten_
  g12/Student%20Support%20Services.htm>
  - NWT program support guide: Programming for student success, 2008
  - NWT Individual education plans: Guidelines for development, 2006
  - NWT Individual education plans: Teacher resource kit (Toolbox, 2006)
  - NWT Student support plans: Guidelines for development, 2006
  - NWT Student support plans: Teacher resource kit (Toolbox, 2006)

NUNAVUT

Legislation

- Nunavut Education Act (revised 2009), section on "Inclusive Education"
  <www.edu.gov.nu.ca/apps/UPLOADS/fck/file/
  EdAct/EA004c-CSFNGuide.pdf>
- For a summary of recent changes, see
  <http://www.edu.gov.nu.ca/apps/UPLOADS/
  fck/file/EdAct/EA002c-Change.pdf>

Key points

- Teachers provide basic adjustments and support for student learning programs.
- The school team develops an individual student support plan (ISSP) for students who

require more significant adjustments or supports. Parents participate in developing this plan.

- Nunavut's inclusion philosophy emphasizes educating students in the regular classroom in their home community. Assistants are provided to meet students' unique needs. Rules exist for determining which students cannot be in a regular instructional setting and for finding them alternative supports or placements.
- There are established dispute resolution methods relating to student support. First stage mediation is by district education authorities (DEA). If that is unsuccessful, a review can be requested by a review board.
- DEAs, the school staff, and the review board make decisions in accordance with Inuit Qaujimajatuqangit (IQ).
- Annual assessments of ISSPs are required under the DEA's direction, and made in accordance with IQ by staff with specific training.

Contacts and resources

- Department of Education <www.edu.gov.nu.ca>
- List of schools and principals and regional school operations offices are available at the Nunavut Department of Education website <www.edu.gov.nu.ca>
- Nunavut Literacy Council <www.nunavutliteracy.ca>

YUKON TERRITORY

Legislation

- The Education Act, revised 2002 (especially Division 2 – Special Education) <www.gov.yk.ca/legislation/acts/education .pdf>

Key points

- Parents or teachers can initiate special education planning, collaborating with a school-based team that may include a school administrator, a learning assistance teacher, a school counsellor, the student (if appropriate), consultants from the Department of Education, and representatives from other community services, as needed.
- The team recommends classroom strategies and sometimes requests additional assessments.
- When the student's needs exceed what the school can provide, consultants from Special Programs become involved.
- Parents must provide informed consent before any formal consultations or assessments are done by Special Programs, and their written, informed consent is obtained before an IEP can proceed.
- The IEP is developed collaboratively and its regular review is required.
- An appeal initially goes to the board, then to an educational appeal tribunal whose decision is final.

Contacts and resources

- Learning Disabilities Association of Yukon <www.ldayukon.com>
- Special Department of Education programs <www.education.gov.yk.ca/specialprograms/ index.html>
- Special Programs Services: A handbook of procedures and guidelines, 1995 <www.education.gov.yk.ca/specialprograms/ pdf/Special_Program_Services_A_Handbook_ of_Procedures_and_Guidelines_OCR1.pdf>
- Western and Northern Canadian Protocol for Collaboration in Education, Rethinking Classroom Assessment with Purpose in Mind: Assessment for learning, assessment as learning, assessment of learning, 2006 <www.wncp.ca/media/40539/rethink.pdf>

Part II: Diagnostics

CHAPTER

6

Data Gathering

Barbara Fitzgerald and Wendy Roberts

In evaluating a child presenting with school problems, the physician must gather, review, and synthesize information from a number of sources. Depending on the setting in which the child is being seen, much or little of this may be available at the time of the first office visit. In a primary care setting, the school problem may be brought up in the context of a well-visit, and the only information available is the parent's history. The physician would then need to arrange to obtain additional information and review this in a subsequent visit. A paediatric consultant may have time to gather supporting materials before seeing the child; some of these may even arrive with the referral letter. To increase efficiency in history-taking and in identifying and obtaining the documents needed, questionnaires—such as those in Chapter 7—can be very helpful. In this way much of this important but time-consuming process can be done outside the clinical visit, freeing valuable minutes for exploring significant findings.

In this chapter we review how to gather and interpret information in preparation for the assessment appointment. We also present the approach to history-taking for developmental concerns, including interviewing both parents and children, with many examples of questions used for various situations. These sample questions would, of course, not all be used in one visit; instead you should pick and choose according to the child's presenting problem and your review of any questionnaires and reports that have been collected for the visit.

REVIEWING PREVIOUS REPORTS

Most school problems are not acute; there may be many previous indicators of possible developmental concern. You can find telling clues to the problem by reviewing previous community developmental reports, school reports, and noting what types of services the child required in the past. The following sources of information may be useful:

- **Medical information:** Includes birth records, hospital discharge summaries, consultants' reports, lab and imaging reports, interdisciplinary team assessments, hearing and vision testing.
- **Infancy and preschool period information:** Includes early intervention or infant development program reports, preschool development services such as Headstart or early education programs, reports from specific allied health disciplines such as speech-language pathologists, occupational and physical therapists, and psychologists.
- **School-age period information:** Includes report cards, notes from teacher(s) outlining concerns (including resource or special education teachers if applicable), school-based team notes and reports, individual program or education plans (IPPs/IEPs), work samples, psycho-educational assessments, and other school consultant reports.

INTERPRETING PSYCHO-EDUCATIONAL ASSESSMENTS

One of the most important pieces of assessment to review is psycho-educational testing, usually done by a school psychologist and consisting in its most basic form of an intellectual assessment (IQ test) and achievement testing, which describes the child's level of academic performance and allows comparison with what is expected at his or her age and grade.

Other testing, such as adaptive skills and executive function, may be required to define the diagnosis.

Qualifications of school psychologists vary widely. Some will have a PhD and years of experience working with children with academic difficulties; others will have a master of education degree in which they have taken some testing courses, and in some cases schools will use psychometricians, who are trained to administer tests but not to interpret them. Reports also vary considerably in the depth and breadth of the formulation, and physicians may need to have some expertise in interpreting results.

Also, as with any medical test that we order, we must ascertain whether the results received fit with the clinical picture. An example of this is when the psychology report tells us that the child does not meet criteria for a severe learning disability (LD) as defined by the statistical analysis of the test. For example, you may be seeing a child in Grade 3 who is not reading despite intensive remediation. The designation criteria for severe LD may vary from jurisdiction to jurisdiction but are often based on a statistical calculation done by the psychologist. The child may need a certain point discrepancy to meet statistical significance, but functionally, that child has a learning disability and will need support for it. Another example is when the subtest scores on a cognitive assessment vary widely, and the person administering the test has simply reported an average overall score, not taking into account that the child has ADHD or a mixed learning disability, which has led to inconsistency of effort and/or ability and the lowered full-scale score. It is useful to identify the paragraph in which the test administrator describes the child's state and behaviour during the testing, often found just before the test results and ending with a statement about whether the tester thought the results were a valid representation of the child's abilities or whether the results could have been adversely affected by some other factor, e.g., anxiety, fatigue, or illness.

ANATOMY OF A PSYCHO-EDUCATIONAL ASSESSMENT

There are hundreds of different psychological tests. Below is a summary of the basic evaluation along with some specific areas of testing that you may wish to request, depending on what you think may be the child's underlying problem. If the assessment has been done before you see the child, you may ask for supplemental testing where required.

Cognitive (IQ) tests

IQ tests measure intelligence, that is, a child's theoretical potential to learn, or as David Wechsler put it: "the aggregate or global capacity of the individual to act purposefully, to think rationally and to deal effectively with the environment."

Intelligence is a construct that describes a set of mental skills for the ability to learn (and to some extent also measure what has been learned, e.g., vocabulary). Older children with reading problems may have reduced vocabulary and general knowledge, which can affect IQ scores. In contrast, the academic skills a child has learned is termed achievement, described below.

Besides a "full-scale" IQ, reflecting a child's overall abilities, factors or subscores reflecting different aspects of thinking abilities will be described. The names for these may vary depending on the IQ test used, but typically they include a measure of language-based problem-solving and a nonverbal measure that reflects visual problem-solving and visual-spatial functioning. On the Wechsler Intelligence Scale for Children, Fourth Edition (WISC-IV), a commonly used IQ test, these are termed Verbal Comprehension and Perceptual Reasoning. The WISC-IV also includes two other subscores: the first, *Working Memory*, is very important for learning. Working memory defines a neurocognitive process whereby information is stored temporarily and manipulated to be used in complex cognitive tasks such as processing, reasoning, and problem-solving. It is, to some extent, a measure of executive functioning and attention. The second one is *Processing Speed*. Processing speed is a measure of cognitive efficiency. The processing speed index is associated with the child's speed in processing visual-spatial information. Processing speed is also influenced by motivation, concentration, and eye-hand coordination. It will be useful to become familiar with the specific psychological tests most commonly used by school psychologists in your area.

Figure 6–1   Normal Standard Distribution and Standard Scores

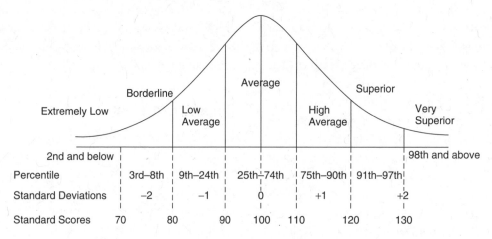

Many tests use standard scores, which have an average of 100 and a standard deviation of 15. The use of such standard scores allows you to see how a child performs relative to peers and to compare the results to other measures using standard scores. Full-scale and factor IQ scores are an example of standard scores. Although psychologists almost always calculate a full-scale IQ score and subscores, the scores are not always included in reports. You may receive only percentiles or an interpretive descriptor (e.g., "average range"). Figure 6–1 shows the normal curve in relation to standard scores.

Adaptive measures

Adaptive scales measure practical daily living skills and are a way to link the IQ score with the child's real-life performance. Measurement of adaptive abilities is not always part of a routine school psychology assessment. This measure is required to confirm a diagnosis of intellectual disability, and the child may not qualify for school services or government financial assistance if it

is not completed. A diagnosis of intellectual disability has serious long-term implications for any person. On the one hand, the diagnosis may confer eligibility for certain types of supports and even has legal implications. On the other hand, there is often a stigma associated with any term used to convey a disability in mental functions, whether it is called *intellectual disability*, cognitive impairment, or the older term, *mental retardation* (which is still ensconced in older legislation and in the DSM-IV; see the Glossary).

Two commonly used adaptive scales are the Vineland Adaptive Behavior Scales, Second Edition (VABS-II) and the Adaptive Behavior Assessment System, Second Edition (ABAS-2). Adaptive scores are reported as standard scores, so they can be compared with other assessment results, e.g., IQ scores. Usually the scores are congruent, but with some conditions, e.g., FASD or ASD, the child's daily functioning is significantly lower than the tested developmental potential as reflected in the IQ score, and this can be helpful diagnostically. The adaptive score may also have implications for the child's safety

Table 6–1   IQ Classifications in Current Use

Classification	IQ score	Percentile
Very superior	≥130	>98th
Superior	120–129	91st–98th
High average	110–119	75th–90th
Average	90–109	25th–74th
Low average	80–89	9th–24th
Borderline	70–79	2nd–8th
Intellectual disability	<69	<2nd

and the level of supervision required at school and in childcare settings.

Achievement testing

These tests measure what a child can do in academic subjects: in other words, what has been learned/achieved in school. They may be easily recognized by the word "achievement" or the name of a school subject like "reading" or "math" in the name of the test. Like IQ, achievement test results are reported as standard scores and percentiles based on age, but here you may also get information based on the child's current grade placement. This is important to note because a child who has been retained may have grade-based scores that seem appropriate for the grade, but when you look at age-based scores, you can see the degree of overall delay.

Comparison of IQ and achievement scores is a way of identifying if a child is working at his or her intellectual potential and is the basis for the discrepancy model of learning disability. A child with borderline ability or intellectual disability will usually have a profile where the achievement scores are similar to the IQ, while a child with a specific learning disability should, by definition, have a full-scale IQ in the normal range but delays in academic achievement in one or more areas. Such children often have uneven profiles in the factor scores; for example, with a reading disability, the verbal comprehension score may be lower than the perceptual reasoning score. The child is still considered to have average intelligence even though one factor score may be low (e.g., verbal comprehension), as long as the perceptual reasoning is in the average range.

THE HISTORY

The medical history is an extremely important component in the evaluation of any child with difficulty in school. For a comprehensive assessment it is necessary to set aside sufficient time by booking a long appointment slot, and review any materials you've received to direct your interview most efficiently. This section describes interview methods and examples of specific questions you can use with children and parents. It is not expected that all the areas and questions in this chapter be used in every case. Clinicians should select what seems appropriate according to what they already know about the child and the family, the possible diagnosis, and the very real constraints of appointment time and clinical load. In busy family medicine or other primary care settings, the interview may need to be broken into shorter segments, each with its own specific agenda. The CADDRA guidelines suggest a way of carrying out this stepped approach.(1) Reviewing the information the parents have completed before the interview allows you to focus on the key points that may indicate some previous issues.

SETTING THE STAGE

- Find out what the parents hope to get out of the consultation and who instigated it. The parents may not think there is anything "wrong" with their child; the request for consultation may have come from the school. On the other hand, parents may have concerns the school does not share. Some parents may be defensive and see the teacher's observations of the child's difficulties as being a reflection on them as being bad parents or having done something wrong during the pregnancy or upbringing of the child. Some parents harbour secret concerns about something they did or didn't do with respect to their child. Ask them specifically if there is anything that they have ever worried about with respect to exposures, injuries, etc.
- Discuss the fact that this type of assessment takes time and that you will need to ask a lot of questions, some of which may seem irrelevant or even overly personal to the parents. There will be questions about family history, family relationships, birth history, etc., and the parents may need reassurance that you ask these questions of all your patients.
- Ask explicitly what the parents' long-term expectations are for their child (e.g., do they expect their child to go on to higher education?).
- Explain the process of your assessment with the parents: review of their concerns, review of school professionals' concerns, review of reports that have been done previously, interview with the child, developmental assessment of the child,

discussion of your formulation and how best to proceed together to ensure their child's success.

INTERVIEWING PARENTS

If you are able, interview the parents without the child present. Any school-aged child who can comprehend what is being said (any child over the developmental age of three years) may be uncomfortable being talked about in front of others. Give the child a task to complete that will help with your assessment: drawing a picture, designing something with Lego, doing an age-appropriate puzzle, etc. If the child must be present (for example, when there is no supervision available), phrase questions in a sensitive manner, modelling this for the parents, e.g., ask about strengths and weaknesses, what areas the child does well in and what areas are "a struggle" or "hard." Remember that even if children do not seem to be engaged in the discussion they may still be listening, and check for their response as well as for the parents'. If a parent tends to use overly critical language in the child's presence, an intervention from you may be needed.

Establish rapport. For some families, this is a quick and easy task. If the parents are feeling defensive, or if they feel the teacher has unfairly singled out their child, then you need to first establish a therapeutic relationship with them. Tell them that the goal of assessment is to determine how their child learns best, so that the child reaches full potential and is happy going to school. Inquire whether either parent ever struggled in school. If they did, and especially if they tell you that they suffered as a result, you can explain that a major goal of assessment is to figure out where the child's strengths lie, to ensure that the child has the best chance to be successful. Explain the concept of brains being "wired differently," how some people learn well by one method and others by another. Ask them how they think their child learns best. Try to ensure that the parents are comfortable with the process you have outlined before you proceed.

Establish whether the parents have concerns, what those concerns are, and whether they have an explanation for them. Review what the teacher's concerns are, either from the material the school provided to you (such as the questionnaire in this book) or from what the parents know. Discuss why the concerns may differ in the school environment versus the home environment.

In addition to the usual paediatric history, these are some specific topics to cover:

- **Developmental history:** See Chapter 7 for questionnaires regarding specific milestones.
- **Early concerns:** Establish if there were any early concerns. Was the daycare provider or preschool teacher concerned? Was the child referred for any early developmental services? Did the parents ever feel that their child was different in some way from other children of the same age?
  - **Support services:** What previous services have been used? E.g., supported childcare, speech-language, occupational, or physical therapy, mental health support.
  - **Developmental trajectory:** Has the child always developed more slowly than other children in areas such as language or motor skills, or was there a sudden change in development and/or behaviour? Has there been any regression (actual loss of a previously attained skill)?
  - **Significant events:** Have there been any significant events that the parents think may have influenced the child? E.g., death of a loved one, mental or serious physical illness in a parent or sibling, extended time spent outside the family with relatives or in foster care, marital separation, significant discord or violence, physical or sexual abuse.
  - **Childcare arrangement:** What was the care situation before school started? Was it adequate? Was English spoken? How many children were there per care provider?
  - **Language:** What language is spoken at home? Do the parents read to the child? What are the parents' literacy levels?
- **Academic history:** How many schools has the child gone to? Why has the child moved schools? What has the child's attendance been like? Has the school given the child a specific

special needs designation? Does the child get extra help at school? Does the child have an individual education program? Does the child ever refuse to go to school?

- **Medical history** (see Chapter 3 for background information on neurodevelopmental conditions associated with learning problems):
  - **Prenatal:** Planned or unplanned pregnancy, prenatal substance exposure, maternal mental health during pregnancy, pertinent information regarding labour and delivery, and postnatal course.
  - **Injuries:** Brain injury specifically or non-accidental trauma.
  - **Serious illness:** Hospital stays, seizures, operations.
- **Review of systems:**
  - **Sleep:** Does the child have sleep difficulties?
  - **Appetite/Nutrition:** Does the child eat items from all the food groups? Is the child especially picky? Are you concerned about your child's nutrition?
  - **Screen time:** How many hours per day does the child spend in front of any type of electronic screen?(2)
  - **Recreation:** Is the child involved in any activities outside school? What opportunities exist for play, especially active play? What activities exist that allow the child to socialize with peers?
- **Family history:** Ask about usual medical history plus the parents' academic history (any difficulties or learning challenges, how far they went in school, reasons for leaving school before completion, etc.), substance use history, and psychiatric illness.
- **Social history:** Ask about family finances. Do they have enough money for food, housing, and clothing at the end of the month? Is their housing adequate? Do the parents work? What types of jobs (e.g., shift work puts extra stress on families)? What is the childcare situation? Can they afford and access extracurricular activities for their children? Do they have support from family or friends? Are they connected to the school or to their religious community? How many

times have they moved? Are there any particular marital stresses? Explore further as necessary.

INTERVIEWING CHILDREN

It is very important to interview the child separately from the parents whenever possible. The child may feel inhibited from discussing certain topics in front of the parents, and you will get an idea of how the child manages in a situation without his or her parents observing. You can obtain very rich information about how a child feels about school, family, friends, perception of the parents' relationship, and whether there are other serious concerns, such as witnessing violence, experiencing abuse, or being bullied. Children can often tell us exactly what their learning difficulty is, so ask them! A child may come right out and say that he doesn't understand anything the teacher says and that is why he fidgets and doesn't pay attention. It is also advantageous to do the developmental assessment without parents watching and putting pressure on the child to get the "right" answer. Where possible, have the parents watch from an observation room—it removes them from the immediate situation yet allows then to see the child's performance. Even when a child comes with a full psycho-educational assessment already completed, you will get very valuable information about learning style, attention, anxiety, etc., by doing some assessment yourself.

Introducing the process

Always be honest with children and tell them in age-appropriate language why you are seeing them today. Children don't like to think that they are different from their peers; reassure them that you are a children's doctor and that you see lots of children who find some parts of school hard or who aren't happy at school, whatever is appropriate for this particular child.

Explain the assessment format

Indicate the length of time to be spent with the child alone and when the physical examination, for which a parent or nurse will be present, will be conducted. If appropriate, a reassurance about "no needles" may provide significant relief.

Confidentiality is critical

The child must be told at the outset that what he or she tells you, the physician, will not be repeated if the child requests confidentiality, unless you are worried about the child's safety. Should that situation arise, you will tell the child that the information must be shared. In some situations (depending on the age and the concern) you may give the child the option of being present when that is done. Some children will prefer to have you discuss a sensitive situation with their parent without being present.

The agenda

Have a clear agenda for the interview, which may include relationship formation, diagnosis, information exchange, support and counselling, progress review, and forward planning, or a mixture. At a first interview, relationship-building is paramount; everything else can be left to later sessions. A minimal psychosocial interview with a child will cover family life (including sufficiency of time spent with parents, fairness of rules, rewards and responsibilities, siblings, financial problems), other problems faced by the child (mood and anxiety, self-esteem, ethnicity, sexuality, substance abuse, long- and short-term plans for the future), and assessment of the other major life areas (school, friends, and recreation).

Counselling style

Remember that "if the doctor asks questions in the manner of medical history-taking, he will always get answers—but hardly anything more."(3) The interview with the child must be an interview and not an interrogation. Listen actively, tolerating silences, creating openings for easy discussion, and responding to the child's body language or tentative offerings (to be explored in depth).

- Third-party techniques can be helpful: for example, you might say, "Lots of children your age tell me they have worries about death/divorce/bullying in school. What about you?"
- Similarly, offering the younger child a chance to make three magic wishes may help by providing an opportunity for the expression of deeply felt desires to change family or school situations.
- Many young children are uncomfortable with looking directly at a physician and answering questions. You may find it helpful to bring out some finger puppets or other small toys for younger children and conduct the interview through them. You will be surprised how much a child might tell a "magic doggy puppet" that they might be uncomfortable sharing with you.

Positives first

The conversation may begin on safe ground by discussing areas of strength, happy memories, favourite activities, and events to which the child looks forward. Children respond to adults who are interested in them. For example, you might approach the child by saying, "I'd like to get to know you a little bit so I can understand how to help."

Talking about a favourite sport, hobby, television program, or movie helps the child to relax and provides a good sample of spontaneous language, which can be evaluated for vocabulary, sentence structure, and discourse planning. Discussion of accomplishments helps to assess self-esteem. Apathy or defensiveness may indicate areas of concern.

School and academic issues

You may wish to use questions like the following to explore school problems:

- Some students really like school and some hate it. How is it for you?
- Which is your favourite subject? Which do you hate the most? Is there anything you find embarrassing?
- How do you feel when the teacher asks you questions? How about being asked to read aloud?
- Are there many students in your school who tease others? Does that often happen to you?
- Some students are embarrassed to get extra help, others like it. What about you?
- When you are in class, do you find you often think about other things than your work? Do you think about home things or school things? (Many children will tell their physician that

they are worrying about a parent's safety or an argument or threat to leave home that they have overheard.)

- What do your parents think about how you do in school? Are they pleased with how hard you work or do they think you could work harder? Did either of them have trouble in school? Do they talk about this with you?

Relationships with peers

You may wish to use questions like the following to explore relationships with peers:

- Do you think you have enough friends? Would you like to have more friends? (Friendless children may not be able to think of any names, or they may supply the names of everyone in the class.)
- Do you have a best friend? How long have you been friends? What do you like to do with him/ her? (E.g., some children may list as a best friend the name of a child who sits in the next desk but with whom the child doesn't really have a friendship relationship. Parents can be of help here—if the name of the "friend" does not sound familiar to the parent, this should be explored.)
- Who do you play with at recess or lunchtime? Are you ever lonely at school?
- What do you and your friends like to play? Are there any kids who won't let you play?
- What sorts of things do you get teased about? What names do you get called? (The assumption that teasing happens to everyone makes it easier to admit to the embarrassment of being teased. You must establish that you can't be shocked by even "awful" names.)
- Have you ever been bullied?
- Do you have better friends at home or at school? What's different?

Activities

Questions such as these can help you find out about the child's activities:

- Everyone likes to be good at something. What are you best at? What does your dad/mom think you are best at? What do other kids think you are good at?

- What groups have you joined? Do you like or avoid groups?
- Do you collect anything?
- Is there something you know much more about than most other people?

Family issues

The questions in the sections that follow on siblings, parents, extended family, and grief should help collect the relevant information about families and relationships that may be affecting the child or be important to him or her. You may start by asking a question such as, "Who is in your family?"

Siblings

To find out about the child's siblings, try asking these questions:

- Tell me about your brother(s)/sister(s).
- With whom do you get on best? With whom do you fight most?
- Does your mom or your dad get more upset when you fight?
- Who gets most upset?
- Who helps to settle arguments between you and your brother(s)/sister(s)?

Parents

The physician should help the child to describe each parent separately, without comparing them. Try asking these questions:

- Tell me about your mom/dad.
- What does she/he do for fun? What do you like to do with her/him?
- Who do you usually talk to if you have a problem?
- Are you the kind of person who tends to keep things inside and not tell anyone?
- Do you have enough time with your dad/mom? What things do you like to do most with your dad/mom? If you could spend a whole day alone with your dad/mom, what would you like to do?
- What do your mom and your dad do when you misbehave? Are the rules at home fair? Do you understand them? Do you always understand

why you are being punished? How do your parents let you know when you've done good work?

Extended family and bereavement and loss

Deaths in the family (including those of pets) need to be explored as bereavements; they are an important source of anxiety and preoccupation that may be missed if losses are not discussed. Children's sadness is often not recognized until a year or two after the death of someone close. Worry about *parental* health and survival often accompanies grief for someone else.

If appropriate, the physician may ask directly:

- Has anyone died in your family that you can remember?
- Who felt most sad? How could you tell?
- Do you still miss/think a lot about him/her? (Or the person is designated according to name or appropriate relationship, e.g., grandfather, aunt, and so on.)
- When do you think about him/her? More at home or at school?

In probing the child's concept of death, the third-party technique can also be very useful.

Pets

Here are some questions to ask the child about pets:

- Do you have a pet? Does it belong to one person or the family? Where does it sleep? (An anxious child often finds great comfort from a pet being in his or her room at night.)
- Have you ever had a pet that died? How did you feel?

Sleep

You can find out about the child's sleep habits and patterns with questions such as these:

- Some people take a long time to fall asleep at night. How long does it take you? (Increased time to fall asleep is one of the most common symptoms of anxiety in childhood.)
- What helps you to fall asleep?

- What do you think about in the dark?
- Do you have dreams?
- Do you worry about the house being safe or one of your parents not being home?

Feelings

Doctors are sometimes guilty of overlooking emotional and mental health aspects of children. Sad and/or anxious feelings can be both contributors to school problems and the result of school problems. It is important to explore how the child is feeling, partly as a gauge of how serious the stresses are that the child faces.

Happiness

Convey to the child that everyone feels happy some of the time and sad some of the time. This will allow the child to feel comfortable about describing sad times. For younger children it can be helpful to draw a scale with a happy face on the right and a sad face on the left, with measures in between. Ask the child where on the scale she is today and where she is most of the time. Sometimes a child will disclose more when looking at the pictures than when talking directly to you. You can also ask:

- When do you feel most happy? Do you usually feel that way? What are you looking forward to at the moment?

Sadness

- What makes you feel sad? Who/what makes you feel better?
- Have you ever felt sad for more than a day or two?
- Have you ever felt so sad that you wanted to disappear? Run away from home? Go to sleep and get away from it all for a long time? Have you thought of hurting yourself or not wanting to live any more? When was that?
- Who else in your family gets sad?
- Do you try to help that person feel better?

Anger

Some of these questions may not be part of your usual history. You will be surprised at how relieved children can be to be asked about things that they will likely never have talked about before:

- What makes you mad/angry/upset? Who do you get mad at the most? What do you feel like doing when you feel like that? Is it frightening when you get really angry? Have you ever really lost control of yourself? What (or who) helps you to feel better? Can you tell your mom or dad that you are mad at her or him?
- What's it like for you when people get mad at one another in your family? How do you feel when your mom and dad have an argument? Does it happen a lot? What do you do? Is it ever your fault? Have you ever been afraid something bad might happen?
- Does anyone in your family change when they drink alcohol? Does anyone get so angry that they threaten to hit somebody else?
- Has anyone ever threatened to leave your family or told you that you would have to leave home?

Worries

Tell the child that everyone worries about things. Explore what her worries are and ask if these worries ever distract her from schoolwork. For example:

- Do you sometimes worry about what things will be like for you when you grow up? Do you think it will all work out?
- Do you worry about your mom or dad? What do you worry about? Do you think about it at school?

Sexuality

Questions about sexuality vary considerably depending on the developmental age of the child. Some typical questions may include:

- Some children wish they were a girl/boy instead of a boy/girl. Have you ever felt that? Are you happy you're a boy/girl?
- Where appropriate with adolescents, you may want to include questions about sexual activity.

Asking about child abuse

Although some children will be careful to deny abuse, many say later that they have never been asked and wish someone had asked. Some know that their family could be destroyed by the ensuing

investigation and have not risked saying anything. Some children have been told by an adult to not disclose abuse. Ask open-ended questions, thus giving the child permission to introduce a variety of topics. Examples are as follows:

- Sometimes children are concerned about things that others do to them or the way they behave, like getting bullied in school or being hit by an adult. Has anything like that happened to you or anyone you know? Can you tell me about it?
- Some children have told me that someone has touched their private parts. Has that ever happened to you?

Ask these questions in a very low-key way; the child needs to feel that you won't be shocked by the answer. A definite "no" is reassuring. If the child hesitates or looks down and doesn't answer, you could say, "Has something happened to you but you don't want to talk about it?" If the child says yes, ask, "Is there anyone who you talk to about this?" This clearly raises serious concerns that will need to be explored further by a social worker trained specifically to carry out these types of interviews.

INTRODUCING THE IDEA OF COUNSELLING

Often if a child or adolescent says to parents or in front of parents that counselling would be a good idea, then parents will agree. Discussing it with the child alone and then asking permission to discuss it in front of parents helps a child to feel comfortable and to trust the physician's ability not to embarrass them or betray their confidence, and at the same time gives them hope that they will get help. These questions can help introduce the idea:

- Would it be a good idea to be able to talk about your feelings and worries a bit more?
- Would you like to talk about these things together with your parents, or separately?
- Talking about our problems helps us understand ourselves and deal with difficult things without being afraid or angry; talking as a family can help everybody understand everyone else better so that you all get along better together. Would

it be all right if I discuss this with your parents when they come back? Is there anything you've told me that I must not tell them? Shall we tell them together? (Many children will ask the physician to tell the parents; some will want to stay in the room, while others will want to leave and join in afterward.)

SUMMARY

A comprehensive approach to data gathering is important. With this information, a single interview can give relief to a child and his parents, leading to hope, reduction in anxiety, better sleep and concentration, improved school attendance, and, incidentally, can also demonstrate the value of counselling. At a follow-up visit, a discussion of the decrease in symptoms after the previous session can be powerful in helping both child and parents to appreciate the role of feelings in presenting complaints and the benefit for the child that follows their expression.

RESOURCES

Augustyn M, Zuckerman B, Cartonna EB. The Zuckerman Parker Handbook of Developmental and Behavioral Pediatrics for Primary Care, 3rd Edition. Philadelphia, PA: Wolter Kluwer/Lippincott Williams & Wilkins, 2011.

Canadian Attention Deficit Hyperactivity Disorder Resource Alliance (CADDRA): Canadian ADHD Practice Guidelines, 3rd Edition. Toronto: CADDRA, 2011. (See Chapter 1 for a description of step-wise interviewing. <www.caddra.ca/cms4/pdfs/caddra Guidelines2011Chapter01.pdf>)

Dixon SD, Stein M. Encounters with Children: Pediatric Behavior and Development, 4th Edition. Philadelphia: Mosby Elsevier, 2006.

Goldfarb DE, Roberts W. Developmental monitoring in primary care. Can Fam Physician 1996; 42: 1527–36.

Roberts W, Humphries T. School problems: A current perspective on assessment. Cdn J Paediatr 1990; 12: 16–29.

Roberts W, Schneeweiss S. Developmental history taking. Cdn J Paediatr 1991; 12: 4–11.

William CB, Crocker AB, Coleman WL, Elias ER, Feldman HM, eds. Developmental-Behavioral Pediatrics, 4th Edition. Philadelphia, PA: WB Saunders, 2009.

REFERENCES

1. Canadian Attention Deficit Hyperactivity Disorder Resource Alliance (CADDRA): Canadian ADHD Practice Guidelines, 3rd Edition. Toronto: CADDRA, 2011. <http://www.caddra.ca/cms4/pdfs/caddra Guidelines2011Chapter01.pdf>

2. Canadian Paediatric Society, Healthy Active Living and Sports Medicine Committee (Principal authors: Lipnowski S, Lelanc CMA). Healthy active living: Physical activity guidelines for children and adolescents. Paediatr Child Health 2012; 17(2): 209–10. <www.cps.ca>

3. Yudkin S, "Six Children with Coughs: The second diagnosis." The Lancet, 1961; 2(7202): 561–3, paraphrasing Dr. Balint, 1957.

CHAPTER 7

Questionnaires

Brenda Clark, Helena Ho, and Debra Andrews

In this chapter we present a short overview on the use of questionnaires in office practice and a set of free-access materials designed for this book that you may copy and use free of charge. These materials are also available as PDF files for download at www.cps.ca.

COLLECTION OF INFORMATION FROM PARENTS AND TEACHERS

The questionnaires and forms in this chapter were designed to gather pertinent medical and educational background information from parents and teachers to facilitate efficient history-taking and subsequent case management. Typically, a member of the office staff would ensure that all the forms and questionnaires are returned and filed.

- Many questionnaires are copyrighted, and there is a cost per use. The following questionnaires were designed for this book and may be copied as many times as needed without charge.
- It is important to remember that these questionnaires are designed to facilitate, and not to replace, history-taking and physical examination. Questionnaires can help identify issues that need more in-depth exploration and set the agenda for the appointment.
- In cases where parents may have difficulty with reading, or speak English as a second language, additional help may be needed to assist them to complete the questionnaires. For example, a nurse or office assistant could read the questions aloud and/or record the responses. An interpreter might need to be present.
- Office staff may have to make a phone call to ensure information is complete.

- A physician's office record flow-sheet may be kept at the front of the chart to keep track of all items requested and received: questionnaires and other documents such as birth records, hospital records, other consultations, and laboratory reports. (See also Chapter 6 on data gathering.)

Which forms should be used?

The **Parent Questionnaire** would be used for all children. One of the two school questionnaires would be chosen by the child's age. The **Preschool/Kindergarten Questionnaire** would best be used for children aged 3 to 5, and the **School Questionnaire** for children aged 6 and older.

- A **consent form** is needed for release of information from schools and other programs. A sample consent form is included for office use or you may use a standard release of information from your institution.
- If questionnaires are being mailed out, a **cover letter** to parents should accompany the two questionnaires and consent form. This letter should be signed by the person responsible for gathering the documents, usually office or clinic staff. The staff person should also fill in the physician's name and address or staple a business card on the right upper corner of the Parent and School Questionnaires.

When should questionnaires be collected?

The **Parent Questionnaire** can be mailed to parents prior to the visit to the consultant paediatrician's office. In the case of a primary care physician, it can be given to parents at their initial visit to be completed at home. Parents will have ample time to reflect and collect relevant information without the pressure of trying to do so in a busy waiting room. They can also check information written in baby books and consult relatives to fill in gaps in the medical and developmental history.

Having the parents return the questionnaire ahead of the family interview will prepare the clinician to focus and elaborate on pertinent points during the history-taking and the physical examination. Part of the discussion should be devoted to answering the specific questions and concerns listed by parents in the questionnaire. It should be noted that once a parent has listed a problem on a questionnaire and sent it back, the parent has given permission to talk about this issue. Referring to the written information on the questionnaire can ease the discussion of potentially difficult or sensitive topics, such as possible alcohol intake during pregnancy or mental health conditions in the family, e.g., "I see here that you've written down that your own brother had some problems with depression. Can you tell me more about that?"

The **Preschool/Kindergarten or School Questionnaire** can be mailed out or given to a parent with the Parent Questionnaire for them to bring to the child's teacher. Any request for information from a school or program must be accompanied by a signed consent to release information.

The information obtained from the school may provide the clinician with an idea of the child's social adjustment and academic performance as well as the resources and services available and what types of assessment have been done already. Further communication with the appropriate professionals listed in the questionnaire may promote understanding and facilitate formulation and implementation of recommendations.

Other questionnaires

Other standardized instruments can be used to complement the material gathered using the questionnaires from this manual. As your experience with assessing children with learning problems increases, you may wish to explore using some of these questionnaires, which fall into two main types.

Broad-based behavioural questionnaires

These screen for a wide variety of conditions and can help identify children who have significant emotional co-morbidity needing additional resources, or who might be better served by a mental health clinic or child psychiatrist. Some of these must be scored and/or interpreted by a psychologist, but a physician can learn how to score and interpret many of them. Examples include the following:

* **Achenbach System of Empirically Based Achievement (ASEBA)** set of behaviour questionnaires has been used for many years in clinical work and behavioural research. Child Behavior Checklist (CBCL) for ages 6 to 18 with the corresponding Teacher Rating Form (TRF) and Youth Self-Report form (YSR) by TM Achenbach and C Edelbrock. 1 South Prospect St., Burlington VT, 05410–3456: www.aseba.org
* **Behavior Assessment Scale for Children, Second Edition (BASC-2)** by Cecil R. Reynolds and Randy W. Kamphaus is an extensive set of rating scales and forms generally used by psychologists, including the Teacher Rating Scales (TRS), Parent Rating Scales (PRS), Self-Report of Personality (SRP), Student Observation System (SOS), and Structured Developmental History (SDH): http://pearsonassessments. com/HAIWEB/Cultures/en-us/Productdetail. htm?Pid=PAa30000&Mode=summary

Symptom-specific scales

These scales quantify a symptom or set of symptoms (e.g., inattention, anxiety, social skills), and are used diagnostically to compare the frequency and intensity of the symptoms with the normal or typical population.

When children present with learning problems, the most frequently used questionnaires would be for ADHD, and several can easily be implemented in physician office practice:

* **Conners Rating Scales for Teachers or Parents.** Contact Multi-Health Systems, Inc., 65, Overlea Blvd, Suite 210, Toronto ON M4H 1P1.

- **Vanderbilt NICHQ (National Initiative for Children's Healthcare Quality) Parent and Teacher Forms** were designed as part of an ADHD tool and are based on the DSM-IV (see below) symptom checklist for ADHD and its co-morbidities (ODD, CD, and anxiety). Downloadable forms and supporting materials may be obtained free by registering through the NICHQ website at www.nichq.org.

- **SNAP-IV Teacher and Parent Rating Scale** is another DSM-IV–based ADHD scale that is available free of charge. It includes a broader question set related to ADHD, and also has items about co-morbidity. It can be downloaded at www.adhdcanada.com/pdfs/SNAP-IVTeacher ParentRatingScale.pdf.

- **Diagnostic Symptom Lists** for attention deficit hyperactivity disorder and developmental coordination disorder are available in the American Psychiatric Association's *Diagnostic and Statistical Manual of Mental Disorders*, 4th Edition (Washington DC: 1994). Note that this version will be soon replaced by the 5th Edition (DSM-V).

- A review of problems with *fine and/or gross motor skills* is part of every good developmental history; however, you may wish to document the extent of the child's difficulties using a screening questionnaire. The **Developmental Coordination Disorder (DCD) Screener** provides information on the quality of motor movements, and the functional impact of motor difficulties. It can be downloaded free of charge on the Can Child website at http://dcd.canchild.ca/en

- With the increasing number of school-aged children presenting with *social skills difficulties*, it is useful to be aware of some questionnaires that specifically address social skills and ASD symptoms. The **Social Communication Questionnaire (SCQ)** by Michael Rutter et al. and the **Childhood Autism Rating Scale, 2nd Edition (CARS2)** are available from Western Psychological Services, Los Angeles CA.

SUMMARY

Questionnaires are an efficient way of gathering a large amount of information outside the office visit time slot. They allow a focused yet comprehensive approach to developmental and behavioural problems. There are many different kinds of questionnaires—familiarize yourself with a few that relate to the kinds of clinical presentations seen in your practice and use them at least a dozen times to get a good feel for their content, and for scoring if applicable, and then decide if they can be implemented in your office.

Always be aware of copyright issues; only reproduce materials in the public domain or those for which you have purchased access. The questionnaires and forms in this chapter may be reproduced without permission. Or visit the CPS website (www.cps.ca) to download them as PDF files.

CONSENT TO RELEASE INFORMATION FROM SCHOOL

Child's name: _____   Birth date (yy/mm/dd): _____

To determine what services your child requires, we require your permission to contact your child's school/preschool.

Name of school/preschool: _____

Contact person: _____

Title/position: _____   Phone: _____

I, _____, parent/legal guardian, consent for the release of any information which the school/preschool may have regarding my child's school function or development, including written or verbal reports to Dr. _____

Signature of parent/legal guardian: _____   Date: _____

Signature of witness: _____   Date: _____

Please return this signed consent from and the completed parent/school questionnaires to:

Dr. _____

Address: _____

PARENT QUESTIONNAIRE

A. General Information

Child's name: _____ ❑ Male ❑ Female

Name at birth if different from above: _____

Resident Address: _____ City/Town/Village: _____

Province/Territory: _____ Postal code: _____

Child's date of birth (yy/mm/dd): _____ Age: _____

Provincial health care insurance number: _____

Alternate health care plan name: _____ Number: _____

Is the child a Registered or Treaty Indian?   ❑ Yes ❑ No

Please attach a recent photograph of your child.

Parents/Legal Guardians:

Name: _____

Address: ❑ Same as child; or:

No./street: _____

City: _____ Prov/Terr: _____ Postal Code: ____

Phone: (H) _____ (W) _____ (C) _____

❑ Biological   ❑ Adoptive   ❑ Foster

❑ Step-parent   ❑ Grandparent

Name: _____

Address: ❑ Same as child; or:

No./street: _____

City: _____ Prov/Terr: _____ Postal Code: _____

Phone: (H) _____ (W) _____ (C) _____

❑ Biological   ❑ Adoptive   ❑ Foster

❑ Step-parent   ❑ Grandparent

Language(s) spoken at home: 1. _____ 2. _____

If English is not spoken at home, indicate the name of an English-speaking contact person:

_____

Phone: (H)_____ (W) _____ (C) _____

List everyone living in the home: _____

_____

Source: Children with School Problems (2012), Canadian Paediatric Society. May be reproduced without permission.
Also available at www.cps.ca.

Child's guardianship status (if applicable): _____

Social worker/legal guardian (if applicable): _____

Address: _____ Phone: _____ Fax: _____

Who suggested this referral? _____

Family physician: _____ Paediatrician: _____

Please list your main concerns:

_____

_____

Do you have any specific questions you would like answered?

_____

_____

Current daycare/preschool/school: _____ Grade/level: _____

Contact name and title/role: _____ Phone: _____

List the preschools, daycare centres, and schools your child has attended. Use a separate sheet if necessary:

Name of program/school	Years attended	Grade/ level	Problems noted	Special programs

Previous assessments:

	Date	Consultant or agency	Is your child currently involved?
Psychology			
Speech-language pathology			
Occupational/physiotherapy			
Audiology (hearing)			
Vision			
Other:			

PLEASE ATTACH ANY AVAILABLE REPORTS OF PREVIOUS ASSESSMENTS TO THIS QUESTIONNAIRE.

Source: Children with School Problems (2012), Canadian Paediatric Society. May be reproduced without permission. Also available at www.cps.ca.

Are you aware of any assessments planned in the next six to twelve months?   Yes ❑   No ❑

If yes, when, where, and by whom? _____

B. Prenatal/Birth History

Total number of pregnancies: _____ Any miscarriage(s)/stillbirth(s)/abortion(s): _____

Duration of this pregnancy (weeks): _____

Did you have any of the following during this pregnancy?

Check all that apply:

❑ Excessive vomiting	❑ Operation(s)	❑ Excessive vaginal bleeding
❑ Infection with fever or rash	❑ Injuries/accidents	❑ Other health problems:
❑ Toxemia (high blood pressure)	❑ Unusual emotional stress	_____
❑ Convulsions/seizures	❑ Prolonged hospitalization(s)	_____

During your pregnancy, did you:

Smoke cigarettes?   ❑ No   ❑ Less than ½ pack per day   ❑ ½ to 1 pack per day

❑ More than 1 pack per day

Drink alcoholic beverages?   ❑ No   ❑ First three months only   ❑ Throughout most of pregnancy

Amount each time (1 drink = 1 beer, 1 glass of wine, or 1 mixed drink):

❑ 1–2 drinks   ❑ 3–5 drinks   ❑ 6 drinks or more

Frequency: ❑ Once per week   ❑ Two or more times per week

Use prescription or nonprescription medications?   ❑ No   ❑ Yes

Use any drugs (marijuana, cocaine, heroin, etc.)?   ❑ No   ❑ Yes

Name of birth hospital: _____ City/Province: _____

How long was labour? _____ hours   Was labour: ❑ Spontaneous?   ❑ Induced?

Type of anaesthetics: ❏ General   ❏ Spinal   ❏ Local   ❏ None   ❏ Other

Method of delivery: ❏ Spontaneous   ❏ Assisted (forceps used)   ❏ Vacuum extraction

❏ Vaginal   ❏ Caesarean (elective)   ❏ Caesarean (emergency)

Position of baby: ❏ Head first   ❏ Breech   ❏ Other

Were there any concerns about your baby (such as fetal distress) immediately before the birth?

❏ No   ❏ Yes   Please explain: _____

Did your baby need any help to breathe right after birth?

❏ No   ❏ Yes   Please explain: _____

_____

How was your baby fed? Were there any feeding problems?_____

_____

Did your baby have any of these problems at birth or during the first month of life? Check all that apply?

❏ Poor sucking   ❏ Injured at birth   ❏ Birth defects

❏ Unusual rash   ❏ Trouble breathing   ❏ Was given medications

❏ Turned yellow   ❏ Turned blue   ❏ Infection (specify)_____

❏ Received blood transfusion   ❏ Kept in incubator (how long?_____)   ❏ Seizures/convulsions

❏ Needed surgery   ❏ Transferred to intensive care nursery   ❏ Was very jittery

❏ Other problems:_____

C. Child's Developmental and Medical History

Early development: When (specify age in years and months, if possible) did your child first accomplish the following:

Age	Milestone	Age	Milestone	Age	Milestone
	Sat without help		Crawled		Walked alone for 10 to 15 steps
	Toilet trained (day)		Toilet trained (night)		Walked upstairs
	Rode a bike without training wheels		Used sentences		Used a spoon
	Spoke first words ("mama," "dada")		Rode a tricycle using pedals		Named 3 or more colours
	Ate independently		Counted from 1 to 10		Named 3 or more body parts
	Used fingers to feed		Put 2 or 3 words together		

When did you first become concerned about your child's development? _____

Do you have any concerns now?_____

Has your child lost any skills he or she used to be able to do? _____

Functional problems: Please check which, if any, of the following concerns you have:

❑ Feeding difficulties

❑ Avoiding eye contact

❑ Limited food choices

❑ Social skill difficulties

❑ Soiling

❑ Shy with strangers

❑ Recurrent headaches

❑ Short attention span

❑ Destructive to property

❑ Mood swings

❑ Frequent temper tantrums

❑ Trouble with police

❑ Withdrawn/In own world

❑ Clumsy/Awkward/Poorly coordinated

❑ Recurrent stomach ache

❑ Resistance to change of routine

❑ Night crying/Nightmares

❑ Snoring

❑ Hyperactive/Impulsive

❑ Defiant/Negativistic

❑ Stealing

❑ Inappropriate sexual behaviour

❑ Resistance to going to school

❑ Unusual/Odd mannerisms

❑ Constipation/Diarrhea

❑ Unusual fears/Anxiety

❑ Trouble falling asleep

❑ Bedwetting

❑ Rocking/Head banging

❑ Aggression toward self or others

❑ Cruelty to animals

❑ Setting fires

❑ Thumb-sucking/Nail-biting

❑ Other: _____

Discipline: When your child is misbehaving, what do you usually do?

_____

Past health problems: Please give age of occurrence and details.

❑ Ear infections	❑ Hearing problem	❑ Tics or muscle twitches
❑ Rash/Skin problems	❑ Eye problem	❑ Casts/Braces
❑ Head injury	❑ Recurrent infections	❑ Surgery (operations)
❑ Meningitis	❑ Allergies	❑ Admissions to hospital
❑ Seizures	❑ Asthma	❑ Other (specify): _____

Details: _____

_____

List any long-term medication, special diets, or large doses of vitamins (taken for longer than two weeks at a time)?

Name/dose: _____ When: _____

Name/dose: _____ When: _____

Name/dose: _____ When: _____

Name/dose: _____ When: _____

Birth parent information/Family history:

Birth mother

Name: _____

Date of birth: _____ Age: _____

Present occupation: _____

Education (highest grade completed): _____

Any learning/behaviour/
emotional problems? _____

Any health problems? _____

_____

Birth father

Name: _____

Date of Birth: _____ Age: _____

Present occupation: _____

Education (highest grade completed): _____

Any learning/behaviour/
emotional problems: _____

Any health problems? _____

_____

Marital status: _____ Are the birth mother and father related? ❑ Yes ❑ No

Describe special circumstance (e.g., other parental relationships involved): _____

_____

Siblings:

Full Name	Date of birth	Gender (M/F)	Grade	Relationship (full, step, half)	Health, learning or behaviour problems

Health conditions in the family:

Check conditions that apply and indicate relationship to your child.

Problem/Condition	Relationship to child	Problem/Condition	Relationship to child
ADHD		Migraine headaches	
Behaviour problems in childhood		Epilepsy	
Learning, reading problems		Autism spectrum disorder	
Speech problems		Thyroid problems	
Developmental delay		Depression	
Repeated a grade		Anxiety disorder	
Genetic syndrome/birth defect		Drinking problems	
Vision problems		Drug abuse	
Hearing problems		Other mental health issues	
Cerebral palsy		Other:_____	

Have there been any major events that may have been stressful to the family (e.g., moving home, physical/mental illness, death, separation/divorce, unemployment, legal or financial problem)?

_____

_____

Additional information that you feel may help us better understand your child (e.g., additional school history):

_____

_____

Name of person filling out this form: _____

Signature: _____ Date: _____

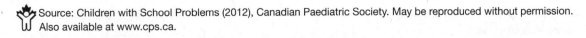
Source: Children with School Problems (2012), Canadian Paediatric Society. May be reproduced without permission. Also available at www.cps.ca.

PRESCHOOL/KINDERGARTEN QUESTIONNAIRE

Child's name: _____ Birth date: _____

Parent/Guardian: _____

To the teacher: Your careful completion of this questionnaire, which will help us to assess this child's needs, is greatly appreciated. Please return to: _____

Name of preschool/kindergarten: _____ Contact name: _____

Address: _____ City/province: _____ Postal code: _____

Phone: _____ Fax: _____

Type of program

	Nursery school/preschool		Half-day		Regular
	Kindergarten		Full-day		Special needs

Date child was enrolled: _____ Who initiated this referral? _____

Please list any specific questions or concerns for which you would like help:

_____

_____

_____

_____

What are the child's greatest strengths?

_____

_____

What are the child's weaknesses or difficulties?

_____

_____

Describe the child's learning style (activity level, organizational skills, impulsiveness, etc.):

_____

_____

Describe the child's behaviour:

_____

_____

Describe the child's peer relationships and social interaction skills:

_____

_____

Which of the following resources are available to your school?

Professional	Consultant or agency	Is this child currently involved?
Special education teacher		
Special education assistant/aide		
Special education program		
Speech-language therapy		
Physiotherapy		
Occupational therapy		
Psychologist		
Community health nurse		
Social worker		
Other (specify)		

Please assess the child in the following areas:

Skill set	Major concern	Minor concern	No concern	Cannot judge	Comments
Gross motor skills					
Posture					
Awkward gait					
Frequently falls					
Easily fatigued					
Tip-toe walking					

Skill set	Major concern	Minor concern	No concern	Cannot judge	Comments
Gross motor skills (cont'd)					
Ball skills					
Playground skills					
Playground safety					
Coordination					
Other (specify)					
Fine motor skills					
Crayon/pencil skills					
Use of scissors					
Easily fatigued when printing					
Hand dominance (switching hands)					
Puzzle skills					
Other (specify)					
Self-help skills					
Undressing self					
Dressing self					
Use of zippers/buttons					
Feeding self					
Washing hands/face					
Helping clean up					
Toileting routines					
Toileting accidents/ soiling					
Other (specify)					
Social skills					
Interest in peers					
Initiation of interactions with peers					
Social responses to peers					
Group play with peers					
Imaginative play					
Solitary play					
Repetitive motor movements or behaviours (spinning, flapping, tics)					
Ability to share					
Turn-taking					

Skill set	Major concern	Minor concern	No concern	Cannot judge	Comments
Offering comfort					
Compliance with rules and limits					
Adjustment to new or changed routines					
Behaviour					
Attention span					
Impulsivity					
Hyperactivity or motor restlessness					
Physical aggression					
Destructive tendencies					
Temper tantrums					
Breath-holding spells					
Unusual fears					
Obsessive interests/ topics					
Ritual behaviours					
Phobias					
Somatic complaints (stomach aches, headaches, pains)					
Difficult temperament/ moods					
Other (specify)					
Receptive language skills					
Following 1-step instructions					
Following 2-step instructions					
Listening in a group					
Listening to stories					
Listening to rhymes and tunes					
Other (specify)					
Expressive language					
Pronunciation					
Speaking in phrases/ sentences					
Taking turns in conversation					

Skill set	Major concern	Minor concern	No concern	Cannot judge	Comments
Expressive language (cont'd)					
Effective verbal communication					
Stuttering					
Other (specify)					
Academic readiness skills					
Knowledge of sizes/ shapes					
Knowledge of colours					
Letter recognition					
Number recognition					
Rote count 1 to 10					
Knowledge of number concepts					
Ability to read and print first name					
Other (specify)					

Has there been a deterioration, loss, or plateauing of previously acquired skills in the past year?

No ❏   Yes ❏ (specify:) _____

General comments: _____

_____

_____

_____

Name of person filling out this form: _____ Title: _____

Signature: _____ Date: _____

Please attach copies of the child's latest assessment or progress reports and include any other information that might help in assessment of this child.

THANK YOU FOR COMPLETING THIS QUESTIONNAIRE.

Source: Children with School Problems (2012), Canadian Paediatric Society. May be reproduced without permission. Also available at www.cps.ca.

SCHOOL QUESTIONNAIRE (6–18 YEARS)

Student's name: _____ Birth date: _____

Parent/Guardian: _____

To the teacher: Your careful completion of this questionnaire, which will help us to assess this child's needs, is greatly appreciated. Please return to: _____

Name of school: _____ Contact name: _____

Address: _____ City/province: _____ Postal code: _____

Phone: _____ Fax: _____

Student's grade or level or placement: _____ Size of class: _____ Date enrolled: _____

Please describe this student's present placement (include type of classroom, special program, and remedial support):

_____

_____

_____

Does the student receive in-class resource help?   ❑ Yes   ❑ No

If yes, how many hours per week? _____ Per day? _____

Does the student receive out-of-class resource help?   ❑ Yes   ❑ No

If yes, how many hours per week? _____ Per day? _____

What are this student's school difficulties and strengths?

_____

_____

Please list any specific concerns and/or questions you would like help with for this student:

_____

_____

_____

Describe this student's social adjustment with adults:

_____

_____

Describe this student's adjustment with other students:

_____

_____

Is this student currently receiving counselling in school? ❑ Yes ❑ No

If yes, please describe:

_____

_____

Please list dates and attach test scores or reports for any previous individual or group testing done for this student:

❑ Psychology: _____

❑ Speech-language: _____

❑ Academic achievement: _____

❑ Hearing/Vision: _____

❑ Other (specify:) _____

Are you aware of any pending evaluations at school? ❑ Yes ❑ No

If yes, when and by whom? _____

Which of the following services/supports does your school provide and/or is currently received by this student?

Service/support	Available?	Consultant or agency (if known)	Currently involved?
Special education program			
Individual education plan (IEP)			
Special education assistant			
Assistive technology			

Service/support	Available?	Consultant or agency (if known)	Currently involved?
Class FM amplification system			
Resource room program			
Speech-language therapy			
Guidance counselling			
Occupational/Physical therapy			
Psychologist			
Community health nurse			
Social worker			
Cultural liaison worker			
Special class			
Other (specify)			

Student performance

Please rate the student's performance in the following areas as you have observed it on a day-to-day basis:

Skill set	Major concern	Minor concern	No concern	Advanced for age	Estimated grade level
Reading					
Word recognition					
Reading rate					
Oral reading					
Silent reading					
Reading comprehension					
Spelling					
Accuracy					
Fine motor skills					
Writing (punctuation, legibility)					
Volume output/speed					
Mathematics					
Computation					
Problem-solving					
Language					
Written					
Word pronunciation					
Comprehension of verbal instruction					
Oral sentence structure and fluency					

Skill set	Major concern	Minor concern	No concern	Advanced for age	Estimated grade level
Language (Cont'd)					
Reciprocal conversations					
Inappropriate use of language					
Knowledge					
General					
Memory					
Immediate					
Long-term					
Art					
Art					
Physical education					
Physical education					
Spatial awareness					
Left/right confusion					

Skill set	Major concern	Minor concern	No concern	Comments
Effort/motivation				
Effort				
Social/emotional				
Interest in peers				
Attempts to engage peers				
Social responses to peers				
Group interactions with peers				
Imaginative play				
Solitary play				
Repetitive motor movements or behaviours (spinning, flapping, tics)				
Ability to share				
Turn-taking				
Offering comfort				
Compliance with rules and limits				
Adjustment to new or changed routines				
Behaviour				
Attention span				
Impulsivity				

Skill set	Major concern	Minor concern	No concern	Comments
Behaviour (Cont'd)				
Hyperactivity or motor restlessness				
Defiance/Noncompliance with authority				
Physical aggression toward others				
Destruction of property				
Runs away from school				
Frequently absent				
Starts fires				
Lies				
Cheats				
History of trouble with the law				
Unusual fears				
Obsessive interests/topics				
Ritualistic behaviours				
Phobias				
Somatic complaints (stomach aches, headaches, pains)				
Difficult temperament/moods				
Other (specify)				

Does your student have access to computers? ❑ Yes ❑ No

If yes, please specify whether in: ❑ Classroom ❑ Computer room

Describe this student's keyboarding skills: ❑ Good ❑ Developing ❑ Absent

Comment: _____

Does this child have any special interests or talents? ❑ Yes ❑ No

Please describe: _____

_____

School/parent relationship:

Are parents aware/concerned? ❑ Yes ❑ No

Please describe: _____

_____

General comments:

_____

_____

_____

_____

Name of person filling out this form: _____ Title: _____

Signature: _____ Date: _____

Thank you for your help in completing this questionnaire. Please attach copies of the child's latest assessment or progress reports and include any other information that may help in assessment of this child.

8

The Physical Examination of the Child with Learning Problems

Debra Andrews

Although the physical examination is the component of a complete assessment least likely to yield significant abnormal findings, it should be done with care. The physician is the only person, with the possible exception of an experienced nurse clinician, who is able to comment on the physical health of the child and interpret the relative importance of various physical findings. Although a neurodevelopmental examination done by a physician may overlap with testing done by educators, psychologists, speech-language pathologists, audiologists, optometrists, occupational therapists, and physiotherapists, no one else's evaluation is going to pick up any physical abnormalities the physician has missed.

In this chapter we review five important reasons for performing a thorough physical examination. These are to rule out physical disease that might interfere with learning; evaluate co-morbid medical conditions; look for minor physical anomalies; describe neurological findings; and rule out contraindications and establish a baseline for possible medication use.

RULE OUT PHYSICAL DISEASE

The first task of the physician is to rule out physical illness. Chronic illnesses such as asthma, inflammatory bowel disease, chronic renal failure, haemophilia, diabetes, or cystic fibrosis will usually be obvious from the history, and the examination will serve to confirm the findings of the history and evaluate severity. Chronic disease may interfere with a child's schooling by causing recurrent or prolonged absences from school. Although it will rarely cause primary school failure, the disease itself may be complicated by involvement of the central nervous system (CNS), as in lead poisoning, or the treatment may cause the problems (e.g., cranial irradiation for leukemia). Some medications used in the treatment of chronic conditions may have CNS side effects (e.g., sedation or exacerbation of hyperactivity).

If disease has been severe enough to retard physical growth, there may be psychological ramifications, as well as effects on gross motor function due to decreased muscle bulk. Cardiac or pulmonary disease may cause increased fatigue and poor stamina, interfering with full participation in school activities and decreasing attention. Some systemic illnesses may affect the special senses, either directly as a result of the disease process (e.g., iritis in juvenile rheumatoid arthritis) or indirectly (e.g., ototoxicity from aminoglycosides used to treat infectious conditions). Determine if the frequency of the child's absences is consistent with the severity of the illness.

Appropriate level of participation must be determined. Chronic illness may affect the way the child interacts with adults, especially if the child is perceived by others as being more fragile or susceptible to illness. It may be that part of the physician's role will be to decide how much restriction of activity is truly warranted.

Neurological conditions are associated with an increased incidence of learning problems. In some cases, the problem may already have been diagnosed, especially if the symptoms are severe or if there are obvious physical findings. Always be alert to subtle signs or an evolving clinical picture. The stigmata of neurocutaneous syndromes usually increase with age, but early on there may be little to note except for a few *café au lait* spots, learning and/or behavioural concerns, and possibly a positive family history. Fragile X and fetal alcohol spectrum disorder (FASD) have a wide range of presentations. The tics associated with Tourette's disorder, unless very severe or frequent, may be suppressed during the general physical examination; they may be more apparent during the history or right after the examination is done, when the child is on the way out of the office and is more relaxed.

Be aware that many genetic syndromes are associated with learning problems. Some are associated with varying degrees of intellectual disability. Others have well-delineated psychometric or behavioural profiles (behavioural phenotype), which can be useful in determining therapy and prognosis. Examples include fragile X, Klinefelter, Turner, Williams, Angelman, and Prader-Willi syndromes. The history or the presence of old, healed scars may be clues to previous anomalies that were surgically corrected. If the child has an unusual combination of major or minor congenital anomalies or dysmorphic features, checking a genetic text or consulting with a genetics/dysmorphology service will clarify the need for further workup.

An important part of the examination is screening for visual or hearing impairment. The child who fails an office screening can be referred for more definitive testing. Although neither hearing impairment nor poor vision by themselves are frequent causes of school difficulties, the physician should not miss any treatable contributor to a child's school problems. Also look for conditions that predispose to middle ear disease, such as cleft palate or allergies, as well as evidence of previous infection (e.g., scarring, perforation, or cholesteatoma).

Note the presence of any physical features that might impact the child's physical or social function in school. Stature, body habitus, and sexual maturity may be important, particularly in questions of class placement. If the school is suggesting retention, there might be additional argument against such a course if the student is the tallest in the class. Children who are overweight may be subject to taunting or isolation from peers.

Commonly, there is no chronic condition, the examination shows no significant abnormalities, and any positive findings are not related to the child's learning problems. Communicate this clearly to the parent, child, and school.

Find out what specific concerns or possible diagnoses caregivers have in mind and be sure to comment on these areas as you do the exam. Parents may not realize that the neurologic examination can help rule out conditions like cerebral palsy or provide evidence that birth-related concerns are not playing a role. It is important to be as explicit about what you are ruling out as about what you are ruling in.

EVALUATE CO-MORBID MEDICAL CONDITIONS

Many children experiencing difficulties in school will complain of symptoms such as abdominal pain, headaches, limb pain, and fatigue. The diagnosis of a functional symptom includes, first, the exclusion of organic causes of the symptom and, second, the identification of psychological processes or pressures responsible for the somatic disorder. A thorough physical exam is the key to differentiating medical versus functional complaints (e.g., increased intracranial pressure versus tension headaches or functional abdominal pain versus ulcer or inflammatory bowel disease), and a comprehensive child and family interview will help to identify the psychosocial factors involved. This is important information for the school, and it may help the teacher to decide whether the child's frequent trips to the nurse's office are due to symptoms that require a medical intervention or whether the better prescription for the child's pain might be accommodations or extra help in the area of concern.

A number of medical problems are seen with increased frequency among children with learning disabilities (LDs) and/or ADHD, especially enuresis and encopresis. Ensure that the appropriate initial workup has been done for these conditions. For enuresis, the physical exam may be non-contributory; for encopresis, the abdominal examination often may reveal large amounts of stool in the descending colon and rectum. Functional eating and sleep disorders are also more common in this population, and physical causes should be carefully excluded.

LOOK FOR MINOR PHYSICAL ANOMALIES

A number of minor congenital anomalies are said to occur with increased frequency in children with learning and attention problems, suggesting a common embryological or gestational mechanism. Most minor anomalies are caused by alteration of mechanical forces affecting the normal fetal tissue development early in gestation, before twenty weeks. These anomalies usually do not alter function but may cause cosmetic concerns. They tend to occur in parts of the body that are complex in structure and subject to wide degrees of phenotypic variation, such as the features of the face, head, and extremities.

It is interesting to speculate on possible associations between these minor dysmorphic stigmata and the minor neurological anomalies postulated to underlie LDs, which must occur simultaneously, between the tenth to nineteenth week of gestation—during the periods of neuronal proliferation (four to twenty-four weeks), neuronal differentiation (fourteen weeks to a peak at term birth), synapse formation and axonal growth (beginning at about eight weeks gestation), and neuronal migration (peak at about eighteen weeks). Anomalies of skin and hair are intriguing if it is recalled that the patterning of hair growth is determined by the direction of stretch on the skin surface at the time the hair follicles develop; this in turn is determined by the growth of the developing brain before the skull bones have formed. The leftward displacement of the posterior hair whorl in 56% of individuals is presumed to be due to the slightly larger size of the left side of the brain.

These minor anomalies are nonspecific, and they also occur in children with no developmental concerns, sometimes as a familial trait; therefore, by themselves they are not diagnostic of LDs or other learning problems. Table 8–1 provides a summary of minor physical anomalies that might be seen during a physical exam. A familial finding can sometimes be useful in helping parents understand genetic contributions to children's problems such as ADHD.

DESCRIBE NEUROLOGICAL FINDINGS

There is a high co-morbidity of learning problems with neurological conditions such as epilepsy or cerebral palsy. If the history suggests a neurological disorder, the neurological examination should be painstakingly detailed.

So-called "soft" signs can be divided into two groups. The first includes *subtle findings* that would be abnormal at any age, such as mild asymmetry of deep tendon reflexes or consistently unilateral hand posturing on stressed gait. The second group is *developmental*, and it includes findings that are normal in young children and that gradually disappear with maturation. The majority of developmental "soft" signs have disappeared by about eight or nine years of age.

Table 8–1 Common Minor Physical Anomalies

Body part	Anomalies
Head	Double hair whorl, abnormal eyebrows, fine electric hair, head circumference above 98th or below the 3rd percentile
Eyes	Inner epicanthal folds, hypertelorism, short palpebral fissures
Ears	Pre-auricular pits or tags (associated with hearing loss); lack of lobulus (adherent lobes); pointed or other abnormalities of shape; low-set, posteriorly rotated, simplified or asymmetrically formed pinnae
Mouth	High arched palate, cleft, submucous cleft (bifid uvula); flattened philtrum and thin upper lip (FASD); overbite or micrognathia
Feet	Wide gap between first and second toe, syndactyly of second and third toe, third toe extends past second, hypoplastic nails
Hands	Single palmar crease, clinodactyly (incurving) of fifth finger, syndactyly, extra digits

Individual "soft" signs observed in an individual child are not very useful, but norms exist for the number of findings common at a given age; an increased number of "soft" signs at a specific age would provide supportive, but not diagnostic, evidence for an LD.

Table 8–2 indicates the neurological "soft" signs that are more common in the population of children with LDs, even up to the age of eleven years. More than two signs observed after eight years of age are considered to be significant.

RULE OUT CONTRAINDICATIONS AND ESTABLISH A BASELINE FOR MEDICATION USE

If medication is to be used, initial measurements and vital signs must be documented. Serial heights and weights help ensure adequate growth and are very reassuring to parents concerned about stimulant-induced anorexia. Some children on consistent stimulant medication may experience a decrease

Table 8–2 Testing for "Soft" Neurological Signs

Procedure	Interpretation
Head rotation with arms drop or spread: Child stands with feet together, eyes closed, arms outstretched in front, fingers widespread. Examiner passively moves head side to side.	Positive (abnormal) if arms drop and move laterally. Negative (normal) if arms remain still.
Finger-thumb: Examiner sitting with hands on knees, palms up, touches thumb to fingers, fifth finger first, two to three times. Child performs first with one hand, then the other.	Difficulties curling fingers, missing, and inaccuracy are positive. Mirror movements on the other hand are positive.
Dysdiadochokinesia: Examiner sitting with hands on knees and facing the child slowly alternates touching front and back of hand to knees with both hands. Examiner asks child to imitate slowly and then faster with both hands, then with each hand individually.	Disorganized performance and slow, awkward turns are scored positive.
Associated movements: When performing unilateral tasks, the other limb moves symmetrically.	Scored positive if it occurs.
Mixed laterality: Examiner asks the child to gently throw and kick a ball and to look at him or her through a rolled sheet of paper or kaleidoscope.	Positive if the child does not use the same side for all tasks.
Strabismus or poor convergence: Use cover/uncover test if necessary.	Score positive if fixed strabismus or if there is lack of ability to converge when following finger.
Raise brows: Facing the child, the examiner raises his or her eyebrows. The child imitates this action.	Score positive if the child is unable to imitate.
Dysgraphaesthesia in palm: With child's eyes closed, the examiner traces five numbers with a finger tip on child's palm.	Score positive if there are three or more errors. (The physician should first confirm that the child is able to read numbers.)
Stressed gaits: Ask the child to stand or walk on heels, toes, or external border of foot (Fogs' test).	Score positive if involuntary associated movements of upper limbs occur.
Finger agnosia: With child's eyes closed, the examiner gently touches the child's fingertips and asks the child to identify which one. It is essential, prior to this test, to ensure that the child is able to name the individual fingers. If not, the test may be modified by allowing the child to point to the corresponding finger on a drawing.	Score positive if three out of ten attempts are incorrect.

Table 8–3 Details of the Physical Examination for School Learning Problems

Exam section	Focus
Measurements	Height, weight, occipito-frontal head circumference. Norms are available for other bodily and facial measurements, which may be required in the process of dysmorphologic diagnosis.
Vital signs	Heart rate, blood pressure.
Special senses	Administer screening tests for vision, amblyopia, strabismus, and hearing if report of specialist's examination is not available or forthcoming.
Regular systemic physical examination	Comment on overall health, nutritional status, facies, and suspected dysmorphism or syndromes, stigmata of neurocutaneous disorders or other skin lesions. Pay special attention to tympanic membranes, upper airway, baseline cardiac examination, abdominal examination for organomegaly and evidence of constipation, Tanner stage for puberty.
Musculo-skeletal system	Gait, muscle bulk and tone, range of motion.
Neurological examination	Standard exam: Cranial nerves (including fundi), sensation, deep tendon reflexes, Babinski reflex, motor strength and tone, cerebellar signs, balance, gait. Extended exam: Motor impersistance, stimulus extinction, associated movements or synkinesia, choreiform movements and tics, rapid alternating movements, praxis (ability to execute voluntary movements on command), gnosis (including finger agnosia), stressed gaits (heel/toe walking, walking on outside of feet, forward and reverse tandem gait, hopping, kicking, catching). Difficulties in these domains can lead to an additional diagnosis of a developmental coordination disorder. Mental status. Neurodevelopmental exam and skill sampling.

in their height velocity (see Chapter 15). Mild changes in pulse or blood pressure are reported in children taking stimulants, but they are rarely of clinical concern.

Table 8–3 provides an overview of a comprehensive physical examination for a child presenting with learning problems, as might be done on an initial visit by a paediatric consultant or as part of a staged assessment in a family medicine office.

SUMMARY

During the physical examination the physician should do the following:

- Rule out physical illness as a cause of learning problems, including considering side effects of medications used for medical illness.
- Evaluate for medical conditions that commonly co-occur with learning problems.
- Look for physical anomalies that might be a clue to a genetic condition or syndrome.
- Describe neurological findings, including both hard signs and developmental "soft" signs.
- Rule out contraindications and establish a baseline for possible medication use.

RESOURCES

von Hilsheimer G, Kurko V. Minor physical anomalies in exceptional children. J Learn Disabil 1979; 12: 462–9.

Peters JE, Romine JS, Dykmann RA. A special neurological examination of children with learning disabilities. Dev Med Child Neurolo 1975; 17: 63–78.

The assessment process: Systematic formulation. In: Levine MD, Brooks RB, Shonkoff JP. A Pediatric Approach to Learning Disorders. Toronto: John Wiley & Sons, 1980: 121–52.

Minor anomalies. In: Lyons Jones K. Smith's Recognizable Patterns of Human Malformation, 6th Edition. Philadelphia: Elsevier Saunders, 2006: 817–34.

Normal standards. In: Lyons Jones K. Smith's Recognizable Patterns of Human Malformation, 6th Edition. Philadelphia: Elsevier Saunders, 2006: 835–63.

9

Medical Investigations of Children with Learning Problems

G. Tyna Doyle and William Mahoney

A comprehensive history and physical examination may be sufficient basis for a sound medical opinion, or it may suggest the need for further tests to verify clinical hypotheses or exclude differential diagnoses.

The physician's role is to rule out physical illness that may be responsible for the difficulties in school. To achieve this, the differential diagnosis needs to be reviewed in light of the history and physical exam findings when considering what investigations to order. (See Chapters 3 and 11.) In this chapter we look at some medical investigations the physician may consider for children with learning problems.

MEDICAL CONDITIONS

The following common medical conditions should be considered in the medical investigations of learning difficulties. These conditions may be the cause of the learning problem (part of the differential diagnosis) or may be additional conditions (co-morbidities) that, once addressed, may improve the child's school performance:

- iron deficiency, with or without anemia
- lead toxicity
- thyroid malfunction
- sleep disorders
- seizures

In general, the history and physical exam will guide what tests are ordered. Even when investigations are indicated, the results are frequently negative or unhelpful. However, this review of systems must be done, as only the physician can exclude these potentially treatable conditions.

MEDICAL INVESTIGATIONS

There are no mandatory investigations for every child with school problems, but some that should be considered. The first step in assessing a child is to ensure that vision and hearing are intact. The child should have a **recent vision examination** completed by optometry or ophthalmology, depending on the presenting symptoms. A formal **hearing assessment** should be completed by audiology, especially for any child with a significant history of otitis or middle ear dysfunction.

Metabolic testing

Recent practice parameters have provided guidelines for investigations in the cases of global developmental delay (GDD) and intellectual disability (ID).(1)-(5) The first thing to determine is if any newborn screening was completed. If universal newborn screening cannot be documented, bloodwork, including metabolic screening, should be considered. This includes capillary blood gas, serum lactate, ammonia, serum amino acids and urine organic acids, and thyroid-stimulating hormone. Routine metabolic screening is not indicated if newborn screening was done, or unless there is a significant family history, developmental regression, episodic decompensation, seizures, hypoglycemia, or physical exam abnormality (e.g., ataxia, severe hypotonia).

Genetic testing

Genetic testing must also be considered, especially in light of the fact that a normal examination does not rule out an underlying genetic diagnosis. This includes a clinical **microarray** (when available) or **routine cytogenetic testing** (karyotype), and possibly **fragile X** testing. A recent review stated microarray testing is abnormal in 7.8% of subjects with GDD/ID (10.6% if associated with syndromic features), and karyotype is abnormal in at least 4% of subjects with GDD/ID (18.6% with syndromic features).(6) One should also consider testing for Rett syndrome in girls with unexplained moderate-severe GDD/ID (7)(8). Microarray is the genetic test with the highest diagnostic yield in unexplained GDD/ID and there is consensus among clinical geneticists that it should be considered first line (9); however, it depends on clinical availability in your area. The Canadian College of Medical Geneticists position statement on the use of array genomic hybridization technology in constitutional genetic diagnosis in Canada recommends that microarray should be first line in GDD/ID, autism, multiple congenital anomalies, or dysmorphic features that are unexplained after a thorough history and physical exam, with the exception of those patients suspected to have a common aneuploidy or triploidy.(10) Testing will be guided by family history, facial appearance, and the presence of any dysmorphic stigmata. Genetics consultation should be completed if any further testing is needed, for example, if there is deterioration in school function or behaviour in a previously successful child. Also, when suspecting a specific diagnosis, other testing may be more appropriate and cost-effective (e.g., Williams and fluorescence in situ hybridization). If in doubt, consultation should occur with the geneticists. Appropriate counselling should be in place before any genetic testing is completed.

Other blood work

Lead levels should be obtained if risk factors are identified, as well as **complete blood count** and **serum ferritin**, if iron deficiency is suspected.

Neuroimaging

Neuroimaging has been recommended in children with GDD/ID, and when there are signs or symptoms of intracranial lesions. It is not indicated for every child with school difficulty. There is debate in the literature regarding the use of imaging in children with global developmental delay. The American Academy of Neurology and Child Neurology Society recommend it as a part of the diagnostic evaluation of global developmental delay.(11)(12) In contrast, the American College of Medical Genetics states that the normocephalic patient without focal neurologic signs should not be considered for cranial imaging.(13) There seems to be agreement that in this population, magnetic resonance imaging (MRI) is preferred to computerized axial tomography (CT). MRI has been found to be more sensitive, with one study stating MRI abnormalities were detected in 65.5% compared to 30% for CT scan in evaluating developmental delay.(14) It is important to remember that MRI often requires sedation, and the risk and benefits need to be considered. Neuroimaging is also helpful when considering other neurological conditions, such as tuberous sclerosis and neurofibromatosis. With suspicion of an acute neurologic event, the decision about the type of imaging is based on the presenting symptoms.

EEG

Electroencephalography (EEG) is not recommended routinely, and should only be completed if there is suspicion of a seizure. Close attention to staring spells on history is important to explore, as absence seizures are in the differential diagnosis.

Sleep investigations

It is essential to identify any sleep disorders, especially in the differential or as a co-morbid condition. A child's sleep problems may be a significant consideration in the explanation for his or her poor attention, as opposed to ADHD— or the child may have both. Also, it has been documented that children with ADHD have increased difficulty with sleep, and if this is better controlled, response to behaviour management and/or medication may be improved.(15)(16) Investigations may include **polysomnography** and/or referral to an **ear nose and throat (ENT) physician** if obstructive sleep apnea (OSA) is suspected.

Regression

Any history of regression is an urgent matter that needs immediate investigation, with input from both neurology and genetics/metabolics. If history or clinical findings suggest a space-occupying lesion or progressive disorder, neurological consultation is recommended.

Pre-existing conditions

There should be a thorough investigation of pre-existing medical conditions in the child with school difficulties; if the child is not physically well, that alone can affect school performance. For example, a child with diabetes who is poorly controlled, or a child with thyroid abnormalities, may be unable to perform because of their underlying medical diagnosis. Order investigations based on significant findings in the history and physical exam, for example, poor growth or pallor.

Contraindications to medication use

Lastly, if considering treatment options for particular diagnoses that include medication options, a review of potential contraindications or risk factors should be undertaken. For example, if there is a history of cardiac symptoms in the child, or a strong family history of cardiac symptoms, one may consider ordering a **cardiac consult,** including electrocardiogram, before starting a stimulant medication for underlying ADHD. A joint statement of the Canadian Paediatric Society, the Canadian Cardiovascular Society, and the Canadian Academy of Child and Adolescent Psychiatry, "Cardiac risk assessment before the use of stimulant medications in children and youth,"(17) gives clear guidelines that include a screening tool for the identification of potential cardiac risk factors for sudden death among children starting stimulant medication, and suggestions for review by a cardiologist prior to starting these medications.

SUMMARY

Medical investigation of the child with learning problems is guided by the history, physical examination, and formulation. Evaluation of vision and hearing is recommended. Common medical conditions that can contribute to poor performance in school need to be considered and investigated if clinically indicated. If more significant difficulties with intellectual development are present, it is appropriate to follow the published guidelines. The following list summarizes a suggested approach for your medical investigations:

- A consult should be requested from an optometrist or ophthalmologist if no vision assessment was completed in the previous two years.
- A formal audiometric examination should be arranged for every child, especially if there is a history of frequent otitis or middle ear dysfunction.
- In the child with GDD or ID, if universal newborn screening cannot be documented, routine metabolic screening should be considered. This includes capillary blood gas, serum lactate, ammonia, serum amino acids and urine organic acids, and thyroid stimulating hormone.
- In the child with GDD or ID, microarray genetic testing is first line. Other genetic testing should be obtained as appropriate. There should be consideration of Rett syndrome in girls with unexplained moderate to severe developmental delay.
- Lead levels and workup for possible iron deficiency may be useful if risk factors are identified.
- MRI of the brain is a consideration in the child with GDD or ID, especially if any abnormalities on physical exam (e.g., micro/macrocephaly, focal motor finding).
- EEG is not routinely ordered and helpful only if there are clinical concerns of epilepsy.
- Sleep study is important if warranted by history.

REFERENCES

1. Battaglia A, Carey C. Diagnostic evaluation of developmental delay/mental retardation: An overview. Am J Med Genet C 2003; 117C: 3–14.
2. McDonald L, Rennie A, et al. Investigation of global developmental delay. Arch Dis Child 2006; 91: 701–5.

3. Michelson DJ, et al. Evidence report: Genetic and metabolic testing on children with global developmental delay; Report of the Quality Standards Subcommittee of the American Academy of Neurology and the Practice Committee of the Child Neurology Society. Neurology 2011; 77: 1629–35.

4. Moeschler JB, Shevell M, et al. Clinical genetics evaluation of the child with mental retardation or developmental delays. Pediatrics 2006; 117: 2304–2316.

5. Shevell M, Ashwal S, et al. Practice parameter: Evaluation of the child with global developmental delay. Neurology 2003; 60: 367–80.

6. Op. cit. Reference 3 (Michelson).

7. Op. cit. Reference 2 (McDonald).

8. Op. cit. Reference 4 (Moeschler).

9. Op. cit. Reference 3 (Michelson).

10. Canadian College of Medical Geneticists. Use of array genomic hybridization technology for constitutional genetic diagnosis in Canada. CCMG Position Statement. 2009.

11. Op. cit. Reference 3 (Michelson).

12. Op. cit. Reference 5 (Shevell).

13. Op. cit. Reference 1 (Battaglia).

14. Demaerel P, et al. Isolated neurodevelopmental delay in childhood: Clinicoradiological correlation in 170 patients. Pediatr Radiol 1993; 23: 29–33.

15. Yoon SYR, et al. Sleep in attention-deficit/hyperactivity disorder in children and adults: Past, present, and future. Sleep Med Rev 2011: 1–18.

16. Youssef NA, Ege M, et al. Is obstructive sleep apnea associated with ADHD? Ann Clin Psychiatry 2011; 23(3): 213–24.

17. Belanger, SA, et al. Cardiac risk assessment before the use of stimulant medications in children and youth. Paediatric Child Health 2009; 13(9): 579–85. <www.cps.ca/english/statements/pp/cps09–02.htm>

10

Developmental and Academic Skills: Screening, Sampling, and Assessment

Barbara Fitzgerald

The role of the physician in developmental assessment is important, even when other professionals may subsequently do more detailed assessments.

First, it can be very valuable to actually see a child work. Physicians may observe the child's attention, motivation, level of anxiety, and pleasure in doing different types of work, and willingness (or not) to try new and difficult things. They can see how quickly children fatigue or how easily they become frustrated. During an assessment, physicians can observe the student's learning style, awareness of task requirements (organization), and approach to problems of different types, and see first-hand whether things like inattention and impulsivity are the main reasons for incorrect answers (as opposed to lack of cognitive ability).

Second, children with behaviour problems also deserve a screen for academic difficulties. Frustration and discouragement about learning challenges can present as behavioural issues in the classroom. It is not uncommon for behavioural disorders to be diagnosed when the underlying problem is a learning disorder.

Sometimes important parts of the history emerge during the assessment process when the child isn't being formally questioned. The developmental assessment is key to the formulation of a working diagnosis. This can provide significant relief to the parents and can mean that school supports start right away, instead of months down the line when other assessments are completed. An example of this is with the child who presents with significant difficulties learning to read and who may be doing poorly in all academic areas as a result. If the assessment finds well-developed nonverbal reasoning skills, the parent and child can be reassured that

the child appears to have good cognitive skills, but is at risk for a learning disability. Direct observation and assessment are preferable to exclusive reliance on school reports. Parents will appreciate a physician's direct observation of academic skills as lending credibility to subsequent recommendations the physician might make for school programming.

LEVELS OF ASSESSMENT BY PHYSICIANS

Depending on the type of physician (family medicine/generalist or specialist) and the focus of clinical practice, clinicians will vary the depth and detail with which they use assessment tools in children with academic difficulties. It is important for every physician to have a "tool kit" that they use to provide some standardization of their own assessment. This tool kit should cover all domains of development to ensure that underlying treatable conditions are discovered, investigated, and treated or supported. Early diagnosis makes a tremendous difference in the outcome of developmental conditions. For example, children with learning disabilities are more likely to drop out of school and engage in risky behaviour if their learning disability goes unrecognized and unsupported. Parents and teachers may come to think of them as "bad" or "lazy" children, instead of as children who learn differently. Getting support early starts with recognition of the problem, often at the primary care level. The contribution that the primary care physician or general paediatrician makes in initiating a more detailed assessment process is invaluable.

In the ideal world, every child with academic difficulty would present to a physician's office with a full psycho-educational evaluation, speech-language consultation, and occupational and physical therapy assessments. This doesn't happen very often. The tools that are used in developmental sampling, screening, and assessment are not a replacement for formal psycho-educational, occupational therapy, physiotherapy, or speech-language evaluation. A physician's evaluation of each area of development may lead to a working diagnosis and at the very least will allow you to determine what the next steps are. This evaluation also gives a perspective with which to read and interpret other reports. In the same way that physicians ensure that laboratory investigations match their clinical impression (i.e., make sense), they need to ensure that other professionals' findings make sense in the context of the whole clinical picture. Children can perform differently with different people and in different settings. Often it is the physician who will have the broadest context in which to review findings.

- **Level I** (primary care) refers to the shorter office visit for screening by the family doctor or paediatrician. These visits may be short, but the physician has the advantage of already knowing the child and family. The history and physical exam will be directed to elucidating specifics that may not have been asked previously. Formal developmental assessment is not possible in this context. A historical account of strengths and weaknesses combined with observation, and a review of report cards and possibly some questionnaires, will guide the physician to make appropriate referrals for further assessment. If physicians are interested in doing more of the workup themselves and/or if there is a wait time for consultation, another primary care approach might be a staged assessment where the child is evaluated over several short appointments. A very important contribution by the primary care provider is to follow the child after supports and therapies have been implemented to see if these changes are having the desired effect.
- **Level II** (general paediatric consultation) might take approximately sixty minutes. In this first visit, a directed history and physical exam is done, questionnaires and report cards are reviewed, and the child is interviewed. A follow-up visit is usually needed for assessment except in those jurisdictions where fee codes allow for a longer initial assessment of the complex child. The assessment should include developmental and behavioural observations and samples from each domain. From this evaluation, a working diagnosis is generated that can allow for preliminary supports to be put in place at school while further assessments are booked. The general paediatrician may decide to refer to a subspecialty developmental paediatrician at this point, depending on his or her own expertise and the complexity of the child's problems.

- **Level III** (specially trained general paediatrician, developmental paediatrician, paediatric neurologist, or child psychiatrist) is done by a medical specialist who will usually be working as part of, or in consultation with, a multidisciplinary team of teachers and special educators, an educational psychologist, speech-language pathologist, occupational therapist, and physiotherapists, and possibly mental health professionals. Developmental paediatricians will do a formal neurodevelopmental assessment.

SCREENING, SAMPLING, AND ASSESSMENT

Screening involves using a specific tool in a standardized way for early detection of important developmental or medical conditions. Screening tests should be quick and easy to administer and score, with good validity and reliability, and are usually developed for conditions where there is effective intervention and/or treatment, and for which early identification and initiation of that intervention/treatment would result in improved outcomes. **Sampling** involves using tools in a less formal way, often resulting in a description of the child's skills instead of a formal score. The most definitive measures involve **assessment**, where the end result is a formulation of the child's developmental age for a given sector and/or a definitive medical diagnosis.

The tools are divided below by age and by domain. It is not suggested that you use every one. Find the ones that are most effective for you and become familiar with how to use them.

Developmental screening tests

Ages 4 to 6 years (Grades K to 1)

- A simple and very quick tool to use is the Ages and Stages Questionnaire (ASQ).(1) Have the family arrive twenty minutes before the appointment to complete the questionnaire or send it to them to do at home; the scoring takes under a minute. This tool tells you if there are concerns in any particular domain of development. It only goes up to age 60 months (5 years) but can still be useful in slightly older children who are delayed. It is also a good tool (from a medical educational perspective) to have a trainee complete with the parent. Once an organization (e.g., paediatric society or hospital) has purchased this instrument, their members have access to make unlimited reproductions of the materials.

Birth to 8 years (to Grade 3)

- The Parent Evaluation of Developmental Skills (PEDS) is a parent report screener for ages birth to 8 years that can be done in the waiting room. It takes about two minutes to administer and score if used as an interview format, and much less time if the parent has already completed it before seeing the doctor. A ten-item hands-on follow-up screen, the Parent Evaluation of Developmental Skills-Developmental Milestones (PEDS-DM), allows clinical validation of reported parental concerns if needed, and there is a practice algorithm to use for interpreting results. It can also be used for teaching development to trainees.(2)

Both the ASQ and PEDS have excellent test characteristics and have been successfully incorporated into office practice. It usually takes about ten to twelve administrations for most clinicians to become adept at scoring and interpreting these tests, so that they can then evaluate the advantages and challenges of using a given test in their own practice. If possible, it is good to "do a dozen" before making your final decision about the feasibility of implementing a screener, or for that matter any of the following tools.

Tools for sampling and assessment

1. Communication and verbal reasoning

Receptive language

The Peabody Picture Vocabulary Test-Revised (PPVT-R) is a test of receptive vocabulary for single words. The child is asked to indicate which of four pictures corresponds to a single word uttered by the examiner. The test correlates reasonably well with language understanding and verbal intelligence, and it can easily be administered in the office. It also allows for observation of impulsive responses, distractibility, and short attention span. This test also gives you an informal window on how much language stimulation the child is getting. A child with average or low-average intelligence who has a very poor vocabulary is perhaps not receiving optimal language stimulation.

Ages 4 to 6 years (Grades K to 1)

- Ask the child to follow instructions using prepositions such as *above, below, under, between*. Ask the child to answer the questions in **Tool 10–1: Complex Sentences (Ages 4 to 6 Years)**.

Ages 6 to 9 years

- **Complex sentences:** Ask the child to answer the questions in **Tool 10–2: Complex Sentences (Ages 6 to 9 Years)**.
- **Story comprehension:** See **Tool 10–3: Story Comprehension**. Read the story to the child, then ask the comprehension questions that follow.

Ages 9 to 15 years

- **Verbal instructions:** See **Tool 10–4: Verbal Instructions.** Ask the child to follow the instructions.
- **Auditory comprehension:** See **Tool 10–5: Auditory Comprehension and Recall**. Read the paragraph to the child. Ask the child to summarize what you have read. Then ask him or her to answer the comprehension questions.
- **Higher-level language functions:** One of the distinctions in older children and youth is the development of higher-level language skills. Children with cognitive weaknesses can be taught simple vocabulary but will not be able to

manage more complex language. Higher-level skills such as figurative speech and understanding inferences are important communication and social skills in older children. Theory of mind, the ability to see another's viewpoint, becomes increasingly important in older children and can be assessed using these tools. See **Tool 10–6: Yes, No, Maybe: Higher-Level Language Function.** Tell the child that you are going to read a sentence and ask a question about it. The answer will always be *yes*, *no*, or *maybe*. Read the sentence and the question to the child. You may repeat each sentence for the child if necessary.

Expressive language

Ages 4 to 6 years

- By this age, the child should be able to relate a sequence of events (tell a story) about something that happened at school or daycare. This is a step up from just being able to answer questions in a yes/no format. Ask the child to describe what happened at a recent classroom celebration or event. Speech should be largely intelligible to a stranger.
- For more details, see **Tool 10–7: Development of Oral Language Skills (Ages 5 to 12 Years).**

Pragmatics (social use of language)

Observe whether the child uses gestures appropriately, makes eye contact, answers to his or her name, and participates in a reciprocal conversation.

Phonological awareness

Phonological awareness is important for learning to read. The child aged 6 years and older should be able to come up with rhyming words to a word you give them. Starting at age 6 years, the child should be able to substitute letters to derive a new word: e.g., "If I take away the 'b' sound in 'ball' and change it to a 't,' what word do I get?"

2. Cognition

Nonverbal reasoning

Human figure drawing: Drawing a picture of a human figure is a complex task that changes as a child develops. The earliest developmental age at which a child can do this is about 3 and a half, when the repertoire of shapes mastered include the circle and lines needed to construct a simple figure. The number of body parts depicted, proportions, and complexity increase with age and correlate roughly with the child's developmental age, although the accuracy and quality of the drawing will also depend on fine motor skills, attention to detail, and task persistence. There are specific scoring methods that require formal training, but human figure drawing can also be used informally as a way of sampling the child's pencil and paper skills and ability to organize a complex task.(3)(4)(5)

A good time to obtain a human figure drawing is while you are taking the history from the parents. Provide a sheet of plain white paper and pencils or pencil crayons, which will give the best quality result. Ask the child to draw a person. Say specifically that you would like the child to draw the whole person (not just the head and not a cartoon or anime). See **Tool 10–8: Human Figure Drawings** for sample drawings by children of various ages. Note how detailed the drawing is and how many body parts are included. A rule of thumb is that each body part represents about three months' developmental age over a base age of three years. You can get information about fine motor/graphomotor skills by noting the child's handedness, grasp of the pencil, and agility with which the child draws. Look at the accuracy of the lines and any signs of tremor. Behavioural information about task persistence, impulsivity, and planning can also be gleaned.

Observations are very important in the evaluation of nonverbal reasoning. As you talk to parents, get the child involved in play that allows you to observe nonverbal skills. Have the child do a puzzle, colour, draw a picture, or construct something with blocks or Lego. Observe attention span, ability to develop a sequence of play, and adeptness with visual spatial tasks.

Ages 4 to 6 years
- See **Tool 10–9: Visual Matching Exercises (Ages 4 to 6 Years).**

Ages 6 to 9 years
- See **Tool 10–10: Visual Whole:Part Analysis (Ages 6 to 9 Years).** Ask the child to find the shape that is hidden in one of the figures. Tell

them that the shape has to face the same way as the picture.

Ages 9 to 15 years
- See **Tool 10–11: Lock-and-Key Designs (Ages 9 to 15 Years).**

3. Fine motor and graphomotor skills

Ages 4 to 6 years
- The child should have a mature tripod pencil grip and should be able to adeptly pick up small objects with a mature and coordinated pincer grasp. Observe copying of Gesell copy forms, **Tool 10–12: The Gesell Copy Forms.**

Ages 6 to 9 years
- Have the child draw a picture and observe pencil control and detail. Have the child print the alphabet. Up to age seven, letter reversals can be typical. By Grade 3, the child's printing should be developed enough to allow for efficient expression of ideas on paper.

Ages 9 to 15 years
- Observe the child handwriting the alphabet. Look for maturity of pencil grasp, speed of writing, and letter formation.

Sensory issues: Many children who learn differently also perceive the world differently and their heightened or blunted perceptions can have significant impacts on their ability to learn and to socialize. There are screening tools for sensory-seeking or sensory-avoidant behaviours that are usually done by occupational therapists. The physician will get most of this sensory information by asking the parents and child specific questions about under- or over-sensivity to auditory, tactile, visual, smell, taste, and pain sensations. For example, children who cover their ears and say that the vacuum cleaner or a siren outside hurts their ears may be reacting to auditory stimuli in the classroom and actually be struggling to concentrate and learn as a result.

4. Gross motor skills

Posture and gait, including stressed gaits, are included in the neurologic exam (see Chapter 8). Observations should include motor coordination, balance (static and dynamic), and ball skills.

Ages 4 to 6 years
- **Motor coordination:** ascends and descends stairs with alternating feet; hops on one foot; smooth, coordinated running gait with reciprocal arm and leg movement; minimal posturing and overflow signs may be present.
- **Balance:** balances on one foot for more than ten seconds, tandem gait.
- **Ball skills:** throws and catches a tennis ball underhand from two metres, kicks a soccer ball.

Ages 6 to 9 years
- **Motor coordination:** skips, runs quickly, and changes direction easily.
- **Balance:** easily balances on one foot for more than ten seconds, tandem gait forward and backward.
- **Ball skills:** catches and throws a tennis ball from three metres.

Ages 9 to 16 years
- **Motor coordination:** all fundamentals are in place; variability in degree of athleticism for sporting activities; can follow a sequence of motor skills (e.g., hop twice on left side, clap three times, hop three times on right side).
- **Balance:** smooth static and dynamic balance.
- **Ball skills:** throws and catches a tennis ball with good accuracy.

5. Social skills

Since deficits in social learning play a critical role in the child's overall functioning and self-esteem, such abilities should be sampled. While autism spectrum disorder (ASD) that is moderate to severe is unlikely to have been missed in the school-aged child, milder ASD in children with higher levels of language and cognitive skills is quite commonly diagnosed later in life. Language disorders and other learning disabilities may be part of the disorder, and the child may present with learning and/or behaviour concerns. Children with nonverbal learning disabilities can be challenging to distinguish from children with ASD and normal cognitive skill levels. The role of the developmental assessor is to note that social difficulties exist. A Level III assessor that is part of a multidisciplinary team will be responsible for the specifics of the diagnosis.

Observe the child's nonverbal communication such as facial expressions and gestures, eye contact, and also his or her response to your nonverbal communication. Talk about or show pictures of common social situations to see how the child interprets them (e.g., getting into a fight at school, expectations in a restaurant). Try to have a reciprocal conversation and see if the child responds with the appropriate use of questions to statements that you make. Reading a story that has characters with facial expressions and getting the child to interpret those expressions can be revealing. Look for a discrepancy between the child's developmental age and social skills. Ask the child specific questions about common social/emotional conditions: e.g., "Tell me what being a friend means to you." "Tell me why you think people get married." "Describe to me how your mother feels about you compared to how she feels about a child your age in your class or in your building." "Pretend that I am from outer space. I have never heard of being lonely/sad/angry—what does that mean?" Again, look for responses that are less mature or more concrete than the child's overall cognitive/developmental age would predict. A Level III assessor will use specialized tools (e.g., ADOS, ADI-R) to make a formal diagnosis of ASD.

6. Academic achievement

Reading

Reading comprehension (*oral*, child reads out loud; *silent*, child reads silently; and *listening*, examiner reads a story and then asks questions) of short paragraphs provides a critical sample of a school-aged child's developmental acquisitions. How the child decodes words and understands meaning, both at factual and inferential (between the lines) levels, will be of great assistance to the clinician's integration of the profile of school problems and helps to identify a disability. Grade samples follow that assess reading ability and recall of facts. You may want to also ask some comprehension questions about the story that the child reads to you. See **Tool 10–13: Reading Tests.**

Writing

Story writing provides a great developmental challenge to a student, requiring simultaneous exercise of many skills, including organization, spelling, grammar, ideas, vocabulary, sequence of ideas, punctuation, capitalization, quality of handwriting, and quantity of production. Normative values exist for story-writing tasks to be used as a frame of reference for comparison with the patient's story. (BASIS provides excellent comparison samples of stories written by students from Grades 3 to 8.) See **Tools 10–14: Assessment of Handwriting Speed; 10–15: Evaluation of Written Stories Using BASIS; and 10–16: Reading and Writing Skills in School-aged Children.**

Spelling

Spelling should be sampled, using graded word lists and a comparison made between spelling in isolation and within story writing. See **Tool 10–17: Sample Spelling Battery.**

Mathematics

Arithmetic should be sampled, looking at informal computation skills; mathematical applications, such as those relating to time and money; and word problems. See **Tool 10–18: Sample Mathematics Tests.**

7. Memory

Visual/Nonverbal memory

Place five objects on the table in front of you (eraser, pencil, paper clip, block, small toy). Point to the objects in a certain order and ask the child to copy you.

Ages 4 to 6 years
- Should remember four objects in sequence.

Ages 6 to 9 years
- Five objects.

Ages 9 to 15 years
- Six objects.

Auditory memory

See **Tool 10–19: Assessment of Auditory Memory from Repetition of Digits.**

TOOL 10–1: COMPLEX SENTENCES (AGES 4 TO 6 YEARS)

Instructions: Ask the child to answer the following questions.

1. The boy saw the man who was carrying a red ball.

   Who was carrying a red ball?   (Man)

2. The girl who played with my friend came home late.

   Who came home late?   (Girl)

3. The lady saw the man who was wearing a green hat.

   Who was wearing a green hat?   (Man)

4. Before it got dark, the man went to the store.

   When did the man go to the store?   (Before it got dark)

5. The baby ate the candy after his mother called him.

   When did the baby eat the candy?   (After his mother called him)

Age (years)	Expected score
4–6	3–6

6. Before the boy went out to play, his mother gave him some water.

   When did his mother give him a drink?   (Before the boy went out to play)

Source: Levine MD. Pediatric Examination of Educational Readiness (PEER, stimulus booklet). Cambridge MA: Educators Publishing Service, Inc. Adapted by permission.

TOOL 10–2: COMPLEX SENTENCES (AGES 6 TO 8 YEARS, 11 MONTHS)

Instructions: Ask the child to answer the following questions.

1. The car is parked next to the garage.

   Where is the car parked?   (Next to the garage)

2. Before the door was opened, the boy put his coat on.

   When did the boy put his coat on?   (Before the door opened)

3. The boy who liked the girl ran away down the street.

   Who ran down the street?   (Boy)

4. The lion that the tiger bit jumped over the giraffe.

   Who jumped over the giraffe?   (Lion)

5. The horse jumped over the fence after it started raining.

   When did the horse jump over the fence?   (After it started raining)

6. The girl saw the man who was wearing green shoes.

   Who was wearing green shoes?   (Man)

7. The clown who called the little dog ran into the tent.

   Who ran into the tent?   (Clown)

8. The car that was hit by the truck was driven by a man.

   What did the man drive?   (Car)

Age (years)	Expected score
6	4–5
7	5–6
8.11	6–7

Source: Levine MD. Pediatric Early Elementary Education (PEEX 2, Record form). Cambridge MA: Educators Publishing Service, Inc. Adapted by permission.

TOOL 10–3: STORY COMPREHENSION

Instructions: Read the story to the child, then ask the questions that follow.

Ages 6 years to 7 years, 11 months

Passage A (Experiential/Narrative form)

It was a hot day. Mary's mother gave her some money and asked her to go to the store and buy some ice cream. On the way home, Mary stopped to talk with a friend. When she got home, the bag was dripping. Mary was worried. She knew her mother would be angry.

Comprehension and recall:

1. What was the weather like?   (Hot)

2. What did Mary's mother ask her to do?   (Go to the store/buy some ice cream)

3. Why did Mary stop on the way home?   (To talk to a friend)

4. Why was the bag dripping?   (The ice cream melted)

5. How did Mary feel?   (Worried)

Age (years)	Expected score
6	2–4
7.11	3–5

6. Why was she worried?   (She knew her mother would be angry)

Ages 8 years to 8 years, 11 months

Passage B (Decontextualized/Expository form)

A long time ago, horses were brought to America from Spain to work on farms and ranches. Many of these horses escaped. They formed large herds and were so tough they were able to survive on just small amounts of grass and water. After a while there were millions of them. Today in some parts of the American West, these wild horses are crowded together. This is causing big problems for them. Many are now very thin and unhealthy.

Comprehension and recall:

1. Why were the wild horses first brought to America?   (To work on farms/ranches)

2. What did many horses do after they arrived in America?   (Escaped)

3. How were the escaped horses able to survive in the wild?   (They could survive on small amounts of grass and water)

4. Where are these horses now found?   (The American West)

5. What problems are many of these horses now having? (Too crowded/unhealthy/thin)

Age (years)	Expected score
8.11	3–4

6. Why are the horses getting so thin?   (Not enough food/grass)

Source: Levine MD. Pediatric Early Elementary Education (PEEX 2, Record form). Cambridge MA: Educators Publishing Service, Inc. Adapted by permission.

TOOL 10–4: VERBAL INSTRUCTIONS

Part A (Condensed syntax)

Instructions: Using the images on page 96, ask the child to follow the instructions below. You may repeat the instructions.

1. Put your thumb in a big circle and then use your pencil to touch the other one.

2. Draw small- and middle-sized circles inside two big circles.

3. Put a circle around the small X that's furthest away from the small square.

4. Make a dot inside the four dots and then make a circle that goes only around it.

5. Make a circle in the big square and then make a square in the middle one.

Part B (Active working memory)

6. Before you make four X's above the middle square, draw a line connecting two circles.

7. Draw five squares at the top of the page if there are more than fourteen dots.

8. Put three dots above the thick line after you've made a square and a circle underneath it.

9. Make small circles under the small X's and small X's under the big circles.

10. Draw four circles next to the shortest line, but first draw one X and two dots underneath it.

Age (years)	Expected score
9–12.11	5–8
13–14.11	7–9

(0=incorrect; 1=correct. Score Parts A and B together.)

(Continued on next page)

Source: Levine MD. Pediatric Examination of Educational Readiness at Middle Childhood (PEERAMID 2, Response book and Record form). Cambridge MA: Educators Publishing Service, Inc. Reprinted by permission.

TOOL 10–4: VERBAL INSTRUCTIONS *(CONTINUED)*

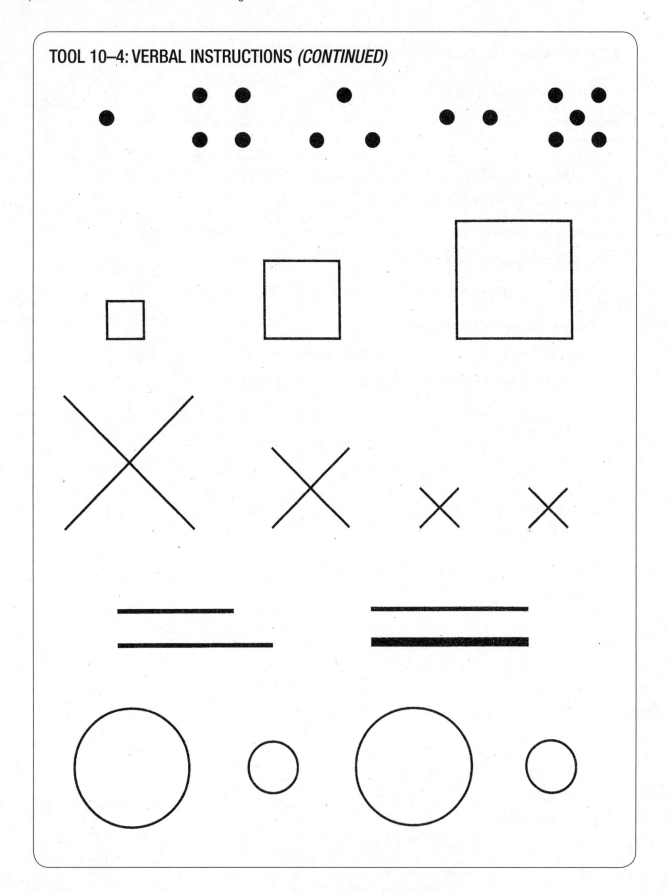

Source: Levine MD. Pediatric Examination of Educational Readiness at Middle Childhood (PEERAMID 2, Response book and Record form). Cambridge MA: Educators Publishing Service, Inc. Reprinted by permission.

TOOL 10–5: AUDITORY COMPREHENSION AND RECALL

Ages 9 years to 12 years, 11 months

Passage A (Experiential/Narrative form)

Jim and Tanya had a great time! Jim always liked his pizza with plenty of cheese and mushrooms. So did Tanya. Their parents told them to clean up as soon as they were finished. They were asked not to leave anything at all on the table. For once, their parents wanted to be sure the kitchen would look neat when they got home. But just as soon as Jim and Tanya ate as much pizza as they could eat, they sped off and watched TV. Their dog, Rusty, could not have been happier. When their parents returned, the table was pretty clean, but there were sliced-up mushrooms on the floor next to an empty, chewed-up pizza box.

Comprehension and recall:

1. What have Jim and Tanya done in the past?   (Eaten pizza/made a mess)

2. Did they finish all their pizza?   (No)

3. What did their dog do?   (Ate the leftover pizza)

4. Why were there mushrooms all over the floor?   (Dog didn't eat/like mushrooms)

Age (years)	Expected score
9–12.11	3
(Score 1 point for each complete answer)	

Passage B (Decontextualized/Expository form)

Swans and geese are like each other in many ways. They both are good swimmers, and both are able to fly very long distances. Adult swans and geese build nests in the spring and are very good parents. But swans and geese are different in some important ways: Swans usually are larger and have longer necks. The fathers help the mothers build their nests. Often the newborn babies, which are called cygnets, ride on their mothers' backs when they're tired. Mother geese build their own nests, and their babies, which are called goslings, always provide their own transportation. Geese start laying eggs when they're two. Swans start when they're three.

Comprehension and recall:

1. What do baby swans do when they're tired?   (Ride on mothers' backs)

2. What can't young swans and geese do when they're a year old?   (Lay eggs)

3. Are geese usually larger than swans?   (No)

4. Who builds a swan's nest?   (Both parents)

Age (years)	Expected score
9–12.11	2–3

(Continued on next page)

TOOL 10–5: AUDITORY COMPREHENSION AND RECALL *(CONTINUED)*

Ages 13 years to 14 years, 11 months

Passage C (Experiential/Narrative form)

The Greeks had many great stories that are now called myths. One of them was about a young boy named Hermes who was a musician and an adventurer. One night when he wanted some excitement, he stole a herd of twelve cows owned by Apollo. To hide their tracks, he made cow shoes from the bark of fallen oak. The next morning Apollo offered a reward for his cows. Later, some people heard about a boy who had just made an amazing musical toy called a lyre from the shell of a tortoise and some fresh cow gut. They wondered where the cow gut came from and accused Hermes of stealing the cows. Hermes confessed. Luckily, ten were still alive. He apologized to Apollo and played a beautiful melody for him on his new musical instrument. Apollo said he could keep the cows but he would have to give him the lyre. That's how Hermes got his own herd.

Comprehension and recall:

Age (years)	Expected score
13–14.11	2–4

1. Why did Hermes steal the cows?   (Wanted excitement)

2. Why did Hermes make shoes for the cows?   (To hide their tracks)

3. Why did the people think Hermes stole the cows?   (Because he made the lyre from fresh cow gut)

4. Why did Apollo let Hermes keep the cows?   (He wanted the lyre)

Passage D (Decontextualized/Expository form)

The brown pelican may soon become an endangered species. We are doing to the brown pelican what we have done to countless other species—wiping them off the face of the earth. In this case, we are using chemical warfare! This bird's tolerance for pesticides is very low. The liquids are sprayed on plants. But *most* of the deadly poison finds its way into the rivers that flow into the sea, where microscopic plankton live. The contaminated plankton form an important part of the diet of larger organisms. Often these fish are eaten by seabirds. Brown pelicans used to be a common sight along the coast of California. These healthy birds would lay three or four eggs a year. Now most of the time their nests contain only one.

Comprehension and recall:

1. Why are the chemicals sprayed on plants?   (To kill insects)

2. Do the pelicans eat the plants that have been sprayed with pesticides?   (No)

3. What does the poison do to the pelicans?   (Makes them lay fewer eggs)

4. How do the fish get contaminated?   (By eating organisms containing plankton)

Age (years)	Expected score
13–14.11	2–4

Source: Levine MD. Pediatric Examination of Educational Readiness at Middle Childhood (PEERAMID 2, Record form). Cambridge MA: Educators Publishing Service, Inc. Reprinted by permission.

TOOL 10–6: YES, NO, MAYBE: HIGHER-LEVEL LANGUAGE FUNCTION

Instructions: Read each sentence and question. Repeat if necessary. Start with this example:

Joe might come home early today. Will Joe come home early today?   (Maybe)

1. John said, "Shouldn't you make the knot loose?" Did John think the knot should be loose?   (Yes)

2. Ricky won't go to the party unless Ann goes. Will Ricky stay home?   (Maybe)

3. Bob promised he would buy the candy. Did Bob buy the candy?   (Maybe)

4. It's usually safe to climb that mountain, although it's very dangerous in the fog. Will it be safe to climb the mountain tomorrow?   (Maybe)

5. Maybe the band would have played last night if the drummer hadn't quit. Did the band play last night?   (No)

6. Mary knows whether John plays basketball. Does John play basketball?   (Maybe)

7. Ann knows that Bill plays the piano. Does Bill play the piano?   (Yes)

8. Jim thinks Tom is good at sports. Is Tom good at sports?   (Maybe)

9. They could not believe that Joe was telling the truth. Was Joe lying?   (Maybe)

10. Linda's dog chased the kitten and ran away. Did Linda's dog run away?   (Yes)

Instructions: Say to the child: "Now I am going to ask you some questions that are very hard. So listen to these carefully. I will repeat each one and then ask you a question."

11. Chris will be happy unless his school wins the football game. Will Chris be happy if his school wins the football game?   (No)

12. Nancy's teacher thinks she's bored in class much of the time. Is Nancy often bored during class?   (Maybe)

13. If it weren't for those experiments in class, Richard would enjoy science. Does Richard like his science class?   (No)

14. The teacher who was looking for Mike rode his bicycle home from school. Did the teacher go home on a bicycle?   (Yes)

Age (years)	Expected score
9–12.11	8–11
13–14.11	10–12

Source: Levine MD. Pediatric Examination of Educational Readiness at Middle Childhood (PEERAMID 2, Record form). Cambridge MA: Educators Publishing Service, Inc. Reprinted by permission.

TOOL 10–7: DEVELOPMENT OF ORAL LANGUAGE SKILLS (AGES 5 TO 12 YEARS)

Instructions: The following standards may be used for taking a speech and language history.

Age	Talking	Listening/Understanding	Social skills
Most 5-year-olds:	• say most speech sounds correctly and are easy to understand • speak in sentences that are five to six words long • ask questions using *who, what, where,* and *why* • use the present, future, and past tenses (*She walks to the park. She will walk to the park. She walked to the park.*) • retell a story by naming the characters and talking about what happened • use different types of words, like action (*kick*) and descriptive words (*yellow, cold*)	• follow three directions at a time • understand many concepts, such as colours, location words, and numbers • put things into basic groups, such as fruits, animals, and toys • understand most adult conversation, including sayings like *"Time to hit the sack."* • understand and answer most questions appropriately • like to listen to rhymes and make up their own rhymes	• make eye contact with other children and adults • take turns and wait for their turn during activities • sit quietly and listen to the teacher during circle time • say *hi* or *hello* and *goodbye* appropriately
	Some 5-year-olds may still have trouble: • saying the sounds *sh, ch, j, s, z, v, r,* and *th.* The *s* and *z* sounds may be lisps. • asking questions that start with *when.*	**Some 5-year-olds may still have trouble:** • understanding the words *above* and *below*	

Age	Talking	Listening/Understanding	Social skills
Most 6-year-olds:	• say most speech sounds correctly and are easy to understand • speak in sentences that are six to seven words long • use words like *then, so,* and *but* in their sentences • tell who was in a story, where the story took place, and what happened • tell how to do simple things like making a peanut butter and jam sandwich • tell you what you do with something (*you eat with a fork*)	• listen for fifteen to twenty minutes • understand words like *right* and *left, first, second,* and *third* • understand how everyday things go together (e.g., a pig, horse, and cow are all animals) • begin to enjoy riddles and jokes • break long words into parts, e.g., they might tell you that "snowman" has the word "man" in it • know the sound that each letter makes (*s* says sssssssssss) • know the first sound and some of the last sounds in short words (soup starts with *s* and ends with *p*)	• know how their friends are feeling and tell you how they are feeling • watch other people's facial expressions and body language to know what they are saying • know how to start, maintain, and end a conversation • begin to solve problems with some help from adults • repeat what they have said if someone doesn't understand them
	Some 6-year-olds may still have trouble: • saying the sounds *r* and *th* • using words like *himself, herself,* and *themselves* • using irregular past tense verbs, like *he ate, she fell,* and *they ran*	**Some 6-year-olds may still have trouble:** • understanding time and place words like *before, after,* and *above*	

(Continued on next page)

TOOL 10–7: DEVELOPMENT OF ORAL LANGUAGE SKILLS (AGES 5 TO 12 YEARS) (*CONTINUED*)

Age	Talking	Listening/Understanding	Social skills
Most 7-year-olds:	• speak in sentences seven to eight words long and use connecting words like *because, so, then, before*, and *after* • use all pronouns correctly, including *himself, herself*, and *themselves* • use irregular past tense verbs correctly, like *ate, fell*, and *ran* • tell complete stories that have many details • use specific vocabulary that they have learned at school • tell you what you do with an object (you *eat* an apple) and what group it belongs to (an apple is a type of *fruit*)	• listen to the teacher's instructions when sitting at their desk • are beginning to understand simple metaphors and similes, such as *soft as a pillow* • know they sometimes have trouble remembering things, but are not sure how to make remembering easier • learn new words by listening to books being read aloud, by talking about these new words with an adult, and by using them in everyday activities • tell you how things are different and how they are the same • tell you the middle sound in a short word (*cat* has the *a* sound in the middle) • tell you the sounds in a short word (*dog* has these sounds: *d—o—g*) • play with words by taking away one sound (*If I take away the d in dog, it says og.*)	• are learning how to work with a partner • are learning that respect and personal space (not standing too close) are important • know how to start, maintain, and end a conversation • know how to be a good friend
	Some 7-year-olds may still have trouble: • saying the *th* sound (*thin, that, mother, math*) • saying longer words, like *aluminum* and *cinnamon* • using words like *some* and *much* correctly (For example, they may still say *some spaghettis* or *much bricks.*)		

Age	Talking	Listening/Understanding	Social skills
Most 8-year-olds:	• say all of their speech sounds correctly and are easy to understand • use connecting words like *instead of, or, if*, and *until* (*We can't go inside until it opens.*) • use words like *could, would*, and *should* when they talk about their favourite books, movies, and things that happen • use different types of sentences, such as *The cat chased the dog, The dog was chased by the cat*, and *Was the dog chased by the cat?* • use questions that start with *Why don't you. . .* • describe things using many different describing words (*A horse is a type of animal that is found on a farm. It is large and has a mane. You put a saddle on it and ride it.*)	• know who the pronouns are referring to in a sentence (*My sister's friend gave a present to her on her birthday.*) • know that sometimes they can't remember everything without doing something to help them remember, like saying it over and over or making a picture of it in their mind • understand words that tell position, order, time, quantity, and space and use them to help understand the things they learn in school, like in science class (For example, when a teacher says, "After you add some of the baking soda, make sure you stir the mixture frequently.") **Some 8-year-olds may still have trouble:** • talking about the most important thing rather than the details • coming up with different meanings for one word • reading between the lines or coming up with hidden meanings in what they hear or read	• stay on topic when talking to a friend or when talking in a group • work toward solving a problem in a group • understand that their friends may have different opinions or ideas

(Continued on next page)

TOOL 10–7: DEVELOPMENT OF ORAL LANGUAGE SKILLS (AGES 5 TO 12 YEARS) (*CONTINUED*)

Age	Talking	Listening/Understanding	Social skills
Most 9-year-olds:	• say all of their speech sounds correctly and are easy to understand • speak in long, complete sentences and use words like *if, now, though,* and *anyway* • explain the different meanings of words (a *trunk* is the back of a car or the nose of an elephant) • tell riddles, jokes, and word plays • tell you opposites (*black/white, hard/soft*), synonyms (*sad/upset*), and subcategories (*animals, jungle animals, forest animals, sea animals*) of different words • give the function or the use of a word when asked what it means (*A saw is something that we use to cut wood.*) • tell the main idea of a story or the most important idea of what they learned **Some 9-year-olds may still have trouble:** • using words like *however, therefore*, or *whenever* correctly in their sentences • using figures of speech or phrases with hidden meanings in their own speech	• understand that words have several meanings • understand idioms or sayings (*hard as a rock, blind as a bat, raining cats and dogs*) • understand that some words have many different meanings and can be used to describe feelings (*cold, bitter, blue*) • understand that sometimes they need to do different things to help them remember information like repeating it over and over, picturing it in their mind, writing it down, or drawing pictures	• change what they have said by repeating it, rewording it, or by adding information to it so that other people understand • make adult-like guesses or predictions about what will happen in a story • begin to laugh at themselves when they realize they have made a mistake or said something strange

Age	Talking	Listening/Understanding	Social skills
Most 10- to 12-year-olds:	• tell you what a word means by saying the group or category it belongs to (an apple is a *fruit*, a truck is a *vehicle*) • use the connecting words *if, now, though, otherwise, anyway, therefore,* and *however* • give their opinion • use the words *really* and *probably* often • tell and write stories in an order that makes sense **10- to 12-year-olds are not done learning language! As they get older, they are still learning:** • new words • longer and harder sentences • ways to play with words and language • how to use what they hear and say to change their world	• use key words (*the three main ideas are . . .*) and connecting words (*if, however*) to help them understand • remember information using strategies, such as picturing the information in their minds, breaking information into smaller chunks, and repeating the information • understand words that describe personalities, such as *cold, bitter, blue,* or *sweet* • use what they already know to help them understand what they are learning • learn that changing the stress or pronunciation of a word can change its meaning (*This is a soft ball. This is a softball.*)	• change how they talk depending on where they are and who they are talking to, such as talking to a teacher at school, talking to a parent at home, or talking to friends • know how people are feeling from what they hear and what they see • know when they weren't understood and know how to fix it

Source: Alberta Health Services (HPDIP—Early Childhood). *Talk Box* tables of speech and developmental norms. The *Talk Box* was developed by speech-language pathologists to share ideas and activities for creating language-rich environments for preschool and school-aged children. It is meant to be a resource for any parent, and is not a substitute for a speech-language pathologist. Visit www.parentlinkalberta.ca and click on Talk Box for more information. Adapted by permission.

TOOL 10–8: HUMAN FIGURE DRAWINGS

Instructions: Give the child a blank sheet of paper and a pencil and say: "I want you to draw me the best picture you can of a person. Draw the whole person, not just the head." If the child stops or asks for help, do not suggest that he or she does more. Say: "Do the best you can." Stop when the child indicates he or she is finished. Compare the drawings to the reproductions supplied here.

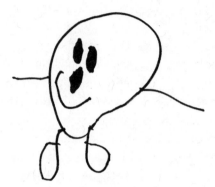

Scores at age 4 years.* Note arms and legs are attached directly to head ("lollipop people") and features are not yet well developed.

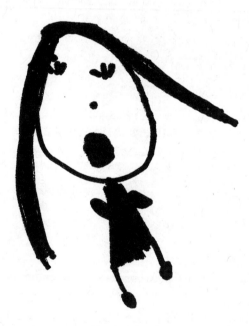

Scores at age 6 years, 3 months. Person now has a body connected to head by a neck, and details such as hairstyle and skirt denote this is a drawing of a girl.

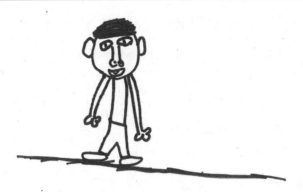

Scores at age 8 years, 6 months. Increasing attention to body proportions (head is smaller than trunk, arms are appropriate length), emerging detail (pupils in eyes, three-dimensional nose and mouth, clothing).

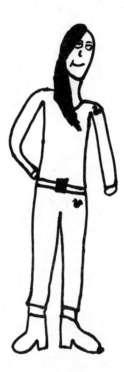

Scores at age 10 years, 6 months. Head, arms, and legs are in good proportion to trunk, and clothing is detailed and complete. Also note three-dimensional nose and mouth, and depiction of shoulders, elbow, and ankle joints.

* For more information on scoring, see Welsh JB, Instone SL, Stein MT. Use of drawings by children at health encounters. In: Encounters with Children: Pediatric Behavior and Development. 4th Edition. Philadelphia PA: Mosby Elsevier, 2006: 98–121.

TOOL 10–9: VISUAL MATCHING EXERCISES (AGES 4 TO 6 YEARS)

Instructions: Point to the underlined figure and say: "Here is a set of designs. I am going to point to one. Can you point to the one that matches?"

Practice: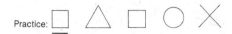

1.   363   <u>393</u>   393   Ɛ93   3P3

2.   b   <u>q</u>   d   q   P

3.   (diamond)   (diamond)   (parallelogram)   (parallelogram)   (diamond)

4.   (asterisk)   (asterisk)   (asterisk)   (asterisk)   (asterisk)

5.   (box figures)

6.   (triangle figures)

7.   ⊓Ɔⴑⴖⴑ   ⴖⴑƆⴖⴑ   ⊓Ɔⴑⴖⴑ   ⴑⴖƆⴑⵊ

8.   ⵊⴖⴑ   <u>Ɔⴖⴖ</u>   Ɔⴖⴖ   ⵊⴖⴑ   ⴑⴖƆ

9.   dad   <u>dab</u>   bab   dab   pad

10.   (triangle figures)

Age (years)	Expected score
4–6	4–10

TOOL 10–10: VISUAL WHOLE:PART ANALYSIS (AGES 6 TO 8 YEARS, 11 MONTHS)

Instructions: Ask the child to find the shape that is hidden in one of the figures. Tell them that the shape has to face the same way as in the picture.

Age (years)	Expected score
6	3–5
7	5–6
8.11	5–6

Source: Levine MD. Pediatric early elementary examination (PEEX 2, Response book and Record form). Cambridge MA: Educators Publishing Service, Inc. Adapted by permission.

TOOL 10–11: LOCK-AND-KEY DESIGNS (AGES 9 TO 14 YEARS, 11 MONTHS)

Instructions: Say to the child: "Take a look at these shapes. Make believe that they are blocks and see if you can find one that fits together with the shaded one on the left to make a perfect square. You can turn the shape around in your mind to see if it fits." When the child chooses the appropriate one from the example, ask him to put a circle around it. Tell the child that in some rows there is one that will fit and in some rows there are two. Score 1 point for each correct answer.

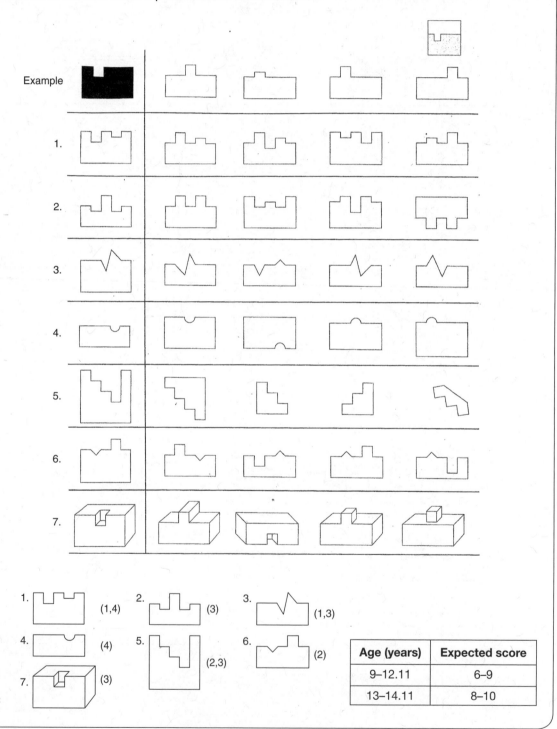

TOOL 10–12: THE GESELL COPY FORMS

Instructions: Give the child a blank piece of paper and a pencil. Show the child one figure at a time, pre-drawn on another sheet, and say: "Make one like this on your paper." Start with the circle. If the child is unable to copy the forms, demonstrate how to draw the first three only, then say, "Now you make one."

Vertical stroke Y N   Horizontal stroke Y N   Circular scribble Y N

Gesell Copy Forms Items

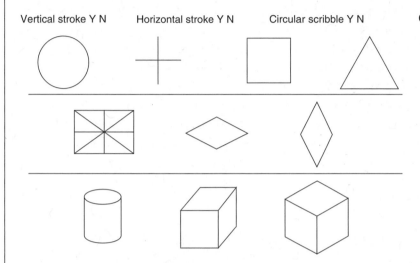

Task/Item Ages:	3	3⁶	4	4⁶	5	5⁶	6
Copy forms							
Scribble	■	■	■	■	■	■	■
Stroke—vertical	■	■	■	■	■	■	■
Stroke—horizontal	■	■	■	■	■	■	■
Circle	■	■	■	■	■	■	■
Cross		▨	■	■	■	■	■
Square				■	■	■	■
Triangle					▨	■	■
Divided rectangle						▨	■
Diamond—horizontal							▨
Diamond—vertical							▨
3-D cylinder							
3-D cube face-on							
3-D cube point-on							

Gesell Copy Forms Performance Level Expectations by Age Band

Note: The age bands in the chart represent data collected 2008–2010 from children whose chronological age ranged between three months below to three months above the stated age band.

■ Black: Solid performance expectation
(70% or more of children in the age band completed item successfully)

▨ Grey: Qualified performance expectation
(50–69.9% of children in the age band completed item successfully)

☐ White: Performance not yet Expected
(<50% of children in the age band completed item successfully)

The Gesell Developmental Observation—Revised is a multidimensional assessment system that evaluates a child's developmental age and rates a performance across five strands of development using nineteen tasks, overt behaviour, and two measures of social, emotional, and adaptive development. Interpretation of the results requires specialized training. Thus, the Copy Forms data chart above serves only to illustrate the results for a single task, and should not be used for scoring or decision-making about a child's overall development. Note: Age norms are approximate and may vary ±six months, with copying being a more advanced task than imitation.

TOOL 10–13: READING TESTS

Background

These reading paragraphs are designed to provide a graded, representative sample of text from Grade 1 to Grade 6. The paragraphs were constructed from vocabulary that was taken from word lists included in informal reading inventories such as those found in the *Handbook in Diagnostic and Prescriptive Teaching*, Boston: Allyn and Bacon, 1979. Sentences were constructed to reflect the increasing complexity of language used by normally developing students as they move through the grades and acquire higher levels of receptive language. The post-reading Cloze comprehension method is familiar to most teachers, and it has been used in educational research for several decades.

Passages were field tested in both eastern and western Canada for appropriateness of level. Results suggested that the passages were reasonably good, broad indicators of reading decoding and recall proficiency for these students.

Instructions

Note: The reading passages and Cloze exercises which follow are not standard administration size and must be enlarged by 200% for use, particularly for early elementary age children.

Ask the student to read aloud the passage at, or one below, his/her grade placement.

A. Decoding

Give the student a page with a paragraph only. Mark omissions (words left out), substitutions (words not read correctly), and additions (extra words inserted). If the student gets stuck on a word, give him/her about six seconds to decode it and then indicate the word if he/she was unsuccessful. Mark these aided words with an "a" above the word.

Count all omissions, substitutions, additions, and "a" (aided words) to arrive at a total number of errors for scores for decoding.

If the student makes more than 5% errors (i.e., greater than 5% of total number of words in error), this passage is too difficult for him/her. (See also Marking.)

B. Recall

Give the student a page with incomplete paragraphs on it. Tell the student: "Here is the same passage you have just read. Some of the words are missing. Try to fill in the blanks with the best word to fit. Don't worry about spelling. Just do your best."

C. Comprehension

Comprehension has not been normed for these paragraphs. You can get a sense of whether the child comprehended the passage by asking him/her some questions related to content. Strictly speaking, the fill-in-the-blanks portion of this test relates more to recall. You can also assess auditory comprehension using the paragraphs extracted from the PEEX and PEERAMID samples. (See **Tools 10–3** and **10–5**.)

Scoring

The child must insert the exact word, verbatim, from the passage. Spelling errors are not counted as errors. If the child is in Grade 1 or 2 and cannot write the word but verbally knows it, score his/her response as correct. Above 45% correct means the student is able to comprehend at that grade level (see Marking).

Marking

Grade 1. Fun at the Farm
44 words

Grade 2. Playing in the Leaves
63 words

Grade 3. Crossing the River
91 words

Grade 4. Sheriff Bacon's Buried Treasure
113 words

Grade 5. Emperor Salmon and Tog
155 words

Grade 6. The Case of Bad Medicine
182 Words

Decoding

The passage is *too difficult* if the child has more errors than the following for his/her grade:

Grade 1 > 3 errors
Grade 2 > 4 errors
Grade 3 > 5 errors
Grade 4 > 6 errors
Grade 5 > 7 errors
Grade 6 > 8 errors

Recall

Number of blank insertions incorrect for grade level meaning inadequate comprehension:

Grade 1 > 5
Grade 2 > 6
Grade 3 > 9
Grade 4 > 11
Grade 5 > 16
Grade 6 > 18

(Continued on next page)

Source: Mann PH, Suiter P. Teacher's Handbook of Diagnostic Inventories: Spelling, Reading, Handwriting, Arithmetic; A Practical Guide with Duplicate Masters. Boston MA: Allyn and Bacon, 1975. Adapted with permission by Angus Lloyd and Associates, Inc.

TOOL 10–13: READING TESTS (*CONTINUED*)

Fun at the Farm

One day I went to the farm.
I went with my mother.
There was a red farm house.
Many animals live at the farm.
We saw little yellow ducks.
We saw a dog playing with a ball.
I like the farm.
It is fun.

Fun at the Farm

One day I went to the _____.
I went _____ my Mother.
There was a red farm _____.
Many _____ live at the farm.
We _____ little yellow _____.
We saw a dog _____ with a _____.
I _____ the farm.
It is _____.

Playing in the Leaves

It was a nice fall day.
Bill and Ann were playing on the grass.
The wind blew.
The leaves fell from the trees.
Some fell on Bill's head.
"I like the beautiful leaves," said Bill.
The friends made a big pile of leaves.
"Let's ask if we can play here tomorrow," said Ann.
Bill said, "Yes, we can make a bigger pile of leaves."

Playing in the Leaves

It was a nice _____ day.
Bill and Ann _____ playing on the grass.
The _____ blew.
The leaves fell _____ the trees.
Some fell _____ Bill's head.
"I like _____ beautiful leaves," said Bill.
The _____ made a big pile of leaves.
"Let's ask if _____ can play here tomorrow," _____ Ann.
Bill said, "Yes, we _____ make a bigger _____ of leaves."

Crossing the River

One cold day, Bill and his cousin went on a journey.
They walked along a gravel path until they
reached a stream.
A sign beside the stream said "danger no crossing."
Bill and his cousin wanted to get to the other side
of the stream.
They needed to find another way to cross the stream.
The boys walked along the stream for fifteen minutes.
Luckily, they saw a bridge.
They used the bridge to cross safely over
the stream.
Bill and his cousin did not want to freeze in
the icy stream.

Sheriff Bacon's Buried Treasure

One peaceful day, Sheriff Bacon was relaxing at
his desk.
He received an alarming phone call.
An evil spy, in search of a great fortune, was
designing a map to find the Sheriff's buried
treasure.
Knowledge about the spy and his plan spread
through the western town.
The Sheriff gathered a search party of people
who had the courage to stop the spy.
The search was a success.
With the help of some guides, the search party trailed
the spy to an island where he was arrested.
The spy was silent.
He was taken to a cell and locked up forever.
In the end, Sheriff Bacon buried his treasure in a new
hiding place.

Crossing the River

One cold day, Bill _____ his cousin went on a _____.
They walked along a _____ path until they
reached _____ stream.
A sign _____ the stream said "danger ____ crossing."
Bill and his _____ wanted to get to _____ other side
of the stream.
They needed to find _____ way to cross the _____.
The boys walked along ___stream for fifteen minutes.
_____, they saw a bridge.
_____ used the bridge to _____ safely over
the stream.
_____ and his cousin did _____ want to freeze in
_____ icy stream.

Sheriff Bacon's Buried Treasure

One peaceful day, Sheriff _____ was relaxing at
his _____.
He received an alarming _____ call.
An evil spy, _____ search of a great _____, was
designing a map _____ find the Sheriff's buried
_____.
Knowledge about the spy _____ his plan spread
through _____ western town.
The Sheriff _____ a search party of _____
who had the courage _____ stop the spy.
The search was a success.
With _____ help of some _____, the search party
trailed the ____ to an island where ____ was arrested.
The spy _____ silent.
He was taken ____ a cell and locked _____ forever.
In the end, _____ Bacon buried his treasure _____
a new hiding place.

(Continued on next page)

TOOL 10–13: READING TESTS (*CONTINUED*)

Emperor Salmon and Tog

Emperor Salmon was a great scholar who lived in ancient times.

Nobody liked him much because he was always solemn and serious.

His only friend was a dangerous man named Tog.

Tog had an ivory spear which he used as a weapon.

He always defeated the Emperor's enemies.

Salmon made a magnificent home for Tog with expensive cushions, silk curtains, and a wonderful terrace garden for Tog to play in.

The people did not like Tog and they did not like the emperor so they plotted to get rid of him.

They invited anyone with ambition to come to the kingdom and fight Tog.

Many came and Tog grew tired of fighting constantly.

He asked the emperor to let him retire and be an ordinary subject.

Salmon realized he had no choice but to scare away his enemies so he made up a legend regarding Tog.

People heard the legend and were so afraid of the story, they did not try to fight with Tog.

Emperor Salmon and Tog

Emperor Salmon was a _____ scholar who lived in ancient _____.

Nobody liked him much _____ he was always solemn _____ serious.

His only friend _____ a dangerous man named Tog.

Tog ___ an ivory spear which ___ used as a _____.

He always defeated the _____ enemies.

Salmon made a magnificent _____ for Tog with expensive _____, silk curtains, and a wonderful terrace garden for Tog _____ play in.

The people did _____ like Tog and they _____ not like the emperor _____ they plotted to get _____ of him.

They invited _____ with ambition to come _____ the kingdom and fight _____.

Many came and Tog grew _____ of fighting constantly.

He _____ the emperor to let _____ retire and be an _____ subject.

Salmon realized he _____ no choice but to _____ away his enemies so he _____ up a legend regarding _____.

People heard the legend _____ were so afraid _____ the story, they did _____ try to fight with Tog.

The Case of Bad Medicine

Jack was running down the dark corridor of the drug warehouse.

His heart pounded rapidly against his chest.

He was positive that he was being followed.

As he proceeded down the hallway, he came to a door that was partially opened.

Afraid of being detained by whoever was following him, Jack ignored the DANGER sign and entered the room.

It looked like an abandoned laboratory.

There were various bottles containing different coloured liquids placed on the counter tops.

Suddenly, there was a loud SLAM.

A large blond man, with extensive scars on his face, stood motionless in the doorway.

The man summoned Jack, "Come here you nosey kid."

"Not on your life," replied Jack as he quickly darted behind one of the counter tops.

The man followed Jack, slipped, and knocked himself out cold.

Jack called the police and gave them a detailed account of what had happened.

The police told Jack that they had been searching for this malicious man for months.

The man was arrested and Jack received a medal for his cooperation in solving "The Case of Bad Medicine."

The Case of Bad Medicine

Jack was running down the dark corridor of the _____ warehouse.

His heart pounded _____ against his chest.

He _____ positive that he was _____ followed.

As he proceeded _____ the hallway, he came _____ a door that was _____ opened.

Afraid of being _____ by whoever was following _____, Jack ignored the DANGER _____ and entered the room.

_____ looked like an abandoned _____.

There were various bottles _____ different coloured liquids placed _____ the counter tops.

Suddenly, _____ was a loud SLAM.

_____ large blond man, with _____ scars on his face, _____ motionless in the doorway.

_____ man summoned Jack, "Come _____ you nosey kid."

"Not on your _____," replied Jack as he _____ darted behind one of _____ counter tops.

The man _____ Jack, slipped, and knocked _____ out cold.

Jack called the _____ and gave them a detailed _____ of what had happened.

The _____ told Jack that they _____ been searching for this _____ man for months.

The _____ was arrested and Jack _____ a medal for his _____ in solving "The Case _____ Bad Medicine."

TOOL 10–14: ASSESSMENT OF HANDWRITING SPEED

Ages 6 to 9 years: Copy a sentence

Instructions: Say to the child: "Now I am going to ask you to copy a sentence in the book." Point to the sentence. Say, "We are going to take two minutes, and I want you to copy as much of the sentence as you can. Remember to be careful and do a good job. Copy down everything you see just the way you see it." Allow two minutes for the child to copy the sentence. Observe five parameters: words copied (total number), spacing, letter formation, accuracy, and frequency looking up. Score the child on the number of words copied.

While Ben was walking down the street last night, he saw the brown dog.

Age (years)	Number of words copied
6	3–5
7	7–11
8–9	10–13

Ages 9 to 15 years: Cursive alphabet

Instructions: Say to the child: "I want you to write the lowercase, cursive alphabet (that is, writing, not printing)—the small letters, not the capitals—as if it's all one long word (all connected). Write it as fast as you can without getting it wrong. Don't take your pencil off the page, so you don't have to cross the 't' or the 'x' or dot the 'i' or 'j.' Are you ready? Okay, go!"

Age (years)	Number of seconds to copy
9–10	30–70
11–12	24–45
13+	20–40

Source: Levine, MD. *Pediatric Early Elementary Examination* (PEEX 2, Record form). Cambridge MA: Educators Publishing Service, Inc. Adapted by permission.

TOOL 10–15: EVALUATION OF WRITTEN STORIES USING BASIS

Instructions: Say to the child: "Write about your favourite place. It could be a room, a house, a park, or any other place that is special to you. Describe the place in any way you like, but be sure to include what makes this your favourite place."

Grade 3—Ranges of Criteria

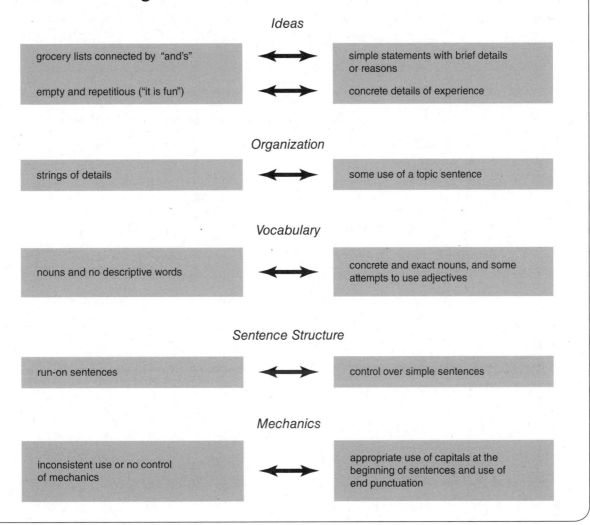

Ideas

grocery lists connected by "and's"	⟷ simple statements with brief details or reasons
empty and repetitious ("it is fun")	⟷ concrete details of experience

Organization

strings of details	⟷ some use of a topic sentence

Vocabulary

nouns and no descriptive words	⟷ concrete and exact nouns, and some attempts to use adjectives

Sentence Structure

run-on sentences	⟷ control over simple sentences

Mechanics

inconsistent use or no control of mechanics	⟷ appropriate use of capitals at the beginning of sentences and use of end punctuation

(Continued on next page)

TOOL 10–15: EVALUATION OF WRITTEN STORIES USING BASIS (*CONTINUED*)

Average Sample—Grade 3

Writing Exercise ☐

my favorite place

my favorite place is Calfornia

I like it because it is pretty

and it has mountains and it never harly

rains and because my dady and my aunt and my

uncle and my grandmother and my cousin lives

there and every time I go swiming and we go

every where and I seen a snake.

·3

Grade 4—Ranges of Criteria

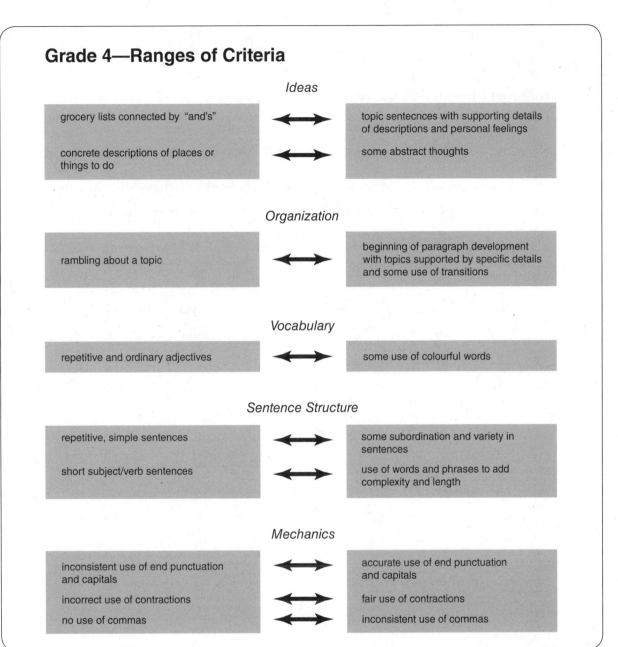

Ideas

grocery lists connected by "and's"	⟷	topic sentecnces with supporting details of descriptions and personal feelings
concrete descriptions of places or things to do	⟷	some abstract thoughts

Organization

rambling about a topic	⟷	beginning of paragraph development with topics supported by specific details and some use of transitions

Vocabulary

repetitive and ordinary adjectives	⟷	some use of colourful words

Sentence Structure

repetitive, simple sentences	⟷	some subordination and variety in sentences
short subject/verb sentences	⟷	use of words and phrases to add complexity and length

Mechanics

inconsistent use of end punctuation and capitals	⟷	accurate use of end punctuation and capitals
incorrect use of contractions	⟷	fair use of contractions
no use of commas	⟷	inconsistent use of commas

(Continued on next page)

TOOL 10–15: EVALUATION OF WRITTEN STORIES USING BASIS (*CONTINUED*)

Average Sample—Grade 4

Writing Exercise

> My favorite place is the park.
> Because people have party's there. I like
> to swing and play on the marry-go-round
> And slide down the slide. and see saw
> and A bunch of people play there.
> The park is fun but some people
> don't like it. But I do. Some parks
> have pools.

Grade 5—Ranges of Criteria

Ideas

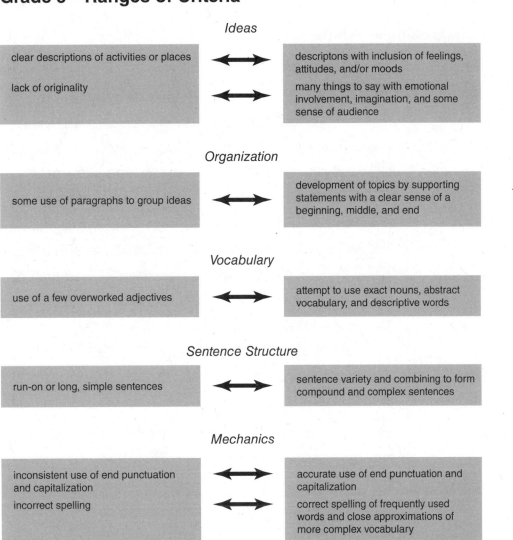

clear descriptions of activities or places	⟷ descriptons with inclusion of feelings, attitudes, and/or moods
lack of originality	⟷ many things to say with emotional involvement, imagination, and some sense of audience

Organization

some use of paragraphs to group ideas	⟷ development of topics by supporting statements with a clear sense of a beginning, middle, and end

Vocabulary

use of a few overworked adjectives	⟷ attempt to use exact nouns, abstract vocabulary, and descriptive words

Sentence Structure

run-on or long, simple sentences	⟷ sentence variety and combining to form compound and complex sentences

Mechanics

inconsistent use of end punctuation and capitalization	⟷ accurate use of end punctuation and capitalization
incorrect spelling	⟷ correct spelling of frequently used words and close approximations of more complex vocabulary
incorrect use of commas	⟷ some correct use of commas

(Continued on next page)

TOOL 10–15: EVALUATION OF WRITTEN STORIES USING BASIS (*CONTINUED*)

Average Sample—Grade 5

Writing Exercise

My house is my
favorite place to be. It is special to me
because my mom and my dad + my Brothers
and sisters live there at night when we
sit down to watch t.V. It is always
cozy It is very pretty inside.
It always stays clean and my mom always
has supper ready for us to. eat. She always.
try to make out with what she has got.
Our house is white chrimmed in black the
porch is gray. That is why my house is my
favorite place to be. The End.

13

Grade 6—Ranges of Criteria

Ideas

lack of originality		inclusion of details and personal responses, and examples of value judgments

Organization

strings of details with one idea or detail following another in seemingly random fashion		well-developed paragraphs with a clear sense of beginning, middle, and end

Vocabulary

ordinary, colourless words and adjectives		some colourful adjectives and use of names for feelings

Sentence Structure

short, choppy, simple sentences or poorly controlled, longer sentences	well-formed subordination and coordination
simple subject/verb sentences	some variety in beginnings
run-on sentences	correct compound sentences and correct use of embedded lists

Mechanics

inconsistent punctuation and capitalization	correct punctuation and capitalization
partial control of commas in a series	correct use of commas in series
incorrect spelling	accurate spelling of most words

(Continued on next page)

TOOL 10–15: EVALUATION OF WRITTEN STORIES USING BASIS (*CONTINUED*)

Average Sample—Grade 6

Writing Exercise

My Favorite Place

My favorite place is my grandma's she
has a big two store house on the highway. When we
go out there, there's lots to do Because
She has such of a big feild we do
lots of fun things. We have lots of
dinners. We have lots of animals to
feed. We also climb lots of trees My
uncle hangs up many tire swing.
We clean the yard almost every
Spring and Fall. We all do lots of fun
things together. We play ball all the
time me and my cousins walk out to
the sandduns where theres kinda like
a pond but good enough to sit in and
get cooled off. We make tracks like
bears at my grandmas in the sand duns.
Then when all the fun over we go home.

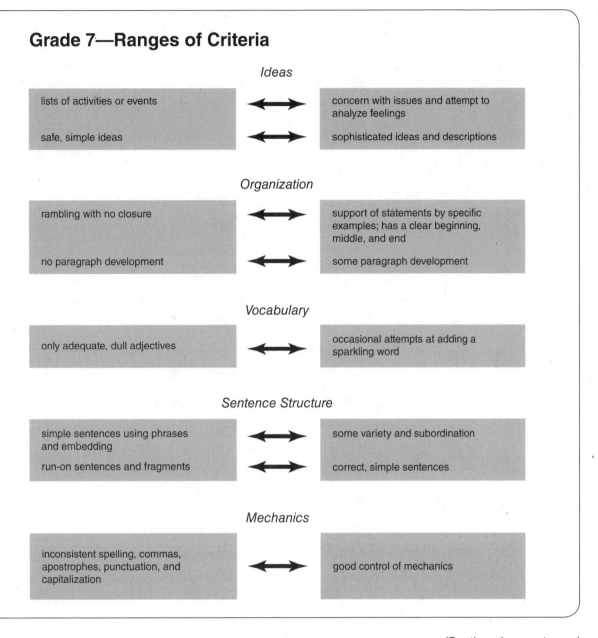

Grade 7—Ranges of Criteria

Ideas

lists of activities or events	concern with issues and attempt to analyze feelings
safe, simple ideas	sophisticated ideas and descriptions

Organization

rambling with no closure	support of statements by specific examples; has a clear beginning, middle, and end
no paragraph development	some paragraph development

Vocabulary

only adequate, dull adjectives	occasional attempts at adding a sparkling word

Sentence Structure

simple sentences using phrases and embedding	some variety and subordination
run-on sentences and fragments	correct, simple sentences

Mechanics

inconsistent spelling, commas, apostrophes, punctuation, and capitalization	good control of mechanics

(Continued on next page)

TOOL 10–15: EVALUATION OF WRITTEN STORIES USING BASIS (*CONTINUED*)

Average Sample—Grade 7

Writing Exercise

My favorite place to go that I
know of is Walt Disney World. Walt
Disney World is in Orlando Florida about
90 miles from where I live. It has
fun things to do there. It has rides,
places to swim, golf, things to look
at, and of coarse they have a motel
to stay in at nighttime. They a Monorail
Train that is fun to ride on. There
is all kinds of stores like t-shirt
shops, suvoner shops, places to buy
food at, and they sell little old
Mickey Mouse caps. I like Walt
Disney World because it is
fun to ride the rides, and do many
other things. Walt Disney World is
beutiful.

Grade 8—Ranges of Criteria

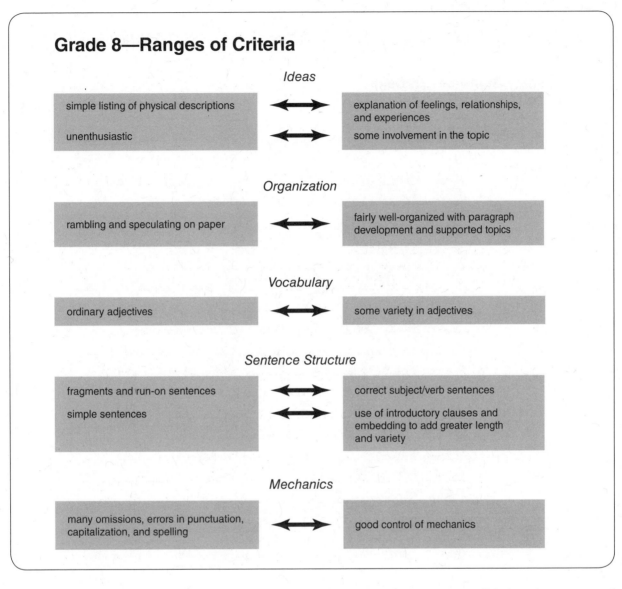

Ideas

simple listing of physical descriptions	←→	explanation of feelings, relationships, and experiences
unenthusiastic	←→	some involvement in the topic

Organization

rambling and speculating on paper	←→	fairly well-organized with paragraph development and supported topics

Vocabulary

ordinary adjectives	←→	some variety in adjectives

Sentence Structure

fragments and run-on sentences	←→	correct subject/verb sentences
simple sentences	←→	use of introductory clauses and embedding to add greater length and variety

Mechanics

many omissions, errors in punctuation, capitalization, and spelling	←→	good control of mechanics

(Continued on next page)

TOOL 10–15: EVALUATION OF WRITTEN STORIES USING BASIS (*CONTINUED*)

Average Sample—Grade 8

Writing Exercise

The living room in my house is my favorite place because it has a pretty frost green paint on the walls, and on the ceiling their is star like sparkles of shiny glass, the ceil is white.

The fireplace is nice and big the bricks come out so you can sit there while getting warm, we have a big, wood, thick mantle that we keep lots of stuff on.

We also have a big picture window that gives us lots of light, we have two picture windows and one regular.

I like the living room because it always nice and warm in there in the winter and in summer it nice and cool, although we don't have an air-conditioner.

We are going to get new carpet before next summer then it will be prettier then usual, and that why I like our living room.

TOOL 10–16: READING AND WRITING SKILLS IN SCHOOL-AGED CHILDREN

Grade	Reading	Writing
Grade 1	• Create rhyming words • Identify all sounds in short words • Blend separate sounds to form words • Match spoken words with print • Know how a book works (e.g., read from left to right and top to bottom in English) • Identify letters, words, and sentences • Sound out words when reading • Have a sight vocabulary of one hundred common words • Read grade-level material fluently • Understand what is read	• Express ideas through writing • Print clearly • Spell frequently used words correctly • Begin each sentence with capital letters and use ending punctuation • Write a variety of stories, journal entries, or letters/notes
Grade 2	• Have fully mastered phonics/sound awareness • Associate speech sounds, syllables, words, and phrases with their written forms • Recognize many words by sight • Use meaning clues when reading (e.g., pictures, titles/headings, information in the story) • Reread and self-correct when necessary • Locate information to answer questions • Explain key elements of a story (e.g., main idea, main characters, plot) • Use own experience to predict and justify what will happen in grade-level stories • Read, paraphrase/retell a story in a sequence • Read grade-level stories, poetry, or dramatic text silently and aloud with fluency • Read spontaneously • Identify and use spelling patterns in words when reading	• Write legibly • Use a variety of sentence types in writing essays, poetry, or short stories (fiction and nonfiction) • Use basic punctuation and capitalization appropriately • Organize writing to include beginning, middle, and end • Spell frequently used words correctly • Progress from inventive spelling (e.g., spelling by sound) to more accurate spelling
Grade 3	• Demonstrate full mastery of basic phonics • Use word analysis skills when reading • Use clues from language content and structure to help understand what is read • Predict and justify what will happen next in stories and compare and contrast stories • Ask and answer questions regarding reading material • Use acquired information to learn about new topics • Read grade-level books fluently (fiction and nonfiction) • Reread and correct errors when necessary	• Plan, organize, revise, and edit • Include details in writing • Write stories, letters, simple explanations, and brief reports • Spell simple words correctly, correct most spelling independently, and use a dictionary to correct spelling • Write clearly in cursive

(Continued on next page)

TOOL 10–16: READING AND WRITING SKILLS IN SCHOOL-AGED CHILDREN (*CONTINUED*)

Grade	Reading	Writing
Grade 4	• Read for specific purposes • Read grade-level books fluently • Use previously learned information to understand new material • Follow written directions • Take brief notes • Link information learned to different subjects • Learn meanings of new words through knowledge of word origins, synonyms, and multiple meanings • Use reference materials (e.g., dictionary) • Explain the author's purpose and writing style • Read and understand a variety of types of literature, including fiction, nonfiction, historical fiction, and poetry • Compare and contrast in content areas • Make inferences from texts • Paraphrase content, including the main idea and details	• Write effective stories and explanations, including several paragraphs about the same topic • Develop a plan for writing, including a beginning, middle, and end • Organize writing to convey a central idea • Edit final copies for grammar, punctuation, and spelling
Grade 5	• Read grade-level books fluently • Learn meanings of unfamiliar words through knowledge of root words, prefixes, and suffixes • Prioritize information according to the purpose of reading • Read a variety of literary forms • Describe development of character and plot • Describe characteristics of poetry • Analyze author's language and style • Use reference materials to support opinions	• Write for a variety of purposes • Use vocabulary effectively • Vary sentence structure • Revise writing for clarity • Edit final copies

TOOL 10–17: SAMPLE SPELLING BATTERY

Instructions: Give the child the instructions appropriate to his/her grade level.

Spelling A

Grades 1–2

"Spell the word 'dog.' Spell 'dog' backward. What does that new word spell?"

Should be correctly spelled and labelled by children 6–7 years old.

Grades 2–3

"Spell the word 'was.' Spell 'was' backward. What does that new word spell?"

Should be correctly spelled and labelled by children 7–8 years old.

"Spell the word 'tip.' Spell 'tip' backward. What does that new word spell?"

Should be correctly spelled and labelled by children 7 1/2 to 8 1/2 years old.

Grades 4–5

"Spell the word 'not' as in 'I will not go.' Spell 'not' backward. What does that new word spell?"

Should be correctly spelled and labelled by children 9–10 years old.

"Spell the word 'live.' Spell 'live' backward. What does that new word spell?"

Should be correctly spelled and labelled by children 9 1/2 to 10 1/2 years old.

"Spell the word 'dial' as in 'dial a telephone number.' Spell 'dial' backward. What does that new word spell?"

Should be correctly spelled and labelled by children 9 1/2 to 10 1/2 years old.

The backward words spelling test may relate to both reading accuracy and comprehension.

Spelling B

"Now these are more difficult words. Some are for Grade 5s, but do the best you can. Spell them as well as you can, or as you think they should be spelled."

Grade 1 words: it, is, the, stop, spot, look.

Grade 2 words: hit, hot, hat, hut, work, talk, girl, went.

Grade 3 words: should, could, phone, house.

Grade 4 words: monkey, elephant, receive, friend.

Grade 5 words: purchase, ethics, delicate, delicious.

Source: Weinberg WA, McLean A. A diagnostic approach to developmental specific learning disorders. J Child Neur 1986; 1 (Appendix A—The diagnostic symbol language battery): 169. Adapted from and reprinted by permission of SAGE Publications.

TOOL 10–18: SAMPLE MATHEMATICS TESTS

Instructions: Give the child the instructions appropriate to his/her grade level.

Senior kindergarten to Grade 1

"How many pennies in a nickel?"

Children who are 5–6 years old should be able to do this item.

"If you had nine apples and three friends, how many apples could you give each friend?"

Children who are 6 1/2 to 7 1/2 years old should be able to do this item. If the child cannot answer this question, then ask: "If you had six apples and two friends, how many apples could you give each friend?"

Grades 2–3

"How many quarters are there in two dollars?"

Children who are 7–8 years old should be able to do this item. If the child gives the answer "four," say, "No, how many in two dollars?" and hold up two fingers.

Grades 3–4

"How many half dollars are there in five whole dollars?"

Children who are 8–9 years old should be able to do this item. If the answer is incorrect, then ask, "How many half dollars in one whole dollar?" and hold up one finger. "Now, how many in five whole dollars?" and hold up five fingers.

Grade 4–5

"If you had to walk one hundred kilometres, and you could walk ten kilometres in an hour, how many hours would it take you to walk one hundred kilometres?"

Children who are 9–10 1/2 years old should be able to do this item.

"Multiply four times four; six times seven; eight times nine."

Children who are 9–10 years old should be able to do these items.

Grades 5–6

"A whole pie is divided into four pieces. One piece of pie equals what fraction of the pie?"

Children who are 10–11 years old should be able to do this item.

Grades 6–7

"Three pieces equal what fraction of the pie?"

Children who are 10 1/2 to 12 years old should be able to do this item.

"What is one-fourth as a percent?"

"What is three-fourths as a percent?"

Children who are 10 1/2 to 12 years old should be able to do these items.

"What is one-fourth as a decimal?"

"What is three-fourths as a decimal?"

Children who are 11 years old should be able to do these items.

Source: Weinberg WA, McLean A. A diagnostic approach to developmental specific learning disorders. J Child Neur 1986; 1 (Appendix A–The diagnostic symbol language battery): 169. Adapted from and reprinted by permission of SAGE Publications.

TOOL 10–19: ASSESSMENT OF AUDITORY MEMORY FROM REPETITION OF DIGITS

Say the digits one second apart and do not inflect the last number. (This requires some practice.) Stop when the child misses three sets of consecutive digits at an age level.

Age	Repeat digits forward	Repeat digits backward
2 1/2	47 63 58	
3	641 352 837	
4 1/2	4729 3852 7261	
7	31859 48372 96183	295 816 473
10	473296 429736 728394	
12		81379 697582 92518
Adult	7259483 4715396 4193582	471952 583694 752618

Source: Stanford-Binet Intelligence Scales. Form L-M, by Termanand LM, Merrill MM, 1972. Austin TX: PRO-ED, Inc. © 1972 by PRO-ED, Inc. Reprinted by permission.

REFERENCES

1 Ages & Stages Questionnaire. Paul H. Brookes Publishing Company Inc., 2011. <http://agesandstages.com/>

2 Parents' Evaluation of Developmental Status. 2011 PEDSTest.com, LLC, 2011. <www.pedstest.com/Home.aspx>

3 Naglieri JA. Draw a Person: A Quantitative Scoring System. San Antonio TX: Psychological Corporation, 1998.

4 Goodenough FL. Measurement of Intelligence by Drawings. New York: World Book Company, 1926.

5 Harris DB. Children's Drawings as Measures of Intellectual Maturity. New York: Harcourt, Brace & World, Inc., 1963.

CHAPTER 11

Differential Diagnosis of the Child Who Is Not Doing Well in School

Debra Andrews and G. Tyna Doyle

Most parents come to their physician's office for an explanation of why their child is not doing well in school, rather than with a specific condition in mind. Teachers may also be unfamiliar with the long list of possible causes for poor school performance or inattention. Physicians can bring their training in differential diagnosis to this problem, defining the presenting symptom(s), narrowing down the list of possible causes, ranking these in order of probability, and developing a problem list and investigation plan that will lead to more definitive diagnosis and intervention.

School failure is a broad term describing a group of more specific symptoms contributing to lack of success in some aspect of school, e.g., inability to read, fine motor delay, poor social skills, and/or inattention. Each of these specific symptoms has its own set of possible diagnoses. In this chapter, we review the differential diagnosis of four common presentations of children who are not doing well in school: academic achievement problems with or without inattention, oppositional behaviour, motor coordination issues, and poor social skills. You will note that the boundaries of these presentations overlap— children may present with more than one symptom, and conditions may have more than one presentation. It helps to begin by choosing the symptom that is of greatest concern and focus there.

Many school problems are multifactorial. Frequently the child's primary problem (for example, an LD) may lead to secondary complaints (for example, depression or functional abdominal pain). Chronic anaemia or a chaotic home life may contribute to inattention and may co-occur. A well-developed problem list will help capture this complexity.

It should include all symptoms and findings from the history, physical exam, and reports from other professionals, described at the highest level of understanding. If a diagnosis is known, that diagnosis should be what is reported on the problem list; otherwise, list the symptoms, symptom complexes, or findings that need further exploration, focusing on the differential and the plans for workup.

Thorough assessment is the key to accurate diagnosis and better understanding of the relative importance of each contributory factor, which will lead to the most effective intervention.

THE DIFFERENTIAL DIAGNOSIS OF POOR ACADEMIC ACHIEVEMENT

Children may do poorly on specific academic tasks because of a **primary learning problem,** i.e., there is a problem with some aspect of the learning process itself, such as a specific reading disability, or because of intrinsic **performance factors** affecting demonstration of previously attained skill, such as attention, anxiety, fatigue or illness. Performance factors often account for variability in results because these factors may not be present all the time.

Issues of general intellectual function

When a child is doing poorly in school, it is important to understand the child's learning potential. Cognitive ability is usually a good predictor of academic achievement, and IQ testing is often the first step in the evaluation process. Children may have trouble in school at either end of the developmental continuum: there are certainly different expectations for the child with lower versus higher cognitive skills, and unique considerations as to why a particular child is not succeeding.

Intellectual disability

A child not achieving at a rate commensurate with peers may not have the potential for such achievement because of *intellectual disability* (ID), previously termed *mental retardation* (see the Glossary). Severe to profound ID (IQ scores less than 35 on standardized psychological assessment) is easy to recognize and is diagnosed early in life. There is a greater likelihood of such children having an identifiable medical cause (e.g., chromosomal anomaly or syndrome) for their delays, and some medical workup to define etiology may be useful if not already completed (see Chapter 9 for medical investigations). Mild (IQ 50 to 70) to moderate (IQ 35 to 50) ID may be less obvious, particularly in the presence of strong family support, and may go unrecognized until school entry. (See the figure in Chapter 6 for IQ ranges.)

Children with cognitive abilities in the "borderline" range (IQ 70 to 80) are often described as "slow learners." Their disability is subtle. They need more time and repetition to master academic tasks and may put in great amounts of effort just to pass each grade. As abstract reasoning becomes more of an expectation, they fall further behind despite their efforts. Children with ID may have been described as having "global developmental delay" or GDD on preschool assessments because of concerns about prematurely labelling a child, but at school age, more definitive testing can and should be done, leading to clarification of the cause of the learning difficulty.

Key presenting features of ID

Features include history of delayed milestones in a number of domains. Slow progress in academics across subjects, slow rate of processing of instructions, much need for repetition and rehearsal, poor memory skills, and an observed tendency toward concrete interpretation of language are suggestive findings. Children with ID may gravitate toward younger children on the playground because the level of complexity of their games, language, and social interaction may be more congruent with the child's own functioning.

Giftedness

Gifted (see the Glossary) children with full-scale scores significantly above average (IQ 120 or greater on a standardized psychological assessment) may also be underachievers. Some very bright students are bored and unmotivated by the standard grade curriculum and its associated teaching methods, and they may daydream in class, resembling the child with inattentive type ADHD. LDs may coexist with giftedness, producing classroom test scores and achievement that are "only average." Such children may not qualify for enrichment classes if entry depends on achievement as well as potential, but a more challenging program may be just what is needed to motivate them. Gifted children may excel in language-related skills (with advanced vocabulary and sentence structure) or in nonverbal tasks (showing excellent artistic and constructional abilities) or both. They commonly have an obvious desire to learn and achieve in all areas. Unrecognized or unfulfilled giftedness may predispose children to behavioural and emotional disorders.

Key presenting features of giftedness

In giftedness, rapid developmental progress, including advanced milestones, may be seen. Learning occurs with little teaching or scaffolding; children may teach themselves to read or do math operations before school entry. There may be special talents, e.g., in music, art, or science. Often there are intense interests in learning about specific topics, but unless there is a co-morbid ASD, usually once a subject is mastered, the child moves on. Some gifted children exhibit uneven development with relative or actual deficits in motor or social skills. Gifted children may gravitate to developmental peers (other "smart" kids) or adults, or may camouflage their abilities to be able to fit in socially.

Learning disabilities

Unlike children with generalized cognitive delays, children with specific learning disabilities have an IQ in the average range or above, indicating at least an average learning potential. They will have specific academic delays—in language-based LDs, these will be the linguistic and phonological aspects of reading, spelling, and written expression, and for nonverbal LDs, math reasoning and written output. See also Chapter 1 for a more comprehensive discussion of LDs.

Key presenting features

Children with LDs may present uneven performance, with average abilities in some areas and unexpected difficulty in learning an academic subject or subjects. For language-based LDs, there may be indications of a broader problem with language, e.g., a history of language delay, or the child may only have phonological difficulties. Children with nonverbal LD may have associated social interaction difficulties, behavioural rigidity, visual-spatial and visual-motor problems, ADHD, and/or anxiety.

Medical issues

Possible underlying medical issues need to be evaluated in any child having difficulty in school; if found, consider the impact on the child's school functioning. This is especially true of any vision and hearing deficits, which may also influence the supports the child receives in school.

Physical illness in the child

A sick child may not learn in school for a variety of reasons. Frequent hospitalizations, doctor's appointments, or the necessity to stay home because of illness may reduce school attendance to the point where it is impossible to make up missed work. For such children, academic instruction arranged through a hospital school program or individual tutoring may help prevent repeating a grade. Note that attendance is included on most report cards and is a handy way to identify significant absenteeism.

In some cases, it is the parent's perception of the severity of illness that determines whether the child attends classes or stays home. Children with asthma, asymptomatic heart disease or innocent murmurs, graduates of the neonatal intensive care unit, or survivors of life-threatening medical conditions may seem to their parents to be frail and more susceptible to acquire new illnesses, leading the parent to keep the child safe at home—the so-called vulnerable child syndrome. Note that survivors of neonatal intensive care or traumatic brain injury are indeed vulnerable—to true learning and attention difficulties.

Children with organic causes for pain or fatigue may fail in their schoolwork because their symptoms interfere with concentration. Medications such as first-generation antihistamines and decongestants, antitussives, muscle relaxants, and some analgesics may cause sedation, inattention, or behavioural side effects. Many central nervous system conditions will influence school performance, some because of co-morbid LD or ID, others through affecting the child's mental status. For children who have had brain irradiation for malignant disorders, poor concentration and LDs may be the price of their survival. Problems with attention and executive function may follow concussion even when the child seemed "fine" after the injury. Seizure disorders, especially of absence type, are a consideration when the child presents with inattentiveness in school; also, temporal lobe epilepsy may cause memory loss. Side effects of anti-epileptic medication can affect school performance. Loss of previously attained skills suggests a progressive neurological condition, and documentation of such losses with schoolwork samples is critical. A child who truly shows deterioration of his or her mental abilities requires a full neurological workup. Regression, including worsening school performance, in a child with a known seizure disorder suggests poor seizure control.

Chronic lead poisoning and iron deficiency anaemia both affect behaviour and attention.

Other medical conditions associated with learning problems include fetal alcohol spectrum disorder, chromosomal anomalies such as fragile X including carrier status in girls, Turner, Prader-Willi, and 22q11.2 deletion syndromes, where the pattern of school difficulties may be consistent with evidence of learning problems on psychometric testing and cognitive abilities that may be found in the low-average range. Children with neurofibromatosis and Tourette's disorder often have significant learning problems.

Sensory impairment

Visual and auditory impairments will contribute to poor school performance in children without LDs, and such impairments may multiply the effects of LDs or other developmental conditions. Regular school screening may be insufficiently reliable for the child who is having classroom problems; either confirm normal function in both areas by screening in your own office or refer to other professionals as appropriate.

In the majority of cases where a child has problems reading and visual acuity is also a concern, merely prescribing adequate glasses will not solve the reading problem. Likewise, most students who have impaired listening skills have normal peripheral hearing. Audiology assessments may demonstrate specific skill deficits and result in recommendations for an FM system, preferential seating, or specific strategies for the classroom. In children with a visual impairment, a vision consultant may suggest ways to use technology or modify classroom materials. Many school systems have these resources.

Attention deficits

Problems in concentration with or without hyperactive/impulsive behaviour, weak organizational skills and work habits, messy handwriting, incomplete assignments, difficulty making and keeping friends, and poor academic attainments may reflect the specific neurodevelopmental disorders that are collectively referred to as ADHD. ADHD has its own differential diagnosis (which includes most of the conditions described in this section) and is co-morbid with many developmental conditions. Special consideration should be given to secondary causes of inattention such as sleep disorders, especially obstructive sleep apnea, which commonly presents as a mild to moderate attention deficit and can be missed if a sleep history is not obtained. Review screen usage and the possibility that sleep is being disrupted by the child's choice of watching television, playing games, or connecting with friends through social networking late into the night. Skipping meals, especially breakfast, also can have a negative effect on school performance, impeding attention. Absence-type seizures may sometimes present as inattentive spells, and a detailed description of "zoning out" will help clarify the need for further investigation or referral. As noted above, hearing should always be checked if there is any question of hearing loss; even a unilateral loss may have some effect on school performance.

Psychiatric disorders

Depression and anxiety are not uncommon in children, and both may interfere with school performance. It is often hard to determine which came first: the school difficulties or the symptoms of behavioural or emotional distress. Problems in school achievement can lead to a secondary depression, with loss of motivation and concentration. Performance anxiety can both affect test-taking and be fuelled by poor test performance. Generalized anxiety can present as an attentional difficulty, with the child worrying instead of working. Children with obsessive-compulsive disorder (OCD) may also present as inattentive when the child is mentally preoccupied with an obsessive thought; performing compulsions steals time from schoolwork and affects work completion.

Emotional and behavioural difficulties may reflect factors outside school, particularly family issues, of which the teacher may not be aware. Adjustment disorders in response to life stresses are common and identified by the temporal relationship of the symptoms (changes in mood, anxiety level, and/or conduct) and the timing of dysfunction at school with the onset of the stress.

Exploring the family history for psychiatric disorders is just as important as checking for family members with developmental and educational difficulties: the physician must evaluate the mental health of the family just as much as that of the child. Using the Parent Questionnaire in Chapter 7 can be very helpful in exploring this.

A family history of affective disorder can be a clue to look for depression in children, who do not always show vegetative symptoms such as apathy, anorexia, or insomnia, and who may instead act out, eat too much, or sleep too much. Dysphoria (or lack of pleasure in life), withdrawal from usual activities, or alienation from friends are other important clues. During the child interview, emotional flatness and lack of engagement may be noted, and it can be difficult to find any topic of conversation in which the child expresses interest. Your usual praise and positive feedback for performance may be ignored.

Family history of anxiety disorders, including panic attacks and phobias, likewise increases the level of suspicion for an anxiety disorder in the child. Children with anxiety may have somatic complaints such as abdominal pain, headaches, and sleep disturbance, and may even have findings on physical exam (e.g., tachycardia, sweaty palms, and muscle tension, especially in the neck and shoulders). Anxious children frequently need repeated reassurance during examination that medical procedures won't hurt and that physical findings are normal.

Family issues

The psychosocial history must include details of family structure, marital status and custody arrangements, approximate income, occupation, educational level and health of all family members, and significant events and stressors in the life of that family. It may help to ask a family to describe a typical day to get a good understanding of their daily routines to be able to determine what family issues could be impacting a child's school performance. The presence of these issues does not, of course, exclude the possibility of a neurologically based learning disorder, but also needs to be identified for appropriate formulation and management.

Separation and divorce

All children know about families where parents are no longer living together; this may even be their own experience. The early stages of separation and divorce create fear and uncertainty in children, including fear of the loss of a beloved parent and fear that parents who have stopped loving one another may also stop loving their child(ren). Children also have practical fears about where they will live/sleep/go to school, along with uncertainty as to when and whether they will ever see the noncustodial parent again. Because children are aware that divorce exists, marital discord, even if mild in the parents' eyes, may be very frightening to their child. It is hard for a child to do well at school when preoccupied by concerns for the permanence of home and family. Parents in marital turmoil or single parents may have too many of their own concerns to be able to help their child do homework or review for a test. They may be too stressed or depressed to respond sympathetically to their child(ren)'s difficulties.

Remarriage of a parent and the often-complex blended families that result may also produce significant stress. The child's position within a family, previously well-defined, may now be unclear and in a state of flux. Family members may have a hard time adjusting to someone who is not their "real" mother (or father, son, daughter). The new parent may have expectations and child-rearing techniques that differ considerably from the child's previous experience. Holidays may be stressful and include a group of "strangers," who constitute the extended family of the step-parent.

Family breakdown may provoke or rekindle separation anxieties, often producing typical school phobia, with the child refusing to leave home to attend classes. Usually there is tacit approval for the child's remaining at home, with some degree of secondary gain by the parent. Over-attached parents may have their own emotional agenda, which must be addressed if school attendance and performance are to improve.

Illness within the family

Chronic illness of a family member is another stressor that may cause a child to worry (e.g., whether the sick person is in danger of dying). Hospitalization of a parent means that parent is not home to help with homework, and the spouse may be overwhelmed with concerns for the partner, as well as by all the usual household chores. If the illness is in a sibling, the time and attention given by the parents may generate strong feelings of jealousy, which may become guilt if the sick child dies or suffers complications. Siblings of handicapped children may be involved in caregiving and pay for these increased responsibilities with academic underachievement. Care for any sick relative may limit the child's ability to devote time and effort to schoolwork.

Parental substance abuse

Alcoholism and street drug use by a parent may produce a chaotic and potentially an abusive home, which may deprive the child of routines such as bedtime, meals, and study time, leading to chronic fatigue and hunger and a student who is unprepared for class. Parental substance abuse all too frequently leads to unemployment, poverty, and domestic violence, which are always terrifying and interfere with the child's school performance.

Child physical or sexual abuse

Be alert to the possibility of school failure as a symptom of physical or sexual abuse. The medical history may have revealed behavioural problems, including new fears, nightmares, sexualized behaviours, and enuresis, but the child is unlikely to share his or her experiences until alone with the physician. A thorough physical examination may reveal ecchymoses or other evidence of inflicted injuries or signs of sexual abuse. Children with developmental conditions may be even more vulnerable to such occurrences, with each factor multiplying the ill effects of the other.

Poverty

Families in or approaching poverty often lack the material resources (computers, books, school supplies, transportation to libraries and museums, etc.) available to more affluent households. If family nutrition is poor, the child may go to school hungry, with consequent inattention and poor work habits. Parents who are poor are more likely to have a lower level of education, and they themselves may not have experienced parental academic and emotional support. In the absence of such modelling, they may not place much emphasis on the education of their own children. Their older children and teenagers may be required to seek after-school jobs to help support the family, cutting into time available for doing homework. Such children may even miss significant amounts of school.

Household moves

Frequent changes of school, whether resulting from family relocation for employment or from eviction and homelessness, are known to reduce school attainment. Lack of continuity prevents teachers from familiarizing themselves with a child's learning problems and interferes with remedial programs. A move of any kind, even if likely to bring long-term improvement in a family's situation, is also a major

life stressor for all members of a family and may result in adjustment problems.

Educational issues

Having explored issues of health and home, move now to investigate aspects of the educational experience that can affect a child's school performance. Schools are designed to educate children in groups; students are placed together by age to form a grade with specific expectations and curriculum. Instruction is geared toward the typically developing student and achievement norms for that age and grade. It is usually expected that children will arrive at school eager to learn and that all learning from previous grades will have been well-mastered. Children with learning problems do not fit neatly into this model. As well, despite shared approaches, policies, and curriculum, there is much variation from one classroom to another. Individual student and teacher characteristics, the student mix, the physical layout (e.g., location in a portable), and many other factors contribute to what happens in each classroom, and should be explored.

Motivation

Poor motivation for learning is frequently blamed for underachievement, but this is unwarranted. Young children have a basic drive toward mastery and achievement—poor motivation is learned. Most children in the early grades want to do well, and they will not stop trying until repeated failure eventually leaves them despairing of success. Avoidance of specific tasks is frequently an indication of particular difficulty in those areas and may be a coping mechanism, perhaps a face-saving strategy to avoid having others see their poor performance. (See also the upcoming sections about differential diagnosis of noncompliance and oppositional behaviour.)

Many younger children for whom school-related tasks are not intrinsically motivating will still work hard at academics to please important adults in their life who have indicated that they want their child to do well in school. However, if the family does not value and reward academic success, or gives little priority to academic activities at home, the child is less likely to care about school performance.

Inappropriate expectations

Sometimes parents or teachers may deny or be unaware of a child's limitations or may compare a child to high-achieving siblings or parents. Parents who themselves were excellent scholars or athletes may be overly critical of a child who is not a similarly high achiever. Some children will try to meet such expectations but continued lack of success can be emotionally exhausting and result in behavioural acting out or depressed mood.

When a child is working as well as may be expected, based on comparing cognitive level and academic performance, you can help defuse the situation by having a frank discussion with the parents, as well as modelling support and encouragement for the child. It will sometimes be necessary to remind all involved of the child's assets and to reflect that there is more to life than academic or athletic success alone.

Lack of exposure

When a child's home behavioural expectations and leisure activities differ greatly from activities expected in the classroom, he or she may struggle with school requirements and appear to have a learning problem, particularly in the early grades. For a variety of reasons, some families may not spend much time at pencil-and-paper prewriting activities, listening to stories, or sitting still for crafts or discussions prior to the child's school entry. Some families may express clear priorities in their enthusiasm for sports or fitness-related activities, and a child with such a background may be at a relative disadvantage when formal schooling is begun. Such a child should only be considered to have an actual LD if there is failure to master the relevant skills given adequate exposure and practice time.

Children for whom the language of instruction is not their primary language may experience difficulties in school. Besides the obvious challenges for the child, parents may not be able to assist with homework and reading practice. Consideration should also be given to cultural attitudes toward school.

Instructional issues

Just as students have different learning styles and aptitudes, teachers vary in their teaching methods and in their ability to convey information to particular types of students. The fit between teacher and pupil influences progress at schoolwork. Teachers who are able to recognize each student's strengths and emphasize positive attributes enhance their students' self-esteem and fuel their enthusiasm for learning. Many students can name an influential teacher who made the difference or turned around a pattern of school failure into one of success.

As in any profession, there may be some teachers who have weak skills. In such a situation, the effects are usually felt by the entire class, so that concerns of one parent may be echoed by others. Sometimes a particular student with poor achievement or behavioural problems may be criticized as lazy, unmotivated, or "bad" by school staff who have a poor understanding of the child's difficulties. If there are concerns about the child's safety, including emotional well-being, the physician must unhesitatingly act as an advocate for the child with the appropriate authorities.

In a school environment with increasing emphasis on inclusion, a regular classroom teacher may be asked to provide special needs programming to a number of different students with little specific preparation or training for the variety of special needs. When dealing with these complex issues, however, it is prudent not to be too quick to side with either the parent or the teacher; reserve judgment and explore both sides of the story. Often teachers are quite willing to discuss programming options for students, and the physician can be instrumental in getting a productive dialogue going between home and school.

It is impossible for all teachers to get along perfectly with all students. Should a severe mismatch occur, the wise teacher will recognize what is happening and try to deal productively with the situation. If this cannot be done and it is felt that a student-teacher relationship cannot be repaired, a change in teaching assignment can be a positive strategy.

THE DIFFERENTIAL DIAGNOSIS OF NONCOMPLIANCE AND OPPOSITIONAL BEHAVIOUR

Oppositional defiant disorder (ODD), as described by the DSM-IV, is "a recurrent pattern of negativistic, defiant, disobedient, and hostile behaviour toward authority figures" such as parents or teachers that persists for at least six months. At least four of eight behaviours described in the DSM criteria must be present, developmental level must be taken into account, and there must be significant impairment in social, academic, or occupational functioning to apply this diagnosis. Unfortunately, the diagnosis of ODD is often treated as an organic entity rather than a behavioural pattern. The label of ODD tells you what but not why. Oppositional behaviour has its own differential, and working through the possibilities will help with choosing an appropriate intervention.

It is useful to look at **parent (or caregiver) factors** and **child factors** in analyzing noncompliant and oppositional behaviour. Parenting is hard work; parents must understand their child's developmental profile and temperament and must present instructions to the child in a clear and consistent way. Optimally, children need more than one caregiver so that one is able to spell the other off, allowing for the rest and emotional recovery needed to maintain the firm consistent approach that benefits most children. Whether actually a single parent or acting as a single parent because the partner is working away or ill, single caregivers are at higher risk of being exhausted by caregiving duties. Shift work and military deployment may be risk factors. Any health condition that affects the caregiver's physical and/or emotional energy level may decrease the ability to engage with the child and provide positive attention, as well as to intervene firmly and consistently when children require discipline. Examples include parental depression, PTSD, sleep disorder, multiple sclerosis, and fibromyalgia.

For the child with school problems who is refusing to comply with instructions, first consider if the task that the child is being asked to perform is within his or her capabilities. Children will frequently try to avoid tasks that are known or perceived to be too difficult. You may have access to test results from the various developmental sectors to try to sort this out. Children who have experienced repeated failure may have learned to expect continued failure and try to avoid things they have not been able to do. Children who are anxious or perfectionistic, or who have negative mood (dysthymia, depression), are more likely to express feelings that a task is too hard even before attempting it.

Problems of attention and executive function will affect compliance. The child needs to recognize that an instruction has been given to comply with it; children with ADHD may not even have registered that the teacher has spoken. Do not immediately label noncompliance as oppositional; ensure that the child has at least attended to the instruction and had an opportunity to comply before suspecting ODD. Deficits in any of the executive function skills of shifting cognitive set (moving one's attention from one mindset to another), organization and planning, and separating one's emotional response to a problem—from the thinking response to the problem itself—can lead to noncompliance and/or meltdowns.(1) So can problems with emotional regulation, as seen in children with anxiety, dysthymia, or ASD, for example (see Chapter 14 for behavioural management). Impaired language processing can make it difficult for children to understand what they are being asked to do. Children who are rigid thinkers, which can be associated with anxiety, nonverbal learning disabilities, obsessive compulsive disorder, and ASD, have trouble with the changing expectations of school and social situations.

A systematic approach to a child's learning problems will usually uncover the reasons for the noncompliant behaviour. The ODD diagnosis may be used when the behaviours are severe and have persisted despite addressing identified contributors as above. Parent training, and/or help from a mental health therapist or psychologist may be needed to provide intervention of sufficient frequency and intensity for the child and family.

THE DIFFERENTIAL DIAGNOSIS OF MOTOR INCOORDINATION

The child who is awkward or clumsy, who has difficulty mastering new motor tasks, and seems delayed compared to age peers may have a neurological or neuromuscular disorder, or there may be performance factors impairing the child's ability to demonstrate age-appropriate skills. As learning motor skills involves procedural memory, opportunity for practice is important.

Developmental coordination disorder (DCD) is a motor skills disorder that affects 5% to 6% of school-aged children and results in a child being unable to perform common everyday motor tasks.(2) Children with DCD usually have intellectual abilities in the average or above average range; in the presence of an intellectual disability, the impairment may be significantly greater than one would expect from the ID alone. Children with DCD do not have an identifiable medical condition to explain their motor difficulties, so DCD becomes a diagnosis of exclusion, and its differential is the differential of motor incoordination.

Baxter describes *apraxia* as "the inability to coordinate complex activities even though the individual components can be carried out, while *dyspraxia* indicates a milder form." He goes on to say, "This concept not only applies to motor function in the limbs, but also to eye movements, facial movements, and oro-buccal functions such as eating and articulation."(3) Dyspraxia is a hallmark of DCD, which might be considered the equivalent of a learning disability in the motor system. ADHD, LDs, and speech-language disorders frequently co-occur.

Medical conditions that must be ruled out include cerebral palsy, childhood stroke, and the sequelae of acquired traumatic brain injury, especially children who are less severely affected or who have hemiparesis. Chronic neurologic conditions such as Tourette's disorder, muscular dystrophies, intracranial lesions (especially of the cerebellum), and collagen vascular disorders may present initially with dyspraxia. Rarely degenerative disorders of the nervous system, such as subacute sclerosing panencephalitis (SSPE), can present as a coordination difficulty. Medication effects may cause motor clumsiness. Adventitious movements such as tremor and chorea can affect quality of motor skills.

Performance factors affect whether a child is able to use the skills he or she has in a given situation. Any illness may affect effort, which in turn affects the quality of the motor output, important

when the skills being tested involve speed and accuracy. ADHD and anxiety are common performance factors. In ADHD, the child's impulsivity and inattention to proprioceptive feedback may result in written work that is rushed and sloppy, with variable letter formation and spacing. Children with anxiety may not attempt tasks or may be so preoccupied with getting writing or drawing exactly right that they exceed time scores on test items. With both diagnoses, children may not practise—with ADHD because repetitive tasks are "boring" and not intrinsically motivating, and with anxiety because the child fears making mistakes or is unhappy with the quality of his or her own work. Anxious children also may fear motor tasks where balance or speed is a factor; they are afraid to take the training wheels off the bike or to mount a ladder for the slide at the playground.

In asking about motor milestone attainment, it is important to ensure the child has had sufficient opportunity to master a task. Failing to learn to tie shoes by age eight is not a delay if the child has only had Velcro fastenings. Provide a chance for the child to try the task before ascribing a delay.

THE DIFFERENTIAL DIAGNOSIS OF SOCIAL INTERACTION PROBLEMS

Social skills are important in overall development. Good social skills in childhood predict peer approval, school adjustment, coping strategies, attention, mental health later in life, school placement and job opportunities, and overall quality of life. Social skills have recently garnered much attention. Autism spectrum disorders (ASDs) are in the public eye and are at the forefront of everybody's mind. Now many children who have some social awkwardness or poor social skills are referred for a query of ASD. Many of the developmental disorders that are seen with children having difficulty in school have some impairment of socialization. In ASDs there is an underlying inherent disorder of socialization manifested by impairments associated with the "autism triad" of language/communication, reciprocal social interaction, and repetitive and restricted behaviours and interests.

To understand the underlying reason why the child is struggling socially, friendships should be explored. The pattern of friendships, rather than the number, is most important. Children with ADHD are frequently found to exhibit social difficulties in a degree comparable to ASD.(4)(5)(6) Such children are often disliked and rejected by their peers immediately. They may have little further opportunity to practise adequate social skills, which may then interfere with the development of *theory of mind* (see the Glossary) skills.

The differential diagnosis of the socially impaired child is vast; not all children who have social difficulties have autism. Children with ASD often are distinguished by their long history of impaired reciprocal social interaction and language delays; their "repetitive and restricted behaviours and interests" will often seem unusual compared to age peers. Eye contact may be poor, or they may have overlearned the need to make eye contact and stare, instead of having the natural gaze shift back and forth that usually occurs in a conversation. Verbal "high functioning" children with ASD may engage in one-sided conversations that never really explore the opinions and feelings of the listener and intrude to talk about their topics.

Children with ADHD have many of the same impairments. Their short attention span often interferes with the ability to stay on task and interact with a peer. They may not notice social cues. They are often gregarious and better at making friends than keeping them. Impulsivity can also lead to bad decisions and being unable to wait their turn, which can often be interpreted as rude. They intrude into others' personal space. On exam, eye gaze may be impaired because they are looking all over the place and not just at you. Conversation may be reciprocal, but language can be very tangential and rambling without much regard for whether you are following their gist.

Anxiety can result in children being socially awkward and not having friends. This may be due to generalized anxiety, or specific social phobia. Children with anxiety may want to have friends but are unable to overcome their anxiety to reach out to their peer group. They may hover on the edges of group activities watching what is going on but not joining in. Eye contact may be poor when confronted, but often they will watch faces when they think no one is looking back.

Mood disorders can also interfere with relationships. Depression is uncommon in very young children and usually represents a change in affect and social engagement from previous adjustment levels. A history of the child's past friendships and relationships is important here. Depressed children will present with a flat affect and are often hard to engage in conversation during examination. They find it difficult to describe interests or enjoyable experiences.

Children with Tourette's disorder can have a number of associated social effects, from co-morbid ADHD, OCD, and anxiety to the actual tics themselves, which may be perceived very negatively by peers. The impairment of socialization is important when considering treatment options for children with Tourette's.

Specific speech and language impairments can also have an important role in social relationships, especially when there is pragmatic language impairment. Intelligibility of speech is very important; other children may be impatient and may not spend the time to try to interpret what a child with significant speech impediment is trying to say, leading to social isolation. The affected child's messages are often misinterpreted, which may lead to frustration and even aggression. The speech impairment may lead to false assumptions about low cognitive ability. The child may eventually stop trying to engage others and give up on friendships.

Extremes of cognitive ability affect socialization affect social skills. Intellectual impairments are associated with social difficulties, as social skills mirror development of cognition. Children with ID may not have the same interests as age-matched peers and gravitate to younger children. They may prefer to stick to familiar activities, leading parents and teachers to describe them as having restricted interests and to refer for an autism workup. For children with high cognitive ability, finding common interests with their peer group may also be difficult. Remember that children who are performing two to three standard deviations above the norm may look as different from "typical" age peers, as do those who are two to three standard deviations below, particularly in the elementary school age group. Gifted children love learning and investigate many topics that might seem odd to others, leading to concerns about ASD. Generally topics will vary over time; when one area is mastered, the gifted child will move on, while a child with autism often continues to have the same interests even though they are not socially or academically useful. When a child's intellectual abilities fall outside the normal range, it is extremely important to consider how the child functions when with developmental peers (i.e., children at the same intellectual level). For gifted children, look also at their ability to show empathy, to take another's point of view, and to hold a back-and-forth conversation. As ASD can occur in both children with ID and gifted children, an extended interdisciplinary assessment may be needed to sort this out.

Consider as well cultural issues in the family, language used at home, the child's exposure to peers outside the home and opportunities for socialization, and any victimization or bullying that may have led the child to prefer not interacting with peers.

When evaluating social skills, the first step is to characterize the level of social impairment and explore any relationships that the child has made. Try to understand the nature of those relationships from the child's point of view. Collect history from both the home and school. This will be critical for exploring the role of social anxiety and will give you an understanding as to how the child is perceived in the classroom and what types of peer relations are exhibited. Look for specific symptoms of the above conditions, such as the restricted interests/behaviours with ASD, poor attention and impulsivity with ADHD, tics with Tourette's, and so forth. Many of these disorders are co-morbid, and it is important to identify the components to help address what is impeding the child's social progress.

SUMMARY

- Most of the common presentations for children who are not doing well in school are non-specific.
- They have a broad differential diagnosis and the potential for co-morbidity.
- They require a thorough workup, which will narrow the differential and guide further assessment and intervention.
- Many children will have a number of problem areas that require assessment and formulation regarding how the components interact.

REFERENCES

1. Greene R. The Explosive Child: A New Approach for Understanding and Parenting Easily Frustrated, Chronically Inflexible Children. New York: Harper, 2005.
2. CanChild Centre for Childhood Disability Research. Overview of DCD. <http://dcd.canchild.ca/en/About DCD/overview.asp>
3. Baxter P. Developmental coordination disorder and motor dyspraxia. Dev Med Child Neurol 2012; 54(1): 3.
4. Clark T, et al. Autistic symptoms in children with attention deficit-hyperactivity disorder. Eur Child Adolesc Psychiatry 1999; 8(1): 50–55.
5. Greene RW, et al. Toward a new psychometric definition of social disability in children with attention-deficit hyperactivity disorder. J Am Acad Child Adolesc Psychiatry 1996; 35(5): 571–78.
6. Buhler E, et al. Differential diagnosis of autism spectrum disorders and attention deficit hyperactivity disorder by means of inhibitory control and "theory of mind." J Autism Dev Disord 2011; 41: 1718–26.

12

Part III: Management

Sharing the Formulation: Feedback to Parents and School

Ana Hanlon-Dearman and Wendy Roberts

This chapter discusses an approach to formulating a description of a child's developmental strengths, challenges, and needs into a diagnostic description that can be shared with parents and schools. Practical suggestions for communicating this information in both contexts are offered, along with a sample formulation.

FORMULATION

With increasing research into the genetics and neuroimaging of learning and brain development, the physician's ability to define the medical etiology of learning difficulties has improved. However, in many cases it is still difficult to identify a specific diagnosis of a child's learning difficulty. In most cases, you will arrive at a formulation of a child's learning strengths and difficulties reflecting etiologic and environmental contributors, rather than a specific diagnosis. It is important to communicate this formulation clearly, emphasizing the importance of functional abilities, particularly when a specific diagnosis or cause of the child's learning problems is not known. For the parent, the etiologic evaluation process can offer the opportunity to understand both the learning problem and its prognosis. It should also be explained that the functional description of a child's learning needs, including their learning strengths, is often the best way to support case management; an etiologic description may be helpful in aiding understanding and prognosis, but generally does not change management. If the parents come to the physician's office with a specific question (e.g., "Is it the teacher's or my fault?" "Does he have dyslexia?" or "Is she autistic?"), this should be answered as clearly as possible through the sharing of the formulation.

Diagnoses in the area of development and behaviour are often less discrete than in other areas of medicine. This ambiguity makes some clinicians uncomfortable; however, the more such feelings are understood, and the more standard patterns of data collection and assessment become predictable and familiar, the more expertise will develop in formulating profiles that lead to useful management plans.

At times, physicians come under pressure from parents or teachers to make certain diagnoses, particularly if medication is desired or a placement is difficult to access. For example, a diagnosis of attention deficit hyperactivity disorder (ADHD) is often felt automatically to justify the use of stimulant medication, and many referrals are made to obtain this specific diagnosis. This type of hidden agenda should be discussed openly with parents, as needed.

Many children with school problems will not be given a definitive diagnosis by the physician. Their various symptoms may cluster into familiar clinical patterns, but because the observations are not standardized, the physician alone cannot make a diagnosis of specific learning disability (LD) with a single visit. Some groupings of symptoms may meet DSM criteria for diagnosis of psychiatric disorders, which can then be made by physicians with appropriate training and experience. Multi-axial taxonomies can be used or more informal assessment can define significant behavioural and developmental co-morbidities, psychosocial factors, and physical problems that need to be identified and shared with parents, to develop an appropriate management plan.

In some situations it is wise to follow the child over a number of months or years, describing the profile of strengths and weaknesses, delaying or avoiding definitive diagnostic labels. It is generally preferable to describe the profile of strengths and weaknesses to be found in any child with developmental or behavioural problems, the likely influence of life events, or other exacerbating or ameliorating factors, and the assets and liabilities identified in the family, school, and community, rather than to attempt a definitive diagnosis suggesting a certainty that exceeds the reliability of the database.

If the physician's opinion on the presence or absence of a specific diagnostic entity is required for the child to be placed in a specific program or for medical treatment to begin, a formal diagnostic statement should be recorded.

The preferred type of diagnostic formulation, occupying one or two paragraphs in a written report, not only summarizes the information from questionnaires (see Chapter 7), parents' history, and the examination of the child, but takes it to a higher level of insight through integration of the information and the application of the clinician's awareness of clinical groupings of symptoms and possible disorders.

FEEDBACK TO PARENTS

After a comprehensive evaluation has been completed, it is necessary to provide feedback to the parents. There may be occasions when bad or difficult news is best given to the parents alone first; however, whenever possible and developmentally appropriate, the child should be present. Most children seem satisfied with, "We've had our time together alone, now it is your parents' turn to talk with me."

The parents should be encouraged to take notes while you talk with them, and they should be encouraged to record any questions they may wish to ask at that time or at a later date. Some physicians may be helped in the organization of their written reports by making their own notes during the feedback phase of the interview.

Ideally the parent should receive a copy of the physician's report, written in plain language or with specialized terminology explained, which can be shared with the school in whole or part at the parent's discretion.

The integrated formulation leads naturally to comprehensive recommendations and program planning. It is particularly important that, if the news to be shared at the interview does not include a specific diagnosis, action plans are suggested at the same time and your commitment to continuing to support the child and family made explicit. Parents must be encouraged to comment on the formulation presented to them, their perceptions of what it will mean to the child and to the school, and whether they feel it is accurate and helpful. If further investigations or tests are required, or further consultations recommended, these should be carefully explained. Plans for follow-up should be agreed upon.

After reading the physician's formulation, parents and members of the community team can share their own appraisals of the child, discuss their perspectives, and coordinate and integrate their contributions to the management plan. This is also a starting point for conversation with the physician so that further information can be shared, a different perspective offered, misperceptions corrected, or follow-up plans made.

FEEDBACK TO THE SCHOOL

The school principal, resource teacher, or special needs educator generally acts as the case manager. Contacting the principal is often the most efficient way to access the system, both for parents and for the physician. Know the philosophy of the local school system and be familiar with the facilities that are available (see also Chapters 2 and 5). Your goal is to be able to suggest practical options and to avoid impractical recommendations that can never be implemented—such recommendations not only raise false hopes for the family but they lead to difficulties in your relationship with the school. You should keep up-to-date with the terminology and the current issues in the local educational system.

Communication with the school may take a number of forms. For example, you may ask for the school's assistance in the following ways:

- Can we discuss this student further? How do you see this student's difficulties?
- Can we discuss available solutions and what is possible within your system?

Try not to give your opinion until asked to do so, and be frank about the limits of your expertise. It is suggested that both parents attend school conferences whenever possible. Remember that the student, by about age ten, also has some rights and responsibilities and may want or need to be included in all or some of the conferencing process.

Participation reinforces the degree of each parent's involvement and concern. It allows parents to hear the information and then recall it more accurately. It also permits all who are involved to problem-solve together more effectively. Since parents may be intimidated by teachers and may be outnumbered by them at some formal conferences, the presence of both parents can provide mutual support.

Parents should be encouraged to bring a support person to meetings if they feel this will improve their ability to participate. Many boards of education and LD associations provide helpful pamphlets that explain conference procedures. Some provincial resources are listed in Chapter 5; encourage parents to explore and take advantage of such resources.

Make sure that written communications with the school respect the confidentiality of the student and family, and that such communications are written in plain language. When it is necessary to use medical terminology, it should be explained simply. The source of information needs to be clear. If subjective information related by a parent is included, it should be clear that you are reporting what the parent has said (e.g., state, "Mrs. White reported that . . ." to clearly label the source of the opinion), and that you are aware of alternative interpretations.

The most important parts of the physician's report are the formulation and the comments or suggestions derived from it, which should be clearly expressed and realistic. Avoid an authoritarian, dictatorial, or adversarial stance. Objective advocacy and teamwork are the goals to be achieved. However, in strictly medical issues, an assertive statement is appropriate (e.g., the need for ensuring the child takes medication as prescribed, with appropriate rationale).

Make sure the teacher knows what type of feedback you would like to receive about changes in symptoms or the benefits or side effects of medications. Behavioural rating scales may facilitate this process, but be careful not to overload the teacher—who is also busy—by selecting locally available and standardized forms that are quick and easy to fill out so that the teacher does not have to spend time learning how to score a new instrument. Classroom teachers and special educators appreciate telephone contacts with their students' physicians (see the two opening questions proposed earlier).

Some teachers may wish to use e-mail for correspondence—be very careful about confidentiality and security issues before agreeing to this route. You should consider including parents on all correspondence about their child in order to ensure openness of communication and avoid misunderstanding. Check both school and clinic/hospital policy and get appropriate consent forms before proceeding. Encryption of messages should be considered to protect confidentiality.

Accepting invitations to participate in case conferences at schools is an excellent way of increasing familiarity with the system and strengthening the physician's standing within it. In some cases, physicians can participate in such meetings via secure web conferencing or telehealth technology, making attendance more feasible.

SAMPLE FORMULATION

The following is a model for a summary by a physician:

Daniel was seen for an assessment of his difficulty in school. Like other members of his family, he was diagnosed as having a developmental language disorder before he started school, and difficulties in all areas of written language were noted from the start. His hearing is normal, but he seems to have weak phonemic analysis skills and his reading is similar to that of a child in Grade 2. His arithmetic skills appear to be good. There is no history of acting-out behaviour at school or at home.

Due to a series of moves from one province to another, Daniel has never experienced prolonged or intensive remedial education, and he has become despondent about his chances of ever becoming a functional reader. He is beginning to think of himself as "stupid," and this makes him very sad, as does his difficulty making friends, which has also been exacerbated by frequent home changes. He has learned to cover up his poor reading, and he is ashamed to let peers or teachers know how far behind he really is.

Daniel's assets include a quiet but friendly personality, good oral communication skills, his interests in fishing and carpentry, and a supportive family. His father, a cabinet-maker who had somewhat similar difficulties in school, is determined to help Daniel do better. Both parents will participate in anything the teacher suggests may be useful. Another asset is that the family will not be moving for at least the next three years.

Daniel does not meet current criteria for attention deficit hyperactivity disorder (ADHD), and there is no indication for stimulant medication. His classroom behaviour and failure to complete assignments are not related in any way to allergies.

No further medical tests or consultations are indicated at this time.

In summary, the family history and Daniel's profile of strengths and weaknesses suggest a specific reading disorder, perhaps exacerbated by many changes of school. Now that Daniel will be in one place for the next three years, he should receive as much individual and small group help with all aspects of written language as possible, subject to identification as a student with special needs. Toward this end, a psycho-educational examination may well be helpful.

SUMMARY

Points to remember for providing feedback to parents and schools:

- Formulate a profile of the child's strengths and weaknesses along with etiologic diagnoses (if present) and comprehensive recommendations.
- Discuss your formulation and recommendations with parents and include the child when developmentally appropriate.
- Provide a copy of your report to parents respecting confidentiality and written in plain language.
- Engage with the school and family to provide realistic suggestions for program planning.
- Remember that objective advocacy and teamwork are goals of feedback.

13

Educational Interventions

Ruth Neufeld and Debra Andrews

Management of learning problems is primarily the responsibility and the mandate of schools, but physicians always have a role in the diagnostic workup—if only to do the basic history and physical examination to rule out possible medical factors. Families often want advice about what more they can do to supplement what the school is doing, and may bring their questions to your office. How much you will be involved in prescribing specific treatment will depend on your interest, experience, and the availability of multidisciplinary assessments either in your community or at a tertiary centre. Find out about billing practices from colleagues who are doing this work, so that you can be compensated as well as possible.

Many physicians say they feel uncomfortable making recommendations for children with learning problems because they perceive their training to be inadequate. In some cases, it may not "feel like medicine" to them. Although prescribing medication is a more familiar role, many doctors shy away from prescribing medications that alter behaviour. This is unfortunate because, like physical examination and diagnosis, this function is also the physician's responsibility.

An overview of educational, behavioural, and medical interventions for those with learning problems is provided in the next three chapters, emphasizing the physician's role. In this chapter we present an overview of educational placement and specific remediation strategies. Understanding these interventions will help you to explain educational recommendations to children and their families.

DEMYSTIFICATION

Simplifying the diagnosis and sharing it with all those involved, using appropriate language and concepts, is the first step in management. No effort should be spared to remove the mystery, fear, and confusion usually attached to anything concerning "brain function."

For the child, there should be emphasis on strengths and abilities as well as a discussion of the child's weaknesses and what can be done to help. Although some people feel that using a label such as "learning disability" can be problematic, many children have already labelled themselves with much more unflattering terms, and they are relieved to know that their brain is not damaged and that they are not stupid, lazy, worthless, or bad. A complex notion such as LD may need to be explained using a concrete example:

> "Everybody knows some people who are smart but at the same time are not very good at gym or cannot sing in tune in music class. A learning disability is when a person has more of some kinds of smartness or skills than other kinds. She may be smart enough overall, but when asked to do a job that depends on a weaker skill, it may seem to her that she is not smart at all."

It may be worthwhile to ask the child's thoughts on what was causing the trouble in school and what others have told the child. Having a better idea of what is causing their learning difficulties in school often brings children a sense of relief—it is not as bad as they thought. With that sense of relief, some improvement in self-esteem and renewal of hope for the future may occur. One should not, however, generate false hopes of a complete and immediate "cure." Children with any kind of learning difficulty often require lengthy and intensive remediation, and they need to be warned of this.

Parents may also have fears relating to the diagnosis, and especially to the cause of the learning difficulties. They may bring these fears to the conference with the physician overtly or sometimes as an undeclared agenda. They may feel guilty in regard to perceived faulty child-rearing techniques or that injury possibly occurred during pregnancy. It is best to identify and discuss such concerns openly.

Review all potential etiological factors and help the parents to put them into perspective. Genetic factors are frequently important and should be presented in a sensitive way, as they may elicit feelings of guilt, frustration, or embarrassment. Presenting the positive traits a child may have inherited, as well as the weaknesses, may help parents to accept this information more easily.

Although genetic factors may determine a range of potential ability, the environment and the child's experiences will determine the child's position within that range. Parents who are frustrated with their child's poor progress may come to the conference with feelings of anger and blame toward the school and other professionals. Be careful to remain neutral while the parents vent their feelings, and remember your role as the advocate for the child. In most cases, actions taken by school officials were entirely appropriate for what was known at that time.

The feedback conference may be the first time the parents have been provided with a complete picture of their child's difficulties, and this can be quite overwhelming. Allowing parents adequate time for questions and clarification is important. Some of the findings may need to be reviewed at a follow-up visit. Parents often report improvement in their child at follow-up, which they may attribute to their own improved understanding of the child's condition.

Professionals dealing with the child may have their own hypotheses and treatment biases. Teachers especially may feel some degree of guilt and/or frustration that they were not able to identify the problem sooner or overcome the problem through their own efforts. They may feel that the parents blame them for the child's difficulties and that their teaching abilities have been challenged. They may have concerns that the child's difficulties stem from something going on in the home, or they may attribute problems to allergies, diet, or poor vision. Some teachers may be reluctant to accept formulation about their student from a physician. It is helpful to get such issues into the open for frank discussion. Furthermore, simply sharing assessment findings with the teachers may be a significant intervention in itself.

CLASSROOM PLACEMENT

In most cases, a physician evaluating a patient without the input of a psychologist or educational specialist would do best to stay away from recommending specific educational settings—unless you are very experienced in the field and familiar with local resources. This does not mean that you must leave all recommendations to teachers and psychologists. There are some general principles that apply to most students with learning problems:

- **Small group or one-on-one instruction benefits most students.** A smaller class or group size means fewer distractions. The student's attention and rate of progress can be monitored more easily, and the program plan can be individualized. If you have tested the child yourself, you can describe the child's response to the one-on-one situation and extrapolate this to the classroom. Both one-on-one and small group assistance can be delivered in a variety of ways depending on the needs and preferences of both the child and teacher. For example, some children who need to feel a part of the group may prefer to receive their assistance in a less conspicuous manner.
- **What has worked or failed before will probably do the same again.** Recommendations quickly

lose their credibility if they have been tried already and found to be unhelpful. This generalization, however, does not have to mean that a particular setting will never be helpful. The analysis of what went wrong may provide the clues to making the same sort of setting work more successfully the next time. The same approach applies to specific program recommendations.

- **It is best to describe the ideal setting rather than a specific teacher, classroom, or school.** A type of placement may be suggested, but this can never be a medical decision. An adversarial stance will not be persuasive and may put school staff on the defensive. Physician recommendations for resources that are unavailable are rarely well received. A clearly presented case, grounded in well-substantiated facts, is more likely to influence the school's decision.

OUT-OF-SCHOOL INSTRUCTION

Parents are often told that they should work with their child at home. This may be beneficial in giving the child extra practice with skills learned at school and demonstrating to the child that the parent thinks schoolwork is an important and valued activity. However, some parents make poor tutors because they find it hard to remain emotionally detached from their children, and their feelings of anger, frustration, and/or disappointment interfere with the remedial activity. You may wish to suggest ways to modify the parent's approach, such as using paired-reading techniques (see below for a description of paired-reading) to minimize correction and to give the child more of a sense of control. However, it is better for schoolwork to be left to the school if it seems that trying to work together at home is causing significant friction in the parent-child relationship. Sometimes giving the family "permission" *not* to do homework can help relieve this stress, but if you are considering this, it may be wise to discuss the rationale for your suggestion with the school staff. Homework should be limited to ten minutes per grade, as there is information that little learning occurs past this time.(1) This includes "makeup work" as well as extra practice.

In addition, some parents mistakenly think that if a little bit of homework and studying is good, then more must be even better, to the point of excluding any activities not related to school. The child then has no time for fun. Students whose out-of-school time is crammed with phonics worksheets, mathematics drills, and prolonged sessions of reading practice may come to resent having to do so much schoolwork and lose interest in academics altogether. Discuss the idea of work-life balance with the parents—children need this, too!

Parents may ask your opinion about hiring a tutor to work with their child after school or over the summer holidays. Because one-on-one instruction is ideal and allows a program to be developed specifically for the child, this may be supported if it is within the family's means. However, simply spending more time teaching in the same way rarely improves performance and often results in boredom. A good tutor will put together an individualized program and will collaborate closely with the classroom teacher. Parents should be gently discouraged from hiring a tutor who is not prepared to accept direction from a special education teacher.

Parents may ask you about commercial tutoring franchises. These programs often promise rapid gains but vary in quality. Encourage parents to talk to other parents who are familiar with the local options. Successful commercial reading programs are usually based on two components: an intensive one-on-one approach, most often involving phonics, and strong incentives, usually highly attractive material rewards that excite many students who have given up and have "turned off" school.

Many parents are interested in helping their child by purchasing educational technologies such as interactive learning gaming systems or an application (app) for a tablet or smartphone. These products and devices can range in price from free to many hundreds of dollars. More importantly, they can also vary in quality from poor to excellent. As consumers of these products, parents need to understand the root of the child's learning concerns so that they can evaluate whether or not the technology will help meet their child's specific need. Associated professionals such as speech-language pathologists, occupational therapists, and psychologists, as well as special education teachers, may have developed expertise in various technologies, making them key resources for parents thinking of purchasing a technological support for their child. There are a number of parent-generated websites that also evaluate applications, such as www.bestkidsapps.com and www. apps4kids.net, but again, it is only when the parent truly understands the child's individual needs that they will be able to navigate these sites like an expert.

SPECIFIC REMEDIATION

Educational remediation is the province of the educators, but physicians who are familiar with the options will be more able to help the child and parents and be in a better position to communicate with the school. Associated disciplines such as speech pathology, occupational therapy, and psychology, along with special education teachers, provide invaluable support and expertise. Many such professionals will happily share their practical "pearls" of information with you. Recognizing what these disciplines have to offer and suggesting their involvement may be one of the most important recommendations you can make.

Children with exceptional educational needs should have their programs described in writing. In many school boards, the preparation of a document, variably called an individual program plan (IPP), individual education plan (IEP), or personal program plan (PPP) depending on your province, is required for any student who qualifies for special education supports (see Chapter 5). Putting together a good program plan is time consuming, but the process often forces clarification of many issues and serves as a reference document for the professionals involved, as well as the parents. A well-written program plan should completely list the child's strengths and weaknesses, with supporting documentation, including psychometrics, achievement test scores, and medical reports.

Each problem area should be listed, with specific remedial objectives and implementation strategies, including techniques and curriculum. One helpful contribution you can make is to check the medical section for completeness and accuracy in listing medical diagnoses.

Arrangements for evaluation and review should be stated. All involved should sign their agreement if this is part of the process, and parents should understand the legal status of the plan. At the conference, parents should not feel shy about asking for clarification of anything they do not understand or about questioning if other options are available for their child.

Problems with spoken language

Children with oral language problems make up a large proportion of students experiencing difficulties learning to read. They may have generalized difficulties with receptive and expressive language development or very specific problems with, for example, word-finding or auditory discrimination. Many children with language delays have a specific deficit in phonemic awareness; that is, they are unable to analyze the component sounds within words. This may also occur as an isolated finding, with other language skills intact. (See the section about deficits in phonemic analysis skills and phonics, below.)

Children with receptive language difficulties (including secondary-to-poor listening skills or attention difficulties) should have instructions and other information repeated, paraphrased, or simplified if they do not understand the first time. They should not be constantly reprimanded for not listening. When possible, gestures, demonstrations, visual schedules, or other visual cues should be used to enhance understanding of orally presented information and verbal instructions.

Such children may have problems with the language of literacy, with its grammatical complexity and rich vocabulary, or their difficulties may be with analytical skills such as inferring and predicting. They cannot easily take advantage of many contextual clues available to other students when they tackle a reading passage; therefore, they may need to have such skills specifically taught. For a student with language delay to notice the pattern or structure of a passage may require that the teacher spend much longer on this aspect of reading and review it many times, spending significantly longer on any one story or unit than might be spent with the rest of the class. The use of repetitive stories and predictable books may be helpful.

Children with word-finding problems may not be able to call up the particular word that fits in a passage, even when they have a good sense of the story and may be able to visualize what is going on. In some cases, teaching multiple bypass strategies may be more useful than attempting direct remediation.

Children with severe language problems probably should not be placed in second-language immersion programs, especially if the new language is not one spoken by the parents. These children have difficulty enough dealing with the demands of language in their native tongue, and there will be little opportunity at home to use and practice second-language skills. On the other hand, bilingual education programs supporting the child's first language, the one that is spoken at home, may support overall language development and connect the child with the family's cultural heritage. Discussing this openly with parents leads to the best plan.

If language problems are suspected, input from a speech-language pathologist in the diagnosis and in formulating suggestions for the student's program plan is critical. For children enrolled in second-language immersion programs, it may be important to test the child in both languages being considered when making such decisions.

Deficits in phonemic analysis skills and phonics

To understand remediation for reading disabilities, one may simplify the process of reading into three main component skills: word identification skills, including phonemic analysis and visual memory; fluency; and comprehension. (See also Chapter 4 for a discussion of reading readiness and Chapter 19 for indications of the physician's role and parental actions to encourage children to read.)

Phonemic analysis includes the ability to recognize "like" and "different" sounds (e.g., rhymes), as well as to identify and separate the component sounds (or *phonemes*) and to note their position within a word. It also includes the skills of synthesizing or blending the component sounds into a word (important for reading) and of breaking or segmenting words into their individual sounds (used for spelling). *Phonics* is a method for teaching reading that emphasizes

sound-symbol relationships and labelling a phoneme (sound) with a letter or combination of letters (symbol). For example, "buh" is the sound made by the letter "b." *Phonetic decoding* ("sounding out") also requires the ability to blend the sounds to form a word. An increasing body of research identifies the child's skill in phonemic analysis at kindergarten as the best single predictor of decoding skills in the mid-elementary years.[2]

Children who are unable to decode phonetically may cope early on if they have excellent visual memory skills. However, this deficit usually catches up with them in the later grades, when sophisticated vocabulary words (most of which follow phonetic rules) increasingly are found in school assignments, especially in subjects such as science and social studies. Students who lack phonemic analysis skills may resort to guessing based on word contour, initial letter, or context of passage. Such strategies are rarely sufficient.

Tests of phonemic awareness, such as the Lindamood Auditory Conceptualization (LAC-3) Test[3] and the Test of Phonological Awareness Second Edition: PLUS (TOPA-2+)[4], help to identify children who lack these skills. Such deficits are the most common causes of specific reading disability, either as an isolated deficit or as part of a generalized language delay or disorder. Another group of poor readers demonstrates the ability to perform the tasks on these tests, but these readers do not use phonetic decoding in their reading. These students are likely not to have received instruction in this area, or they may even have been actively discouraged from using a phonetic approach. Both of these groups of children benefit from intensive specific remediation in phonemic analysis, starting with learning the letter sounds and identifying their positions in words, and progressing through blending and segmentation. The Lindamood Phoneme Sequencing Program for Reading, Spelling and Speech—Fourth Edition (LiPS-4) (www.lindamood-bell.com) is a curriculum designed for use by special education teachers.[5] This program is used for remediation in phonemic analysis skills, starting at a very basic pre-reading level and using visual aids and articulatory feedback cues. Early intervention is key. Evidence shows that the largest gains in reading occur when phonemic awareness skills and phonics are taught in kindergarten and Grade 1.(6) This is the rationale behind the Response to Intervention initiative in the United States.

Phonics is a useful strategy for decoding words encountered in a sample of text, but it can be painstakingly slow, resulting in loss of continuity. Extraction of meaning from the passage is lost because the child cannot remember the beginning of the sentence. It then follows that the rate at which one can analyze sounds is also critical. Some exciting LD research points to a deficit in the ability to segment sounds in speech presented at a normal rate. When speech was artificially slowed down using a computer, children who had been unable to learn to analyze the sounds were then able to do so. Commercial software based on this experimental technique is available for use in classrooms.(7)

At first, word decoding and passage comprehension are separate processes, but soon readers combine phonemic knowledge with their understanding of language, as well as their general fund of knowledge and use of context to correct their initial phonetic approximation of a word. This "sense-making" feedback loop becomes increasingly operative in mature readers.

Deficits in visual memory and sight-word vocabulary

Because letter-by-letter decoding is slow, most children move quickly to decoding chunks of sound (blends, digraphs, and syllables). Eventually whole words are committed to visual memory. Building up a sight-word vocabulary allows increasing speed and automaticity in reading a passage. However, a sight-word approach alone is rarely successful in teaching a child to read. There are too many sight words that are not sufficiently distinctive to the eye, and a great many differ by the addition or omission of a single letter or inversion of a pair of letters.

Readers with poor visual memory but good phonic skills may benefit from a "word family" approach by which they add sight words to their vocabulary in groups of related words (such as *bake, make, rake*) rather than individually. They must be taught the rules for regularly irregular words that cannot be

sounded out. Children who make frequent reversals in reading and spelling can be taught mnemonics for "b" and "d." Paper with a left and top margin helps with the student's orientation and reinforces the left-to-right, top-to-bottom progression of English print. The automatic movement of the cursor on the word processor also helps in this regard.

Deficits in reading fluency

The automatic word recognition needed for fluent reading comes from reading practice. Evidence supports the use of *guided or repeated oral reading* techniques to improve students' fluency and reading achievement.(8) Many of these techniques use repeated readings of the same passage for a certain number of times or until a predetermined level of proficiency is attained. Because most of these programs use peers, tutors, or one-to-one instruction, a student receives an increased amount of oral reading practice compared to round-robin oral reading (where students take turns reading paragraphs from a passage). Another guided reading technique is *paired reading*, which provides social support in the form of a parent or peer tutor whose job it is to give encouragement and assistance with decoding without trying to instruct the child, thus avoiding nagging and arguments. The learner first selects a passage, and then the skilled reader and the learner read the passage aloud in unison. When the learner gives a prearranged signal, the skilled reader stops reading aloud, while the learner continues to read aloud independently. When the learner makes an error, the skilled reader models the word correctly and resumes reading in unison. A commitment to using the technique regularly (for ten to fifteen minutes per day, five days per week, for a minimum of six to eight weeks) is most likely to bring about results.(9)(10)

Good readers use every opportunity to practice, not only reading recreationally but reading boxes, labels, signs, and advertising on television. Unfortunately, many poor readers avoid reading outside school hours, feeling they have been "punished enough." Incentive programs that offer prizes for reading a given number of books may motivate weak readers to practice more often. Please refer to Chapter 19 for more strategies on encouraging reading.

Deficits in comprehension

Comprehension is directly related to decoding skills. Students who make many errors on a passage will generally have difficulty in understanding what they have read, although some students with excellent language skills and background knowledge may be quite good at extracting meaning. Such difficulties often catch up with students in the later grades.

Comprehension will be best when students read at their *instructional level*, that is, the grade-equivalent materials on which they make fewer than 5% errors. Less than 90% accuracy in decoding defines the *frustration level*. Parents can use this information to select a book at the child's level when there is no one to advise them. Have the child try to read a page or short selection of text, then count up the total number of words and divide this by the number of words that were difficult for the child. If the result is more than 10%, the book is too difficult for the child to read unassisted. Choose another book for the child to read or choose to read this book to the child.

Cloze passages are exercises in which certain words in a passage are substituted by blanks, which the student must fill in by use of the context. (See also Chapter 10 in which this method is used as a way to screen for comprehension.) The idea is to help the student to read past the difficult word to try to extract meaning from the rest of the passage. Teachers may use this method in the classroom or for homework assignments. Parents may often use this method when reading to a child, not realizing that they are using a "method."

Both explicit instruction and incidental learning of **vocabulary** can be used to improve students' reading comprehension. They should be exposed to vocabulary words multiple times and in different contexts. Computer instruction can also be an effective way to teach new vocabulary.(11)

Multiple **comprehension strategies** can be taught to students with learning problems. All students with learning problems should be encouraged to check periodically that what they are reading is making sense. They may also need to read study questions *before* they begin a chapter to know what information they are seeking. Having the student ask the reporter's five "W" questions (who, what, when, where, and why) is a simple strategy for ensuring that the main points have been noted. Other strategies include summarizing the main or most important ideas of the passage and developing a graphic representation of relationships and meanings within the text.

Some readers are able to decode quite accurately yet still fail to understand or remember what they read. This may be due to inattention, poor overall language skills, memory problems, or failure to link the verbal information contained in the words themselves with a nonverbal image of what the words portray. Most mature readers construct mental pictures of what they have read, and this helps with the text. Students who fail to do this may be helped to improve their comprehension by using curricula that emphasize visualization techniques (e.g., Nanci Bell's program for visualizing and verbalizing).(12)

All students should be taught a *variety of strategies* and taught never to rely on just one. Students who can neither decode phonetically nor remember sight words need as many chances as possible to discover the word's meaning. Curricula that entirely exclude phonics deprive students of the most reliable way of approaching an unknown word, while those that focus only on phonetic rules draw the child's attention away from the fact that words and passages are supposed to mean something. Fluent adult readers draw on both of these strategies to deal with unfamiliar words, using phonics to discover how the word sounds and using context to help with the meaning. Marie Clay's Reading Recovery program (www.readingrecovery.org) is an example of a remedial curriculum that combines both of these approaches.(13)

Bypass strategies for reading

Older students whose reading level is significantly below grade level and/or who read very slowly may need adjusted expectations. Often they are working at their instructional level in their remedial reading class, yet are given textbooks in their content areas (e.g., science or social studies) that are at grade level. This volume of reading may be impossible for them to handle; they are unable to finish reading the assigned chapters and thus are not exposed to all of the material on which they are to be tested.

Providing alternative materials that are easier to read, using materials on DVDs, CDs, or text-to-speech technology that read the text to the student (such as e-readers), and teaching note-taking and skimming skills that help them to locate the key information in a passage without having to plod through word by word, may all be of assistance. The school can provide this technology. Some study skills involving reading, such as finding the main idea, outlining, and dealing with subject-specific new vocabulary, are best addressed in the resource-room setting, where actual materials from the student's regular classes can be used to demonstrate the effectiveness of such techniques. Students with reading disabilities also benefit from extra time to complete examinations.

Written output problems

Children may have problems with written work for a variety of reasons, including poor fine motor skills, poor spelling ability, expressive language delays, organizational problems, and attention deficit hyperactivity disorder (ADHD). Most students with learning problems need specific instruction in editing their work, and modern technology can be invaluable in assisting them to work through multiple drafts. This is particularly effective in combination with a serial proofreading strategy in which the individual components of written work (spelling, punctuation, capitalization, grammar, organization) are corrected one at a time instead of simultaneously. As with reading, incentive programs for developing typing skills and writing journals, stories, reports, and letters may be necessary for students with learning problems to gain sufficient practice with written expression.

Children with fine motor problems may benefit from programs that enable them to demonstrate their knowledge without excessive writing or typing. Some may even need to be granted permission for oral examinations or use of speech-to-text software. Bypass strategies including recording lectures, having the teacher share a written or electronic handout or summary of the most important

points, or assigning a note-taking buddy (or scribe) have worked to shift the focus from the mechanics of writing to the actual subject content. Early introduction of technology can allow students to concentrate on spelling and content as opposed to letter formation, and it saves them from tedious recopying when working through successive drafts. The use of technology can be part of a student's program plan.

For some students, learning cursive handwriting is such a nightmare that it may be useful to seek permission for that student to continue to print. For others, learning cursive writing actually helps because it forces the left-to-right counter-clockwise directionality and eliminates mirror-image reversals. Children with fisted or other maladaptive pencil grasps can sometimes be helped with a simple rubber pencil grip (sold in many stationery stores) or they may need to be retrained in how they hold their pencil. Input from an occupational therapist can be very helpful, if available.

As noted, modern technology can be especially supportive of children with written output difficulties. Information on various technologies and software programs can be found online: http://sites.wiki.ubc.ca/etec510/Supporting_Written_Output_Challenges_with_Technology.

ADHD

Many classroom accommodations and strategies promote on-task behaviour. For example, seating a child close to the teacher maximizes saliency of the teacher's presence by eliminating distractions (often other students) from the student's visual field—thus presenting the teacher as "larger" and "louder." Cuing the child that instructions or other important information is coming up by using a general statement such as "Are you ready, class?" or giving a private signal (to an individual student) may decrease the number of times that student needs repetition. Providing repetition freely, without making inattention a "moral" issue, helps to avoid stigmatization of individual students.

Many students with ADHD have problems with executive functions such as organizational and study skills, and may need such skills to be taught.

It is unwise to assume these skills will be acquired naturally or without effort. Students with impaired attention tend to work better one to one or in small group settings that minimize distractions and allow for better monitoring of the student.

Passive learning style

Many students with learning difficulties lose motivation and become passive or avoidant learners. After years of failure, they learn that effort is not rewarded. They stop trying to reason things out and approach many academic tasks superficially.

In mathematics, passive students may not follow operations through to their logical conclusions. For example, they might subtract yet fail to notice that the answer is more than what they started out with. Their estimating skills are often poor.

When reading texts, passive students may not notice the relationship of what they are studying to material in previous chapters. They fail to connect lessons to prior knowledge, and it does not even occur to them to do so. To become more actively involved in learning, such students may need specific instruction and supervised practice in self-questioning and self-monitoring skills. (See also the upcoming section on organization, studying, and homework.)

Intellectual disability and autism spectrum disorders

To learn academic skills, students with intellectual disability (ID) require more repetition and a longer period of time to progress in their learning. Children with mild to moderate ID are capable of learning basic literacy skills. Skilled teachers need to provide explicit instruction and intensive practice in the component skills of reading, including word identification (both phonemic decoding and sight-word decoding), fluency, vocabulary, and comprehension. Students make the most gains when the teaching and practice are both meaningful and motivating to them. When teaching decoding skills, words are most meaningful (and therefore most likely to be successfully decoded) when they are in the student's oral vocabulary. A behaviour modification program using tangible reinforcement may be helpful in keeping students with ID on-task and motivated(14) (see Chapter 14 for more on behaviour modification programs). Once a reward system has been successfully implemented, reinforcers can often be provided less frequently and become less tangible. Short-term gains may be too small to measure by norm-referenced tests, which may lead to discouragement and frustration for the student's parents. Therefore, instructors may need to develop criterion-referenced measures to document a student's progress. A number of students with ID will learn reading decoding skills fairly well but have much more difficulty with reading comprehension.

Similarly, students with autism spectrum disorders (ASD) are often skilled at decoding but tend to struggle with reading comprehension. Understanding narratives is typically difficult for such students, because this often relies on the ability to make inferences. Specific instruction in vocabulary of emotions may aid in the understanding of narratives for children with ASD, since knowledge of a character's emotions equips the student to make inferences about the character's motives.(15)

ROLE OF PHYSICIANS' ADVICE TO STUDENTS

Students may be more willing to take advice from their teacher or parent if their doctor reinforces the advice. Consequently, you may serve a useful role in "backing up" appropriate suggestions, when the student is being seen in the office either for follow-up or for other reasons. Because of your knowledge of the human body, you might use physical analogies, outlining how the nervous system benefits from practice at a particular mental task in the same way a muscle is made stronger by regular exercise. When a muscle is not used, it atrophies. The mental and motor "programs" in the brain are enhanced by rehearsal in a similar way. Most children can think of physical skills they have improved through practice, and they can be encouraged to view thought processes and academic learning as shaped by the same type of effort.

ORGANIZATION, STUDYING, AND HOMEWORK

In order to experience school success, students with learning difficulties not only need to learn basic skills and concepts, they also need to "learn how to learn," especially as the onus for learning content material shifts from their teachers to the students. Teaching meta-cognitive skills and use of external organizers can make learning more efficient and effective. Learning occurs not only at school but also at home. Homework and home study are necessary to complete assignments and to prepare for examinations so that students can receive credit for their learning. Strategies and tools exist to enhance a student's learning at home as well as at school.

Organization and study skills

Many students with learning problems, especially those with a mixed LD/ADHD picture, have poor executive functioning, particularly if a complex task requires integration of component parts into a coherent whole. They may do well when performing any of the components individually, but the level of a component skill drops when it becomes a step in a larger, more complex task (for example, a child might earn a grade of 100% when spelling words learned in lists, but may misspell the same words when writing compositions).

In the early grades (Grades 1 to 3), the emphasis is on the component skills, the so-called "basics." The teacher does most of the organizing, guiding students through more complicated tasks, step by step, and ensuring that they are not overwhelmed by having too many assignments due at the same time. By Grade 4, the emphasis has shifted from "learning to read" to "reading to learn," and from the mechanics of handwriting to the written expression of ideas and demonstration of acquired knowledge. For this shift to be successful, the component skills must be sound and at grade level. If the component skills are not fluent and automatic, the student may expend so much time and energy on one aspect of the task that completion of the whole assignment becomes impossible.

Many school curricula do not emphasize organizational and self-monitoring skills, nor do they teach students how to be good at studying. It is assumed that students will easily develop such skills on their own. In fact, many students never do unless they are specifically instructed in study skills and then drilled in their use. Study skills curricula exist, and they are available to teachers and occupational therapists. These emphasize task analysis, organization, planning, and self-monitoring. Precise study skills may need to be taught, particularly to poor readers, and skills include the following:

- Varying one's reading style for different types of assignments. Understanding the main idea and supporting points in a passage.
- Using outlines, brainstorming, and mind-mapping.
- Using time management and work schedules.
- Employing test-taking strategies.

Volume of homework

Homework can be a burden for many students with learning challenges, especially if they are also expected to complete any work that was not finished in class. Reasonable limits must be placed on the time to be spent each night to ensure there is also time for recreation and rest. Repetitive drills rarely improve the ability to grasp new concepts, and it may be better to have the student work on fewer problems in more depth. Drill may be more useful for improving fluency of a skill after it has been mastered. Time spent on work completion should be considered part of the ten minutes per grade expectation.

Remembering assignments

A homework book, assignment book, or agenda, either written or electronic, may help both the student and the parent to know when assignments are due. For the younger elementary student, a homework book may need to be combined with a behaviour-modification approach to increase the motivation to use it, until it becomes a habitual part of the student's school program. Many schools now provide agendas to all students at the beginning of the academic year.

In junior high school, when the student has a number of different teachers, each with a different agenda and course requirements, the format of the homework book may need to be revised; however, its continued use should be strongly encouraged. Many older students who have never used a homework book before are quite resistant to its introduction, and they will insist that they "don't need it." Some preliminary counselling may be necessary before the student is willing to commit to try a homework book. The student should be reassured that the homework book is not a make-work project designed by teachers and parents to annoy the student. It is a tried-and-true strategy that has been found to be successful by many students.

If the homework book becomes a major point of conflict between a student and parents, it may help to put the onus of responsibility on the student; if the student wants to avoid parental reminders, information can be volunteered before the parent has to ask. Parents should be sure to reinforce such behaviour.

The number of assignments completed can be viewed as a kind of game score, with the previous week's score being the one to beat, and with the parent serving as a silent record keeper. If the student places the homework book and completed assignments in a designated area for parents to check, nagging can be avoided.

Developing home study habits

Regular study habits are important and need to be developed early. Young elementary students may be participating in home reading programs for at least fifteen minutes each day. It is easy to designate this as "homework time," which is gradually increased as the volume of homework increases. If possible, such an approach should be initiated before the student begins to resist homework. Keeping to the rule of no more than ten minutes per grade is a useful guideline.

Parents' enforcement of homework time sends a strong message to the student that homework is an important and respected activity. Involve students in choosing a time that avoids conflict with favourite pastimes or team sports, but remind them

that the later in the evening homework is begun, the more tired he or she will be, and the less attentive and efficient. For students with an attention deficit, this is especially important; such students may need their block of homework time divided into two or three shorter sessions to accommodate their shorter attention spans. The parent should also assist the student in setting up a quiet and well-lit work environment, free of distractions, with all necessary materials close at hand.

SUMMARY

Educational remediation of learning problems begins with *demystification*—a clear explanation of the child's learning difficulties, including specific strengths and weaknesses, with all terminology explained and questions answered. There are a host of educational strategies that may assist with different kinds of learning problems, and physicians' awareness of these approaches can help children and their families to understand, accept, and use them. Organizational skills, homework, and studying should also be addressed.

SELECTED RESOURCES

Assistive educational applications, approaches, and technologies

Apps4kids: <www.apps4kids.net>
Best Kids Apps: <www.bestkidsapps.com>
Lindamood Phoneme Sequencing Program for Reading, Spelling, and Speech, 4th Edition (LiPS-4) <www.lindamoodbell.com>
Reading Recovery Council of North America <www.readingrecovery.org>
Supporting Written Output Challenges with Technology <http://sites.wiki.ubc.ca/etec510/Supporting_Written_Output_Challenges_with_Technology>

REFERENCES

1. Cooper, H. The Battle over Homework: Common Ground for Administrators, Teachers, and Parents, 3rd Edition. Thousand Oaks CA: Corwin Press, 2007: 102.

2. Shaywitz S. Dyslexia. Sci Am 1996; 275: 98–104.

3. Lindamood CH, Lindamood PC. Lindamood Auditory Conceptualization Test (LAC-3). Austin TX: Pro-Ed Inc., 2004.

4. Torgesen JK, Bryant BR. Test of Phonological Awareness, 2nd Edition, PLUS (TOPA-2+). Austin TX: Pro-Ed Inc., 2004.

5. Lindamood PC, Lindamood PD. LiPS: Lindamood Phoneme Sequencing Program for Reading, Spelling and Speech, 4th Edition (LiPS-4). Austin TX: Pro-Ed Inc., 2011.

6. National Reading Panel (NRP). Report of the National Reading Panel: Reports of the Subgroups. Washington DC: National Institute of Child Health and Human Development Clearing House, 2000. <www.nationalreadingpanel.org/default.htm> (Version current at April 30, 2012.)

7. Tallal P, Miller SL, Bedi G, et al. Language comprehension in language-learning impaired children improved with acoustically modified speech. Science 1996; 271: 81–4.

8. Op. cit. Reference 6 (NRP).

9. Topping K. The Paired Reading Training Pack, 3rd Edition. West Yorkshire: Oastler Centre, 1988.

10. Brailsford A. Paired Reading: Positive Reading Practice: A Training Videotape with Accompanying Manual. Northern Alberta Reading Specialists' Council. Kelowna: Filmwest Associates, 1997.

11. Op. cit. Reference 6 (NRP).

12. Bell N. Visualizing and Verbalizing for Language Comprehension and Thinking, 2nd Edition. San Luis Obispo CA: Gander Publishing, 2007.

13. Clay M. Reading Recovery: A Guidebook for Teachers in Training. Aukland: Heinemann Education, 1993.

14. Allor JH, Champlin TM, Gifford DB, Mathes PG. Methods for increasing the intensity of reading instruction for students with intellectual disabilities. Education and Training in Autism and Developmental Disabilities, 2010; 45(4): 500–11.

15. Randi J, Newman T, Grigorenko EL. Teaching children with autism to read for meaning: Challenges and possibilities. J Autism Dev Disord 2010; 40: 890–902.

14

Behavioural Management

Cara Dosman and Debra Andrews

Our behaviour is our output, and includes our actions, emotional expression, and consciously controlled thoughts. Behavioural difficulties manifest as oppositional defiance, aggression, or explosive outbursts, and can be managed with specific behavioural modification strategies. However, strategies by themselves are not enough to produce the most successful outcomes. We must understand and address the underlying causes of behavioural difficulties, such as the child's cognitive skill set and ability for self-regulation. A complex combination of underlying causes is the rule rather than the exception.

To address this complexity, behavioural management generally requires a multi-faceted, often multidisciplinary approach in which specific behavioural, regulation, and cognitive strategies are used simultaneously. At times, the identified factors causing the child the greatest distress must become the current treatment priority. For example, if the outbursts of a child with a learning disability (LD) are accompanied by plummeting self-esteem because of the child's inability to read, *immediate* help may mean decreasing the stress by temporarily reducing school workload and having the parent read to the child, while the *long-term* solution would be remedial intervention to strengthen the reading skills.(1)

In this chapter we review some of the specific factors that contribute to behavioural problems so that you may more thoroughly explore them in your behavioural history. Then we describe general behavioural strategies and the specifics of time-out and behaviour modification programs, and finish up with a brief discussion of self-esteem, mood, and social skills programs.

UNDERLYING FACTORS AFFECTING BEHAVIOUR: COGNITIVE ABILITIES

Behaviour is affected by a child's ability to pay attention, to control impulsivity and motor activity, to process and remember incoming information, to understand and use language, to think flexibly about problems to be solved, to interpret nonverbal communication, and to recognize the thoughts and feelings of others. Children with learning problems may struggle with any or all of these skills both in the classroom and at home, so it is no wonder that they may also have trouble with behaviour.

Developing these skills and using strengths to help compensate for weaknesses builds resilience and adaptive behaviour. Strategies to strengthen and accommodate for weaker skills can be developed and implemented both at school and at home. Schools may use available consultants, such as behavioural specialists, speech-language pathologists, and occupational therapists or psychologists; parents may consult their physician and/or community-based mental health services. Medication for ADHD may improve some of the cognitive skills mentioned and, thus, improve behaviour.

UNDERLYING FACTORS AFFECTING BEHAVIOUR: REGULATION

One of the big changes in how we manage behaviour problems in children is our awareness of the importance of regulation. A good understanding of this area can help you predict which children are more likely to respond to basic behaviour strategies—like time-out and reward systems—and which children will more likely require a more intensive approach, often involving consultation and/or medication.

Regulation is the brain's ability to control our state of arousal. A *calm and alert* state of arousal is needed for a person to learn and interact with others. Stress responses are triggered when we feel challenged or threatened, and lead to varying expressions of emotions. We may feel overwhelmed with strong feelings of anger or fear (*flooded* state). Alertness is heightened when we are anxious or hypervigilant (*hyperalert* state) but decreased when we are withdrawn, depressed, or under-aroused (*hypoalert* state). To get back to the calm and alert processing state that we need for learning and interaction, we must go through a process of *stress recovery*. If we don't recover adequately from stress, this can create a "load condition" in which our stress responses occur much too frequently and remain strong long after the stressor is removed. You may see this kind of heightened stress response in children who have experienced significant trauma in early childhood, for example. There is evidence that such unresolved chronic stress places children at risk for physical disease and continued problems with self-regulation into adulthood, so the development of healthy regulation is important for both short-term symptom relief and long-term well-being.

School-aged children with behaviour problems may have regulatory issues, so this must be explored in your workup. How can we tell if a child has good self-regulation? The medical history will give some clues. Signs include a capacity for deep sleep, recognition of internal body signals (e.g., hunger, elimination cues, fatigue, pain), the ability to maintain an alert processing state and make smooth transitions from one arousal state to another, adaptive expression of all stress response types, and efficient recovery from stress, including the ability to self-soothe. Ask about regulation difficulties in infancy; parents may report that their baby had difficulty in establishing routines for sleeping or feeding, or trouble with colic. Most typically developing children go through a period of tantrums around age two, where they learn the limits of their behaviour and begin to cope with negative emotions and replace them with more socially appropriate

responses. They gradually develop a repertoire of self-calming strategies (for example, upset children may be able to calm themselves by taking a walk or listening to some music), but they may continue to need external help with regulation from their caregivers (e.g., the child may seek out the parents to talk to or to hug the child). This is called *co-regulation*. Older children with regulatory problems may not be able to calm themselves down and have blow-ups and tantrums beyond the expected age. They still need support from a parent or other adult to help them.

STRATEGIES FOR HELPING WITH REGULATORY PROBLEMS

Many child and parent factors influence regulation. For each risk factor that the child *doesn't* have, there is a corresponding *increase* in resiliency toward better outcomes. *Child risk factors* include sleep difficulties (which are common—25% of all children), poor nutrition (e.g., iron deficiency), prenatal factors (maternal stress, poor care, intrauterine growth restriction, exposure to alcohol, drugs, and other teratogens), swallowing difficulties (reflecting vagal nerve dysfunction), other conditions that disrupt physiology (prematurity, genetic disorder, chronic allergies, or other medical conditions), and sensory modulation difficulty (hyper- or hyposensitivity). Helping regulation includes treatment of any specific factors where possible.

Sleep problems should be treated specifically, depending on the cause; an excellent clinician resource is *A Clinical Guide to Pediatric Sleep: Diagnosis and Management of Sleep Problems*, which includes sleep treatment handouts for families.(2) Sometimes sleep medication may need to be considered when there is an underlying condition disrupting sleep and when the child or family is in a "load" condition with excess ongoing stress.

Occupational therapy consultation for soothing sensory experiences could be sought when necessary. Relaxation techniques such as deep breathing or progressive muscle relaxation may help regulation in older children.

Child anxiety and depression are usually responsive to cognitive-behavioural therapy, but medication is required when emotional disruptions are severe enough to significantly limit the child's ability to work on his or her treatment program.

Finally, it is important to ensure daily opportunities for the child to pursue an interest or strength, because these create positive emotion, enhance a perception of safety, help bring the child to a calm and alert state, and build self-esteem.

Parents with their own regulatory difficulties present risk factors for child dysregulation, because these parents will be less emotionally available to help regulate their child. Examples of *parent risk factors* include inadequate food, shelter, or clothing; limited financial or community resources; sleep difficulty; chronic depression or anxiety; substance abuse; domestic violence: malnutrition; or chronic medical conditions. The presence of such parent risk factors may signal the need for parent interventions such as social work, mental health, or medical treatment, done in tandem with the child interventions to promote healthy regulation for both parent and child. Parenting style (authoritative, authoritarian, permissive) and the parent-child relationship also affect the child's emotions, memories, and regulation. Group parent training or individualized parent-child relationship therapy may be required.

EVIDENCE-BASED APPROACHES TO BEHAVIOUR: PROGRAMS, RESOURCES, AND GENERAL PRINCIPLES

Remember that "discipline" is about teaching skills, not about punishment. Focusing on creating a strong parent-child attachment relationship encourages child compliance, caring behaviours, and self-esteem, and helps discipline strategies go more smoothly. In the pyramid model of behavioural intervention(3) (for more see www. incredibleyears.com), most of the intervention time is spent on the parent-child relationship and teaching positive skills (empathy, positive attention, play, listening, talking, teaching appropriate behaviours and problem-solving, specific praise, rewards). The least time is spent on using ignoring, consequences, and time-outs for misbehaviour. These evidence-based principles apply across the

school-age span, both for children with oppositional defiant disorder (ODD) and children with negative behaviours that are less severe and fall within the range of typical development.

There is a strong body of evidence about what works in effective parenting, and there are many available resources. A CME article in *Canadian Family Physician* includes a parent handout on discipline.(4) Parent handouts on positive discipline, time-outs, and tantrums are available through the Canadian Paediatric Society's Caring for Kids website (www.caringforkids.cps.ca). Evidence-based books for parents are available through the Parent Resources section of the Incredible Years website (www.incredibleyears.com). Evidence-based group parent training programs for children with ODD may be offered in the community through family resource centres. Many materials are available through websites and bookstores, such as the Incredible Years, Triple P Positive Parenting Program (www.triplep. net), and Community Parent Education Services (COPE) (www.mcmasterchildrenshospital.ca/body. cfm?id=189).

Talk with the caregiver about following the child's lead in an activity together every day, imitating and describing the child's actions, and giving specific praise for the child's ideas and efforts. To increase positive behaviours, caregivers can give immediate positive attention (specific praise such as "I like that you started setting the table as soon as I asked you to," or giving a smile or hug). Praising positive behaviours should happen at least three to four times more often than identifying misbehaviour. Children are not spoiled by praise, but rather learn from it to compliment and encourage peers, and this social skill makes them more well-liked by others.

Setting up a rewards program (described in detail later in this chapter) can help motivate the child to do something that the child finds particularly difficult, such as doing homework, helping with dishes, or brushing teeth. A home-based rewards program for targeted positive behaviours at school is often one of the first interventions for ADHD. A daily school-behaviour report card can be used for social and academic behaviours impacted by ADHD symptoms. A report template can be photocopied by parents who purchase Russell Barkley's book *Taking Charge of ADHD: The Complete Authoritative Guide for Parents.*(5) Parent handouts on tips for using a parent-school report card can be photocopied and distributed by clinicians who purchase the ADHD toolkit from the American Academy of Pediatrics (www.aap.org). This toolkit also includes parent handouts on tips for managing common problem behaviours for children with ADHD, such as homework and getting ready in the morning. This is also available at www. nichq.org/toolkits_publications/complete_adhd/12HowToEstabSchlHomeDailyRepCa.pdf.

Talk with the caregiver about setting limits that are clear and consistent, and reducing the number of commands to those with the highest priority, so that the caregiver is always able to follow through. Offering the child choices between two options (e.g., "Do you want to tidy up now or in five minutes?") gives the child some control and decreases power struggles. Have the caregiver consistently ignore minor negative behaviours that are not the treatment priority, such as protests when told no, or swearing. As soon as the misbehaviour stops, the caregiver should suggest an appropriate behaviour and then give immediate positive attention to that positive behaviour. For recurring negative behaviours, such as being late for supper or using more screen time than allowed, caregivers can use an immediate consequence, either *natural* (e.g., the food will be cold and the child will eat alone) or *logical* (e.g., the same amount of screen time will be taken away the next day). It is important for the parent to stay calm, remembering that the child's feelings about himself or herself are as important as obeying the commands.

Using time-out

Time-out to calm down is a commonly used strategy to reduce aggression, frequent noncompliance, and arguing. Counting down before a time-out is quite effective, and an excellent tool is 1–2–3 Magic.(6) In implementing time-out without counting down, the caregiver states clearly what the child needs to do (e.g., "Put your video game away in the cupboard before supper."). If the child has not complied, then the caregiver waits five seconds and states the consequence for noncompliance ("If you don't put your game in the cupboard, you will have to go to time-out."). Again, the caregiver waits five seconds. If the child continues to be noncompliant, the caregiver starts the time-out procedure (e.g., "I asked you to put your game in the cupboard and you disobeyed. Go to time-out now."). In school-aged children, time-out should last at least five minutes; it starts when the child is in the time-out area and can be stopped once the child has been calm for two minutes. Once the time-out is over, the caregiver should praise the child for calming down and then repeat the original command.

Meltdowns and outbursts

Some children may react to requests and simple changes and transitions with extreme inflexibility and aggression. Such children generally do not respond as well to standard strategies, and consequences may actually heighten their emotional arousal. Many children with autism spectrum disorders, sensory processing issues, or anxiety fall into this category. These families will likely need the help of a mental health therapist and sometimes a physician (child psychiatrist, paediatrician, developmental paediatrician) for medication. Managing these explosive outbursts requires investigating and treating the underlying cognitive and regulatory causes described above, and prioritizing what issues to insist on.(7) Caregivers must understand that because of the high level of arousal, the child will not be able to think clearly during the outburst. The child needs the adult to help him become calmer and problem-solve. Ross Greene's book *The Explosive Child* is an excellent resource in this situation.(8)

Help caregivers recognize situations that trigger outbursts (e.g., what was the child doing, who was she with, where and when did the outburst occur) and talk about removing any unnecessary contributions to the child's global level of frustration. While beginning to teach the child new skills, start with a very small set of priorities, focusing on safety (e.g., no aggression allowed), to prevent meltdowns and achieve family peace. Caregivers can use rewards and consequences for safety infractions, but since bringing the child to time-out often exacerbates the meltdown, the parent and child may need to go to separate designated areas of the house. Some children, such as those with autism, need "co-regulation" with a caregiver before they can self-regulate through time-outs. In these situations, a "time-in" where the parent stays with the child can help the child calm down. The child may try sensory strategies, according to preferences, to release energy from the emotionally flooded state and calm down (e.g., jumping, silence, using a swing or therapy ball). Once the child has started to calm down, the caregiver can "mirror" the child's feelings (with facial expressions, tone, and words, e.g., "You are so mad!"), empathetically help the child use words to identify the feelings that provoked the outburst (e.g., "I see that you were mad when I told you to get ready for bed. I wonder if that was because you were enjoying playing so much?"), and stay with the child until calm. This mirroring and empathy help the child see himself or herself through another's eyes, tune into another's perspective, and recover from stress to a calm and alert processing state while nurturing the parent-child relationship.

Less important issues (e.g., cleaning one's room, completing homework) may need to be set aside temporarily until outburst frequency has decreased. Important behaviours that are not safety issues will be the ones that caregivers use to teach their child flexibility and frustration tolerance, but not insist on to the point of an outburst. Teaching a child the skills involves helping the child recognize and label the early emotional warning signs of frustration (e.g., "You're looking frustrated. Is there something I could help you with?"); distracting the child to an enjoyable activity; helping the child downshift moods through empathy, humour, or praise; or asking the child to show the caregiver what the child would like to do; and giving a break if the child does not calm down. Then the caregiver can give the child sentences to use to express what the problem is (e.g., "I feel bad right now."), describe the problem for the child (e.g., "You want to go skating today, and your sister wants to go sledding. Let's think of how we can work this out."), think of alternative solutions

and their outcomes, use one of the solutions, and praise the child for working things out. Eventually the child will problem-solve unassisted.

Setting up a rewards program

Tangible rewards programs using checkmarks, tokens, or stickers are a key part of the management of many children, including those with ADHD, oppositional behaviour, or other learning problems. Such methods are particularly useful in encouraging children to work consistently at tasks that have not been intrinsically rewarding. Many popular books on parenting and discipline emphasize these techniques, which are based on general principles of *operant conditioning* (see the Glossary).

Here are some important principles for rewards programs:

Reinforcement (reward) should be immediate, consistent, and predictable. Unfortunately, many parents and teachers are not consistent. The need to monitor more than one child at a time, to enforce more than one rule, or to perform other tasks simultaneously can make it harder for the adult supervisor to notice every instance of a behaviour and reinforce it promptly. If the reinforcement is delayed, its relationship to the causal behaviour may be blurred, and the reason for the reward may even be attributed to some unrelated action.

If the caregiver is attempting to reinforce too many rules, the point may come when the caregiver cannot "keep up" with all the occurrences of the behaviours the child needs to learn. When this happens, the most important rules continue to be reinforced while the reinforcement of those that are not priorities drops off. The child then "gets away with" breaking lower-priority rules.

Avoiding an unpleasant task can be a powerful reward. It is extremely important to know what is, and what is not, reinforcing a behaviour. A common mistake is the assumption that all children are motivated by so-called "positive" rewards such as praise, attention, privileges, stickers, or tokens, and that all children try to avoid such "negative" consequences as being reprimanded, timed-out, or losing privileges. This is an oversimplification.

For some children, the attraction of assumed rewards or the threat of punishment is far outweighed by the desire to avoid stopping something enjoyable and moving on to a less preferred activity. Children will also go to great lengths to avoid humiliation. A poor reader may consistently "act up" during reading group so as not to have to read out loud, preferring to sit in time-out in the principal's office than to demonstrate disability in front of peers.

Students with ADHD frequently are great "escape artists"; their difficulty in postponing gratification may make it particularly hard for them to leave a pleasant activity to come back to it later. Even if the required task is not aversive, it may be less attractive than another activity that has to be interrupted to do the required work. A vicious cycle arises in which apparently simple requests become increasingly emotion-laden as the parent or teacher reminds the child again and again—while the child fails to respond again and again. Finally, the caregiver loses his or her temper with the child, and at times applies consequences that are out of proportion to the infraction. (*Defiant Children* by Russell Barkley(9) is a detailed parent training curriculum for those parents who require further information.)

Attention can be a very potent reward. For most children, positive interaction with a caregiver (being noticed or praised, having the adult's undivided attention) is one of the best reinforcers, leading to an increase in the behaviour that preceded the interaction. Many parents and teachers believe their main role is to correct the child's behaviour; they are generous with criticism but not with praise. They take for granted and fail to reward the things the child is doing right.

Ignoring a child's behaviour usually brings about a decrease in that behaviour—most children (and adults, too) hate to be ignored. However, a child who is being ignored may escalate attempts to get the caregiver's attention by resorting to behaviours the adult will not ignore, as this has worked in the past. The caregiver may then respond with a presumed deterrent—yelling or some other "punishment"—which, in fact, increases the amount of attention the child receives, and the child comes back for more. What was supposed to discourage the behaviour is in fact a reinforcer for that child and that particular behaviour.

Such a pattern is very common in households with busy daytime schedules in which all the family members converge on the home just before dinner, tired and needing support from each other at the end of the day. Unfortunately, there are many tasks that need to be done before everyone can relax, and bad behaviour peaks when dinner is being prepared. If parents are able to schedule time for interacting with their children prior to getting started on the chores—or failing this, if they are able to divide up the work so that one caregiver is dealing with cooking the meal while the other keeps the "troops" entertained—fewer incidents of misbehaviour may occur during this time of day.

One reward gives a clearer message than a number of punishments. Punishment gives the message to decrease a particular behaviour; it does not say what to do instead. The child must go back to his or her repertoire of thousands of behavioural alternatives and select another option. For many students with ADHD, their second (and third and fourth) choice of a behaviour is just as "wrong" for a situation as their original choice. A reward for a positive behaviour says "do this particular behaviour again"—a much clearer and more specific message to the child.

Steps to setting up a behaviour modification program

Setting up a simple behaviour program is much easier than most physicians imagine it to be. It can be an extremely useful tool in your tool kit for working with children with school problems, and can be used for many other common child behaviour problems seen in primary care and general pediatric practices. The following steps serve as a recipe for getting started. The first few times through the steps will likely feel a bit awkward and unfamiliar, but feedback from families will help to fine-tune the process. Sometimes workshops or seminars given by psychologists or other therapists can be very helpful to your understanding of this process, as well as giving an opportunity to discuss ways to improve your approach. You may also wish to contact local clinicians who do this work for advice and tips (see Chapter 21 for developing a resource worksheet). Here are the steps:

1. **Have each parent/teacher list the behaviours to be modified:** The items on the list should be as objective and specific as possible. Vague or moralistic terms (e.g., "Johnny should be more respectful of others.") should be avoided, because different observers may have different notions as to what constitutes a "respectful" attitude. Stick to phrasing that describes a behavioural outcome that is easily identified and quantified (e.g., "Johnny will raise his hand and be recognized before speaking in class.").

2. **Select two or three behaviours to target across all environments.** Different caregivers may have different priorities. Therefore, they will give mixed messages in the way they reinforce the rules. *To ensure that rules are consistently reinforced and to avoid confusion, it is important to come to an agreement* about what those rules are before presenting them to the child. Also, if the caregivers are trying to train too many new behaviours at the same time, it increases the chances of inconsistent reinforcement. It is best to select two or three new behavioural priorities and put the others on hold until the first set of target behaviours occurs regularly.

3. **Establish a behavioural baseline.** It is impossible to tell if behaviours are diminishing if you don't even know how often they are occurring in the first place. Counting the number of occurrences of a particular behaviour over a specified time period during the day will define the starting point of the program and allow measurement of any change.

4. **Add to the list one or two desirable behaviours the child already performs with reasonable frequency.** Rewards serve as the "carrot" to get the child engaged in the behaviour modification program. No child will want to play the game if there is no chance of winning. Often the desired behaviours are so difficult for the child that it is unlikely that they will occur often enough for the child to realize the connection between behaviour and the reinforcers used. Using behaviours the child already knows helps to teach the program.

5. **Rewrite all items on the child's behaviour list in positive terms.** This makes the institution of the program more pleasant for the child. The list is a set of behavioural goals rather than a "list of sins." The child is reinforced for what is done right.

6. **Have parents, teachers, and the child brainstorm to develop a list of possible reinforcers.** Rewards must be meaningful to the child. This means sitting down together and writing out as many alternatives as possible. Privileges at home and at school may serve as reinforcers. Time spent with a parent in shared activity (e.g., a trip to the park or a game of cards) can be a powerful reinforcer, especially for younger children.

7. **Edit the list of reinforcers so that what remains is realistic and acceptable to all parties.** What the child has proposed may seem excessive to the caregiver, while what the caregiver is offering may not seem like enough to the child; some negotiation may need to occur. Nothing should be promised as a potential reward unless it can actually be delivered. The general principle that one should never make promises that cannot be kept also applies to threats. Failure to follow through with consequences undermines the credibility of the caregiver's statements and authority.

   Many caregivers find the need for reinforcement difficult to accept, and they will insist that rewards are "bribes" and that children should be self-motivated toward good behaviour. Although children "should" want to behave or try hard at school, in the real world rewards such as salaries or privileges are invariably used for activities, including many that would otherwise be regarded as pointless or unrewarding. However, some families will prefer to avoid using monetary rewards or purchased items, as this might encourage materialistic attitudes.

8. **Assign a value to each of the items on the child's program.** For many caregivers, this is a major stumbling block. They may spend too

much time agonizing over how many points or tokens to assign to each item or how many times the child must perform a given task to achieve a given reward. The actual number of points is not really that important. What is important is that more difficult or more "valuable" positive behaviours should be worth more than minor ones, and that the scale of points should make sense to the child. Younger children whose number concept is not yet well developed will have an easier time with lower point values, and they are likely to be confused if the program is too complicated. Older children may prefer "lots of points," so be generous.

9. **Set out the details of the program in writing.** This avoids misunderstandings and promotes consistency of reinforcement. Have the child and parent sign the contract, reinforcing that this is an important and formal agreement. You may wish to keep a copy of what has been produced on the child's medical chart for future reference.

10. **Make a visual record of the program to demonstrate the child's progress.** Behavioural change, like physical growth, is hard to see from day to day. Younger children especially, with their undeveloped concepts of time, may have difficulty appreciating that they are making progress without some kind of visual reminder. The visual record can be marks or stickers on a calendar, a checklist, or a more elaborate chart. Accumulating vertical blocks on a bar graph (e.g., for complying with a reading incentive program) can be particularly appealing to young children.

11. **Reinforce promptly and consistently.** The younger the child, the more the child will need to be reinforced as close in time as possible to carrying out the appropriate behaviour. Stickers or check marks on a laminated card may serve as rewards in themselves for younger children, or points may be accumulated for privileges at home or at school for older students.

12. **Make frequent changes in the menu of reinforcers to avoid satiation.** Children tire of the same old rewards and privileges after a while. This is particularly true of children with ADHD. Refer back to the brainstormed list of privileges for possible replacements.

13. **Do not introduce penalties until the program is working.** Many caregivers are eager to apply punishments as well as rewards, and they make the mistake of removing privileges too soon. The child will soon return to a negative cycle, with any gains rendered temporary.

14. **Do not make hasty or arbitrary changes in the reinforcement schedule, especially when the child is angry or upset.** Many caregivers have a tendency to over-punish when the child's misbehaviour has elicited an emotional response. The caregiver retaliates against the child's actions by removing privileges or increasing punishments to unrealistic proportions. Later, the caregiver may feel guilty about having been so harsh and try to make it up to the child by reinstating or even increasing the privilege and/or not following through with the punishment. The child then learns that there are times when parents "don't really mean it." Some children may even recognize the pattern and try to provoke this response in the parent.

It is much better to decide about rewards and punishments when things are calm, as decisions are more likely to be realistic and fair. If changes need to be made, wait until the heat of the moment is past, then decide on the new schedule. The child needs to be aware of the new rules before they are instituted.

15. **Identify and eliminate hidden reinforcers, such as secondary gains and attention from important others, which serve to promote negative behaviours.** For example, for the child who would seek to avoid reading aloud, a combination of recognizing that the behaviour is motivated by a desire to escape and addressing the child's reading difficulties to make reading in front of others more comfortable would likely eliminate the behaviour.

If a newly implemented behaviour program is not working, consider these possibilities:

- **Behaviour was not consistently reinforced:** for example, there may be a single exhausted caregiver with insufficient supports; perhaps an adult tried to reinforce too many behaviours; there may be multiple caregivers who were not consistent; or the behaviour was not sufficiently defined.

- **Reinforcers were poorly chosen and were not reinforcing:** for example, an adult selected what he or she thought the child "should" want or refused to accept what the child did want.
- **Punishment was introduced too soon.**
- **Stressors exist within the environment:** examples are marital discord, child abuse, poverty, physical or mental illness in a family member, and/or other students with special needs in the classroom.
- **Secondary gain for child and/or caregiver resulted in continuing misbehaviour:** for example, attention from important adults or peers, escape from an even more unpleasant or difficult task.
- **The child has more complex psychopathology.**

If a behaviour program that was working begins to lose its efficacy, consider the following possibilities:

- A caregiver has begun to take the program for granted and is **not reinforcing as consistently as before.**
- **A new and inconsistent caregiver** has been added to the household or classroom: for example, a grandparent moves into the home, or the child has a substitute teacher.
- A caregiver has **new competing demands** from another person: for example, the birth of a sibling, the caregiver has a new relationship, or a new student with school problems transferred into the class.
- **New stressors** have been added: for example, the family has moved or physical or mental illness has developed in either child or caregiver.
- The **reinforcement schedule has not been upgraded** in a long time.

SELF-ESTEEM AND THE CHILD WITH SCHOOL PROBLEMS

Self-esteem is not a behaviour, but *a way of thinking that guides behaviour.* All people have a sense of themselves, their worth, and efficacy in the tasks of their lives. A strong sense of being valued by others (family, peers, community) and feelings of mastery and achievement allow us to move through life in a connected and hopeful way. Poor self-esteem is associated with poor effort and a sad mood, but an overly inflated sense of one's own value and contribution is equally damaging. Ideally, we hope that children will develop a realistic idea of their achievements and a solid sense of self so that they are able to receive and use feedback and celebrate true accomplishments.

For the elementary school child, who defines himself or herself by achievements, lack of success in school is equated with lack of success in life. Children this age have a tendency to overgeneralize: when faced with discrepant information, they may ignore what is not congruent with their perception of the "big picture" instead of reformulating their ideas to accommodate the new data. The model of LDs as uneven subskills in the face of good overall cognitive abilities makes no sense to them. It is not only the child with LDs who believes he or she is "stupid" or "bad." Peers, who are at the same developmental level, believe it too, confirming the child's own poor opinion. Teasing and outright bullying, both physical and verbal, are commonly experienced by children with learning problems, who may come to see themselves as others label them.

Children with varying degrees of intellectual disability may struggle with all areas of learning. Participating in integrated classes may encourage socialization but also demonstrates the child's broad range of difficulties for all to see and may decrease the time to work intensively on certain academic skills. Segregated classes may allow more program differentiation, individual support, and a protected environment away from bullies. Unfortunately, students attending "different" classrooms may be ridiculed by other students without special needs. Whatever the setting, there are both advantages and drawbacks, and schools need to foster an atmosphere of tolerance and acceptance for individual differences among all students, especially for this group of students who may have a higher frequency of genetic syndromes or other visible differences, making it even harder for them to fit in.

The "back-to-basics" approach taken by some schools, with greater emphasis on reading and writing skills, may decrease the number of opportunities for children with any kind of a learning problem to shine in other areas, such as sports, music, drama, or art. Their classmates may never see them in any other light than as a person with problems.

Children who also have attention problems may be at the highest risk of all: many of them are unable to negotiate a twenty-minute recess without committing some sort of offence. Their pervasive lack of attention and impulsive behaviour affect all aspects of their life. Even when they get home in the afternoon, they may get in trouble with their parents and siblings.

Teenagers with LDs are better equipped cognitively to understand what an LD is, but they may not want to hear yet another authority figure telling them who they are and what they ought to do. After years and years of failure, they may have given up on that aspect of their life, having cultivated a different image, perhaps choosing to look "cool," as if they do not care. Some may not care. Some may not believe the helper's message. Some are so depressed that they never hear the message at all.

Teenagers with intellectual disability may be much more aware of the ways in which they are different from age peers as the absolute skill gap widens. When they were younger and functioning at a developmental level where parent and teacher approval was most salient, they may have been less aware of peers. Now as they move into a developmental phase where peers' opinions begin to equal and then surpass those of important adults, concerns about self-esteem may arise for the first time.

Ideally, early identification and early intervention, along with a school atmosphere that fosters tolerance—and even celebrates individual differences—should help all children develop a healthy sense of self-esteem. Unfortunately, many children are not seen and assessed until the damage to their self-image has already begun.

Fostering a healthy sense of self-esteem

Healthy self-esteem is a product of feeling valued by others *and* having a sense of true mastery and accomplishment. Self-esteem development programs that focus only on the first component have produced students who expect to be valued for anything that they do and who may have an inflated sense of self-worth and entitlement, and other students for whom no degree of empty praise can compensate for their own sense of a lack of achievement.

Healthy self-esteem for all children, especially those who have developmental challenges, can be fostered in these ways:

- Setting individual, appropriate, achievable expectations for each child.
- Avoiding unfavourable comparisons with other children.
- Seeking and emphasizing the strengths in every student.
- Rewarding effort as well as accomplishment with specific praise.
- Helping children to see gains in achievement.
- Building and celebrating true skills and accomplishments.
- Helping children feel part of a group (family, school, or community) by giving them specific and valued roles within that group (e.g., chores and jobs).

For a parent handout on developing self-esteem in all children, visit the CPS Caring for Kids website (www.caringforkids.cps.ca).

Locus of control: Learning to take responsibility

Locus of control is a useful concept for exploring children's understanding of the reasons for their own successes and failures, and can help you in evaluating and counselling children and families. The locus of control concept explains why the degree of disability does not always correlate with the degree of difficulty and unhappiness experienced in the classroom. Some children who reveal only very mild developmental delays on psychometric testing may be completely paralyzed by their problems. Others, whose developmental delays are much more marked, may be able to persevere, and they may ultimately have a better response to remediation.

A child with an *external locus of control* might feel that the reason he or she did not pass a mathematics test was that the teacher made the test too hard. If the child felt that the grade reflected the amount of studying that had been done, the child would be said to have an *internal locus of control*. (See *locus of control* in the Glossary for more on these terms.)

If the causes of people's behaviour are seen as outside themselves, then they might reason that little or nothing can be done to change their fate. Such an attitude contributes to a sense of helplessness and hopelessness.

Locus of control follows a developmental progression, with a shift from external to internal locus in most children as they grow older and have more influence on outcomes in their lives. Many students with learning problems never experience this progression. Because of repeated failures, they are convinced that nothing they can do will affect their schooling, and they feel powerless to change the situation. Such *learned helplessness* may be the worst enemy of a child with an LD or with ADHD. Children with intellectual disability who are being pushed to do tasks that are above their developmental level may feel that everything is always going to be too hard and there is nothing that they can do about it. Alternatively, expectations may be so low as to interfere with developing independence. In either case, the locus of control is external. Ideally, the level of challenge should be such that the child can begin to see the relationship of effort to outcome, and parents and teachers may need to point out specific, concrete results to build the kind of work ethic that may eventually contribute to success in employment.

To learn to recover from their errors, children with learning problems need to have contact with adult role models who demonstrate the ability to admit to their errors, assess what they did wrong, and regroup to make other attempts to solve their problems, and to practice using such strategies themselves.

For some children, the above measures to foster healthy self-esteem may be insufficient against the residua of years of failure. In such cases, the intervention needed may be more than it is possible to achieve in a few office visits, and referral to other professionals may be needed. School counsellors, psychologists, and social workers may have expertise in counselling students who have learning disabilities.

To summarize, what makes most people happy and satisfied with themselves and what they do in life depends on many factors:

- Perception of competence in being able to do at least one thing well.
- Feelings that their life is under their control and that they can affect their future.
- Feedback they get from others as to their performance.
- Sense of being included in a group or community.

All of these issues must be addressed when dealing with students with any kind of learning problem; these children are particularly at risk for poor self-esteem because they feel incompetent in the main arena of childhood—school. They may experience little control over their lives, and the messages they get from others are frequently negative. They are often excluded from participating in activities within their community because of the level of ability for successful participation, lack of access, bullying and teasing, and the stigma of being different. *Taking measures to improve a child's self-esteem may help to prevent learned helplessness and depression.*

When it's more than poor self-esteem, monitor for depression

If a child's negative mood is more severe and prolonged, consider whether that child may be depressed. Depression frequently accompanies developmental disorders. Risk for significant depression is increased if there is a family history of affective disorder. Children may not present with all the classic vegetative symptoms of depression that are seen in adults. Symptoms may include disturbances of appetite and sleep: both lack of appetite and overeating, insomnia, and excessive sleeping. *Anhedonia* (lack of pleasure) and loss of interest in friends and outside interests are seen in children who are depressed. There may also be angry acting-out.

Physicians who are not comfortable making the diagnosis of depression should refer the child to a paediatrician, developmental paediatrician, child psychiatrist, or mental health professional for further evaluation. Depressed mood may be a consideration in the choice of medication for ADHD.

Always pay attention to worsening mood and suicidal ideation and help direct families to crisis-intervention services promptly so that any suicidal risk can be addressed.

RELATIONSHIPS WITH PEERS

Attending school is about being with age peers. Most children enter school with a cohort of peers who are roughly at the same age and developmental level, they are educated in groups, and progress through school in groups. In our information age where it is impossible to know everything, more and more jobs are team-based, collaborative endeavours, and this approach is also used in schools, where students will regularly participate in group projects and presentations. Children who have difficulty with social interaction will soon make themselves known to teachers, parents, and other students.

If asked, many students with school problems will report having problems getting along with their peers. They might be teased and ostracized for being "different" or "stupid" by children who have a hard time understanding how anyone who is unable to read can still claim to be "smart." Students who have language disorders may have difficulty with the language demands of social interaction. They don't "get" jokes or know when someone is teasing; they may have a hard time expressing their own thoughts and feelings. Many are labelled as "space cadets" by classmates because of their long latency in responding to questions. Children with nonverbal LDs, and many children with ADHD, have trouble with the visual-spatial aspects of social interaction; for example, they misread or ignore body language, especially in dynamic situations with peers. They may also violate other people's body space. Impulsive children are frequently in trouble for social gaffes resulting from their failure to foresee the consequences of their actions or their inability to take another's point of view. At times social interaction difficulties may be the presenting complaint in a doctor's office. For more information on the causes of poor social skills, see Chapter 11 on differential diagnosis.

Such social concerns have led many teachers and counsellors to try to develop curricula and intervention programs to address social skills.(10)(11)(12) Unfortunately, many social skills training programs have not had long-term benefits because students fail to generalize their skills from the classroom, group room, or counsellor's office to the real world of the playground, school bus, or lunch room. The best and most successful programs are those that follow up teaching of specific skills with attempts to practice using those skills in other settings, with the hope that generalization will occur. These successes present a strong argument for doing such teaching at school, where there are ample opportunities for students to try out specific strategies.

For some children whose diagnosis lies on the autism spectrum, the problem with peers may be the primary concern. More intense and specialized programming is needed which takes into account the deficits in reciprocal social interaction, language disorder, and behavioural rigidities, as well as factoring in the child's cognitive level and any developmental or psychiatric co-morbidities. Such programs are beyond the scope of this manual.

SUMMARY

- Look for cognitive and regulation factors underlying the behavioural difficulties, so that you can treat them or make referrals.
- For discipline, remember that the emphasis is on the parent-child relationship and teaching positive skills, with parents spending a smaller proportion of time on identifying misbehaviour.
- Children with severe explosive outbursts may require help from a mental health professional and sometimes medication, and require caregivers to prioritize what issues to insist on, provide empathy (and sometimes help in calming the children down), and teach problem-solving.
- When helping parents with a behaviour modification or rewards program, refer to this chapter for principles, tips for setting up a program, and causes of poor efficacy.
- Self-esteem is a product of feeling valued by others and having a sense of true accomplishment; children with school problems are at risk

for poor self-esteem, and measures to improve self-esteem may prevent depression.

- Parents of children with ADHD, oppositional, and defiant behaviour may be helped by group parenting courses run by mental health professionals. Many parents respond not only to the formal aspects of such programs but also to the informal peer support offered by other parents. Health facilities and tertiary referral centres are likely to have information as to what is available in a given location.

RESOURCES

American Academy of Pediatrics. <www.aap.org>

Centre for ADHD Awareness Canada (CADDAC). <www.caddac.ca>

Canadian ADHD Research Alliance (CADDRA). <www.caddra.ca>

Caring for Kids, the Canadian Paediatric Society's website, has resources for parents on positive discipline, self-esteem, and behaviour. <www.caringforkids.cps.ca>

The Incredible Years. <www.incredibleyears.com>

National Initiative for Children's Healthcare Quality. <www.nichq.org>

Triple P Positive Parenting Program. <www9.triplep.net>

Community Parent Education Services (COPE). <www.mcmasterchildrenshospital.ca/body.cfm?id=189>

REFERENCES

1. Lillas C, Turnbull, J. Infant/Child Mental Health, Early Intervention, and Relationship-Based Therapies—A Neurorelational Framework for Interdisciplinary Practice. New York: Interdisciplinary Training Institute LLC and Janiece Turnbull, 2009.

2. Mindell JA, Owens JA. A Clinical Guide to Pediatric Sleep: Diagnosis and Management of Sleep Problems, 2nd Edition. Philadelphia PA: Lippincott Williams & Wilkins, 2010.

3. Webster-Stratton C. The Incredible Years: A Trouble-Shooting Guide for Parents of Children Aged 2–8 Years. Seattle WA: Incredible Years, 2005.

4. Tidmarsh L. If I shouldn't spank, what should I do? Behavioural techniques for disciplining children. Can Fam Physician 2000; 46: 1119–23.

5. Barkley R. Taking Charge of ADHD: The Complete Authoritative Guide for Parents. New York: Guilford Press, 2005: 253–5.

6. Phelan TW. 1-2-3 Magic: Effective Discipline for Children 2–12. Glen Ellyn IL: Child Management, 1995.

7. Greene RW. The Explosive Child: A New Approach for Understanding and Parenting Easily Frustrated, Chronically Inflexible Children. New York: Harper, 2005.

8. Op. cit. Reference 7 (Greene).

9. Barkley R. Defiant Children: A Clinician's Manual for Assessment and Parent Training, 2nd Edition. New York: Guilford Press, 1997.

10. McGinnis E, Goldstein AP. Skillstreaming in Early Childhood: Teaching Prosocial Skills to the Preschool and Kindergarten Child. Champaign IL: Research Press, 1990.

11. McGinnis E, Goldstein AP, Sprafkin RP, et al. Skillstreaming in the Elementary School Child: A Guide for Teaching Prosocial Skills. Champaign IL: Research Press, 1984.

12. Goldstein AP, Sprafkin RP, Gershaw NJ, et al. Skillstreaming and the Adolescent: A Structured Learning Approach to Teaching Prosocial Skills. Champaign IL: Research Press, 1980.

15

Medical Management

Brenda Clark and Debra Andrews

In this chapter we present information and recommendations for managing medical conditions in children with school learning problems, with a focus on ADHD medication, as this is the most common reason for physician involvement in the management of this population. It is important to realize that this is not the only physician role, nor is it necessarily the most important. Physicians can and should be involved in assessment, and should be primarily responsible for any medical conditions affecting school performance, both directly (e.g., ADHD) and indirectly (e.g., disordered sleep due to obstructive sleep apnea). Depending on experience, physicians may choose to be involved in activities like counselling and program planning (see Chapters 13 and 14 on educational and behaviour management), and because of their ongoing relationships with families and children, their contributions to care are often highly valued by both the parents and the school learning team.

THE ROLE OF MEDICATIONS IN MANAGING CHILDREN WITH SCHOOL PROBLEMS

Prescribing medication is a familiar role for physicians, and it is tempting when seeing a child who is struggling to want to do something therapeutic for that child, particularly when there is good evidence for medication efficacy and safety. However, many parents and professionals are very concerned about the use of medications for conditions like ADHD, and it is imperative that they are used appropriately. Before you pull out the prescription pad, ask yourself the following questions:

- **Does the child have a symptom for which there is a known pharmacological treatment?** ADHD, anxiety, depressed or labile mood, aggression, sleep disturbance, and tics are examples of symptoms for which there are effective medications. Reading and math disabilities, global and specific developmental delays, and poor social interaction, to cite a few examples, do not have medications that will treat or cure them, and are appropriately treated using other interventions.

- **Do the medications I am considering have established efficacy and safety in children? Are they approved uses or off-label? How comfortable am I with off-label prescription?** Many behavioural medications used in children are off-label; that is, there is no established clinical practice guideline for their use, or they may be listed as not approved for use in children under a certain age. Most primary care providers for whom school learning and behaviour problems are not a regular part of their practice should follow established guidelines and seek consultation for more complex conditions.

The rest of this chapter focuses on well-established and commonly used medical interventions, and primarily on the use of stimulant medication for ADHD.

USE OF MEDICATION FOR ADHD

The diagnosis and management of ADHD in children is challenging for primary care physicians due to the limited time they have to address the complexity of clinical presentations, the time needed to counsel and support the family, and the need for long-term multimodal team efforts to achieve successful outcomes. Access to school and community personnel and mental health supportive services to provide continuous coordinated care can become the biggest barriers to successful management. The Canadian ADHD Resource Alliance (CADDRA) has recently published the 2011 version of the Canadian Practice Guidelines for management of ADHD.(1) As well, in November 2011, the American Academy of Pediatrics (AAP) published clinical practice guidelines along with supplemental information for the "process-of-care" algorithm to guide the recognition, evaluation, diagnosis, and treatment of ADHD as a continuous process.(2)(3) Both guidelines provide a broad consensus of recommended practice, along with a review of the literature and resources to guide the process. The AAP guidelines also include levels of evidence for all recommendations. The next sections of this chapter provide a summary of the information presented in these documents. It should be recognized that some of the differences between the two sets of guidelines may reflect a referral bias and different levels of evidence: paediatricians often see mild to moderate ADHD, while child psychiatrists are more likely to be referred the children with more severe problems and more co-morbidity. Please access the full documents noted in the references at the end of this chapter for further information.

Deciding to do a medication trial

In ADHD, as with other developmental conditions, approach to intervention must be comprehensive and highly individualized. Although stimulant medication has the best evidence for efficacy with the core symptoms of ADHD (inattention, impulsivity, and hyperactivity), intensive behavioural approaches improve associated symptoms, such as oppositional behaviour and homework completion, and current recommendations are to use a combined approach (4)(5)(6). Whether and when to start medication is a complex decision. The following issues should be taken into consideration:

- **Has a complete workup been done so that the diagnoses are clear? Have causes of inattention that are not appropriately treated by medication been ruled out?** A complete workup does not necessarily mean a tertiary team assessment; it simply means that inattention has been present over a period of time and has been confirmed by reliable observers and that the differential diagnosis of attention difficulties has been reviewed as it applies to this particular child.

- **Is a treatment plan that addresses all aspects of the child's learning difficulties in place?** Medication should be thought of as a part of a complete treatment plan, and it should not stand alone. Concerns relating to expectations that medication will solve all the problems so that nothing else needs to be done are legitimate. However, this does not mean that medication should wait until all other options have been exhausted.

- **How severe are the ADHD symptoms? Does the child respond to one-on-one instruction, a structured setting, and behavioural measures, or are symptoms so pervasive that the child will have difficulty even in the best of settings and under the best of circumstances?** How a child performs in a one-on-one situation during the sampling of skills may give some indication of the likelihood of response to behavioural interventions in the school. The severity of symptoms as measured by behavioural rating scales is also a helpful indicator. Safety issues where there is a risk of injury to the child (e.g., near-miss pedestrian traffic accidents) or other children and staff (e.g., impulsively throwing furniture or sharp objects like scissors) creates urgency for immediate intervention with a combination of medical and behavioural management.

The degree of functional impairment and the period of daytime coverage required will need to be determined. Some children, generally those with inattentive type ADHD and no behavioural co-morbidity, only need coverage for the school hours, but others with moderate-to-severe ADHD require continuous day and evening coverage to succeed at daily routines, homework, and evening activities. For teens, the issue of symptom coverage when they are driving is an important consideration, as there is evidence that their driving skills are improved when they are taking their medication. The goal of treatment is symptom reduction and better quality of life, but physicians also need to take into account patient concerns and family preferences.

- **What associated behavioural difficulties is the child having? Is there aggression or defiant behaviour? Are there mood and anxiety issues?** The more serious the rule infractions, the sooner the need for intensive intervention, because there is evidence that once children with continuing conduct disorder or oppositional defiant disorder reach their teens, management becomes increasingly difficult.

   When there is a co-morbid disorder present, it is important to prioritize the key symptoms before making a medication choice. It is generally advised that the treatment should address the more severe disorder first; the CADDRA guidelines suggest that depression, bipolar disorders, and substance abuse disorder should be identified and treated prior to ADHD.(7) Referral to a child psychiatrist, developmental paediatrician, or ADHD specialty clinic would be appropriate if there are concerns about a co-morbid diagnosis.

- **What has been tried so far and what has been the response?** Many parents are extremely uncomfortable with medication use and would prefer to do almost anything (even in some cases try expensive and/or untested "treatments" with no proven efficacy) to avoid medication. If parents have reviewed what has not helped and have come to the conclusion that medicine should be tried, they are much more likely to be compliant with its use. (See also the section about enhancing compliance later in this chapter.)

- **Is the child at a relatively stable point in the school year and not in the midst of any significant transitions? Are there any major programming changes that are going to be occurring in the near future?** Transition points are poor times for medication trials because the behavioural baseline is unstable, and it may be difficult to determine whether changes in behaviour following institution of medication are due to the medication or to some other factor.

If the child starts medication and switches into a new program at school, it is hard to know if it was the medication or the new program or a combination of the two that made the difference. The very beginning and the end of the school year are also bad times for a medication trial, as is the month of December (with the upcoming holidays). Of course, if serious behavioural problems have escalated, there may not be the option of trying to tease out the effects of individual components of intervention, and several therapeutic manoeuvres may need to be tried at the same time.

- **Are the parents ready?** Although medication is the most efficacious treatment option for ADHD and should be offered when the diagnosis is made, many parents are not prepared to start medication right away. Parents must feel that they have sufficient time and information to weigh risks and benefits and make an informed choice for their child. They must feel that all aspects of the child's safety and well-being are being addressed—all possible side effects have been reviewed, and a plan for dealing with any problems is put in place. They must not feel coerced or forced, or the medication trial will inevitably fail. Some parents will elect not to proceed, and physicians must continue to support these parents, provide other evidence-based suggestions,(8)–(13) and monitor the child's progress.

Choosing a medication

Age considerations and individual variation

Preschool children

New recommendations have expanded the age range of the use of stimulants for ADHD to include preschool children (aged four to five years), and this raises a number of issues to consider. Physicians may struggle with the diagnosis and management of young children who demonstrate significant behaviours of hyperactivity, impulsivity, and inattention, as the DSM-IV criteria have not typically been applied to this group. There is a wide range of what one could consider "normal" in terms of hyperactive and impulsive behaviours in preschoolers. It may be difficult to obtain reliable, unbiased reports of child behaviours and functioning, as many young children have not had opportunity to participate in structured activities outside the home.

Research in the medical management of young children with moderate-to-severe ADHD is limited, but suggests many young children four to five years of age will have improvement of symptoms with behaviour therapy alone.

Focused checklists can help physicians in diagnostic evaluation, and the Conners Comprehensive Behavior Rating Scale and the SNAP-IV are scales that have been validated in the preschool child. When there is clear history of significant behaviour problems causing functional impairment, current recommendations suggest these children should have evidence-based parent- and/or teacher-administered behaviour therapy as the first line of treatment. If the behaviour interventions do not provide significant improvement, and there is moderate to severe disturbance in the child's function, then methylphenidate may be used (action statement 5, AAP guidelines).(14) The criteria for severe symptoms include symptoms that have persisted for at least nine months; dysfunction that is manifested in both the home and other settings such as preschool or daycare; and dysfunction that has not responded adequately to behaviour therapy. The behaviours that indicate severity outlined in the AAP's guidelines supplemental information include ejections from mainstream preschool, nursery, or daycare; significant risk of injury to self, peers, or adults; suspected CNS injury; behaviours interfering with treatment; or significant family stress as a result of the behaviours.(15) It is important to consider the child's developmental profile, safety risks, and the consequences of the behaviour for school and social participation when looking at the treatment options.

As the rate of metabolizing stimulant medication is slower in this age group, it is even more important to start with a lower dose and use smaller increments. It is appropriate for the treatment of a preschool child to be under the direction of a specialist such as a child psychiatrist or developmental paediatrician.

Adolescents

As the DSM-V will increase the latest age at onset of symptoms causing impairment to twelve years, new recommendations have expanded the age range of medical management to include adolescents through to eighteen years of age. There is no maximum age to treat ADHD. Physicians need to consider the special circumstances posed by this age group when implementing medical treatment programs. Youth in this age group often have multiple teachers from various programs, and each teacher may have little contact time for structured observations of the student. It may be difficult to get information from other community program sources related to behaviour and function. It is even more of a challenge when the target symptoms are related to inattention and organization rather than hyperactivity and motor restlessness. Youth may minimize problem behaviours on self-reports, and their observations may differ from those of adults. Parents need to be informed that untreated adolescents with ADHD are at greater risk of substance abuse, increased risky sexual behaviours, automobile accidents and traffic infractions, and co-morbid diagnoses such as anxiety and depression. Medication coverage should be planned with regard to the times of day when high-risk activities are more likely to occur.

Medication trials

Each child is unique and will respond better or display more adverse effects to one over another preparation. These effects cannot be determined ahead of time, and therefore a "trial" is needed. Individual patient response is known to vary widely, and each patient has a different risk/benefit profile, ranging from those who cannot tolerate or benefit from medication at all to those who have complete remission of symptoms with no side effects.

There is clear evidence for psychostimulants as first-line medication, and the various practice guidelines are consistent in suggesting that a second stimulant be tried if there is insufficient response to the first stimulant tried.

If the child does not respond to stimulant medications, then atomoxetine (Strattera) or second-line medications can be used to augment treatment.(16)

Other off-label second-line medications such as buproprion, clonidine, guanfacine, modafinil, or imipramine may be helpful, but a referral to a child psychiatrist or a developmental paediatrician should be made in these cases. These medications are only used in the treatment of ADHD when first- and second-line choices are not effective, associated with unacceptable side effects, or contraindicated.

Length of trial

Although effects of stimulant medications can be seen almost immediately, there are two reasons for suggesting a minimum three-week trial. First, this helps eliminate a placebo effect, often caused by the hopes and expectations of the parents, teacher, and child that things will be getting better. Conversely, more side effects may be reported in the first weeks. This may be because some anxious parents may be very focused on watching for possible problems, or a concern might be one of the true side effects, which often improve over time, e.g., rebound irritability.

Start low; go slow

This old adage is as useful with stimulants as it is for many other psychotropic medications. If you overshoot the initial dose and the child has a significant side effect, you may lose the parents' trust. As well, the individual response to these medications varies widely and can't be predicted. It is wise to start with a dose below what you expect will be the maintenance dose and titrate upwards. Do not make rapid dosage changes; in general, allow a week between increases. Use questionnaires to monitor treatment effects, and stop when the child's symptoms are below the cut-off for the clinical range. Use the child's real response to stimulant medications and not a theoretical dosage as your guide. Atomoxetine has stricter guidelines for dosing titrations.

In general with stimulants, making changes no more frequently than once a week gives adequate observation time to decide if the change really has made a difference. Changes in behaviour in response to the dose change may often be seen over a much shorter period of time; however, other, often undefined, factors may affect behaviour. Therefore, too short an observation period may give a false picture. With longer-acting medications such as atomoxetine,

you need to wait longer because it may take several weeks before definite clinical effects can be seen. With atomoxetine, it is necessary to titrate the dose to avoid side effects.

Long- versus short-acting preparations

In general, long-acting stimulants are preferred for smoothness of action and ease in compliance in long-term use, and these medications are the basis of both the paediatric and child psychiatry clinical practice guidelines, although there is no clear evidence to support this. Long-acting stimulants vary in overall duration of action and in the proportions of the immediate release and sustained release components, addressing symptoms in the morning and afternoon respectively. Consider the time of day when the attention problems are greatest in making your choice of preparation.

For many younger or smaller children, even the lowest dosage of a long-acting stimulant is too strong for them, and short-acting medication must be used. As well, for some older children who are slow to metabolize, the length of action of a once-a-day stimulant may be too long for that child, extending into the dinner hour and affecting appetite for the evening meal, or even further to the child's bedtime and inhibiting sleep. Insomnia affects attention and is counterproductive to what you are trying to achieve with the medication. Resist the temptation to treat the insomnia with another medication, and focus your efforts on optimizing the timing and dose of the stimulant whenever you can.

In using short-acting stimulant medication, try as much as possible to adapt the medication schedule to provide coverage when the child most needs it. For most children, regular-release methylphenidate takes about half an hour to begin to be effective and lasts three to four hours. Keeping this in mind, you can consider when peak effects will be most helpful to determine the timing of the morning dose. Timing of the next dose depends on the clinical half-life of the medication for that child. Ideally, the mid-day dose should be given before the morning dose has worn off completely, thus avoiding a period in the late morning (often, unfortunately, morning recess) when efficacy is waning and ADHD symptoms recur.

In considering whether a late-afternoon dose of short-acting stimulant is required, review exactly what the child does after school and how much trouble the child is having, not only with the targeted behaviour problems but with side effects such as appetite suppression, sleep disturbance, rebound hyperactivity, and irritability. If the child has homework or structured activities such as lessons or tutoring, medication may be beneficial at those times. A smaller, late-afternoon dose may help extend positive drug effects without interfering with the evening meal or the night's sleep.

For some children, a combination of sustained-release and regular stimulant provides the best coverage, the regular preparation giving a quick onset of action in the morning, and the sustained-release smoothing over the mid-day transition period. Coming up with a schedule that best fits the child may take several weeks, with frequent telephone communication being essential.

Templates for documenting progress of symptoms as well as the side effects of medications are available in the CADDRA Tool Kit available on their website at www.caddra.ca.(16)

Choosing a specific medication

All Health Canada-approved stimulant medications are methylphenidate- or amphetamine-based compounds. They all have a similar profile of effects and side effects with a long history of efficacy and safety. The CADDRA guidelines and the AAP Clinical Practice Guideline Supplemental Appendix have listed the approved stimulant and non-stimulant medications for ADHD.(17)(18)(19) Some medications in the US guidelines are not available in Canada. The CADDRA guidelines are specific to medications that are available in Canada.(20) The CADDRA ADHD medication charts are reproduced in Tables 15–1 and 15–2, and additional information is available on the CADDRA website. The charts provide the latest information on the classes, dosage, titration suggestions, and appearance of ADHD medications, along with photographs that are useful when discussing medication options, as you can show parents what the pills look like. If a parent forgets the name of the child's medication when you are obtaining the

history, you can use the photos showing the colour and size of the medication to help them identify the preparation.

Dextroamphetamine is the only medication approved for use in children younger than six years of age, but there is little research to support the efficacy and safety in this age group. There has been one large prospective multi-centre study that looked at the effects of methylphenidate on young children aged three to five years showing some reduction in symptoms.(21) If the clinical symptoms include anxiety or mood concerns along with ADHD, or the family has a strong preference against stimulant medication, then a non-stimulant medication may be considered before a trial of stimulants.

Some children may experience difficulty with swallowing pills. Although many children can be trained to do this, there are always a few who can't swallow a pill or tablet, limiting treatment choices. Some of the long-acting preparations can be sprinkled on food without changes in the duration of effects (Dexedrine spansule, Biphentin, Adderall). Some preparations can be crushed or dissolved in water. If regular-release stimulants are accidentally bitten by the child, this will not affect efficacy. Regular-release tablets can also be crushed.

Atomoxetine is a selective norepinephrine-reuptake inhibitor and it may take four to six weeks to evaluate its effectiveness. Symptom change is more gradual than with stimulant medications, so parents need to be aware of the difference. Atomoxetine may be considered as the first choice for ADHD in individuals with an active substance abuse problem, co-morbid anxiety, or tics. Side effects of atomoxetine include somnolence, poor appetite, and gastrointestinal symptoms, especially early on in treatment, so only half the treatment dose is given for the first week. Liver dysfunction is a rare side effect, but this discussion needs to be included in the consent for the medication and a process of monitoring needs to be developed.

Alpha-adrenergic agonists include clonidine and guanfacine, which also have long-acting preparations available in the United States. Patients may experience a dry mouth or somnolence, and the maximum effects are also delayed at two to four weeks. These medications need to be tapered over one to two weeks when discontinued to avoid possible rebound in blood pressure.

Further specific information on medications used to treat ADHD can be found in the supporting documents on the CADDRA website.

Table 15–1 Medical Treatment for Uncomplicated ADHD in Children

Brand name (active chemical)	Dosage form	Starting dose	Titration schedule every 7 days		Maximum per day[1] (up to 40 kg child)	
			Per product monograph	Per CADDRA board	Per product monograph	Per CADDRA board*
FIRST-LINE AGENTS – long-acting preparations						
Adderall XR® (amphetamine mixed salts)	5, 10, 15, 20, 25, 30 mg cap	5-10 mg q.d. a.m.	↑5-10 mg	↑5 mg	30 mg	30 mg
Biphentin® (methylphenidate HCl)	10, 15, 20, 30, 40, 50, 60, 80 mg cap	10-20 mg q.d. a.m.	↑10 mg	↑10 mg	60 mg	60 mg
Concerta® (methylphenidate HCl)	18, 27, 36, 54 mg tab	18 mg q.d. a.m.	↑18 mg	↑18 mg	54 mg	72 mg
Strattera® (atomoxetine)	10, 18, 25, 40, 60, 80, 100 mg cap	0.5 mg/kg/day	Maintain dose for a min. of 7-14 days before adjusting to 0.8 mg/kg/day then 1.2 mg/kg/day	Maintain dose for a min. of 7-14 days before adjusting to 0.8 mg/kg/day then 1.2 mg/kg/day	lesser of 1.4 mg/kg/day or 60 mg/day	lesser of 1.4 mg/kg/day or 60 mg/day
Vyvanse® (lisdexamfetamine dimesylate)	20, 30, 40, 50, 60 mg cap	20-30 mg q.d. a.m.	By clinical discretion	↑10 mg	60 mg	60 mg

CB * Doses per CADDRA Board that are over product monograph maximum doses should be considered off-label use. A consensus decision has been made based on clinical use and research data.

SECOND-LINE/ADJUNCTIVE AGENTS – short-acting and intermediate-acting preparations

CB **Indications for use:** a) p.r.n. for particular activities; b) to augment long-acting formulations early or late in the day, or early in the evening and c) when LA agents are cost prohibitive. To augment Adderall XR® or Vyvanse®, short-acting and intermediate-acting dextro-amphetamine products can be used. To augment Biphentin® or Concerta® short-acting MPH products can be used. b.i.d. refers to qam and qnoon and t.i.d. refers to qam, qnoon, and q4pm.

Brand name (active chemical)	Dosage form	Starting dose	Titration schedule every 7 days		Maximum per day	
Dexedrine® (dextro-amphetamine sulphate)	5 mg tab	2.5-5 mg b.i.d.	↑2.5-5 mg	↑2.5-5 mg	40 mg	20 mg
Dexedrine® Spansule[2] (dextro-amphetamine sulphate)	10, 15 mg cap	10 mg q.d. a.m.	↑5 mg	↑5 mg	40 mg	30 mg
Ritalin® (methylphenidate)	10, 20 mg tab	5 mg b.i.d. to t.i.d.	↑5-10	↑5-10	60 mg	60 mg
Ritalin® SR[3] (methylphenidate HCl)	20 mg tab	20 mg q.d. a.m.	↑20 mg	↑20 mg	60 mg	60 mg

[1] The maximum daily dose can be split into once daily (q.d.), twice daily (b.i.d.) or three times daily (t.i.d.) doses except for once a day formulations

[2] Dexedrine® Spansule may last 6-8 hours

[3] Ritalin® SR may help cover the noon period but clinical experience suggests an effect similar to short-acting preparations. An increased dose could be spread out to include q2pm dose with a daily maximum of 60 mg.

Source: The Canadian ADHD Resource Alliance (CADDRA). Canadian ADHD Practice Guidelines, version October 2011. Reproduced with permission. Refer to www.caddra.ca for updates.

(Continued)

Table 15–1 Medical Treatment for Uncomplicated ADHD in Children (continued)

Brand name *(active chemical)*	Dosage form	Starting dose	Titration schedule every 7 days		Maximum per day (up to 40 kg child)	
			Per product monograph	Per CADDRA board	Per product monograph	Per CADDRA board
GENERIC MEDICATIONS						
PMS® or **Ratio®-** **methylphenidate**	5, 10, 20, mg tab	5 mg q.d. a.m. and noon	⬆ 5 mg (add q4pm dose)	⬆ 5 mg	60 mg	60 mg
Novo-MPH ER-C® *(methylphenidate)*	18, 27, 36, 54 mg tab	18 mg q.d. a.m.	⬆18 mg	⬆18 mg	54 mg	72 mg
THIRD-LINE AGENTS						
These medications (impramine, buproprion, modafinil, etc.) should be initially or first prescribed only by a specialist. These are off-label products and described only in the members section of the CADDRA website.						

Source: The Canadian ADHD Resource Alliance (CADDRA). Canadian ADHD Practice Guidelines, version October 2011. Reproduced with permission. Refer to www.caddra.ca for updates.

Managing side effects

All medications may cause side effects, but most of these improve over two to three weeks of continuous use. The most common side effects of stimulant medications are appetite loss, abdominal pain, headaches, and sleep disturbance. It has been observed that stimulants cause slight but clinically insignificant increases in heart rate and blood pressure.(22) Some children may experience mood lability and dysphoria, but hallucinations and other psychotic symptoms are uncommon. Some pre-existing conditions such as tics, sleep disorder, headaches, GI symptoms, low weight gain, or dysphoria may be aggravated by ADHD medications. However, some pre-existing symptoms such as headache and sleep disorder may also improve on treatment.

Those who experience major side effects that cannot be managed by adjusting the dose or timing of medication should be switched to a different stimulant. If side effects persist, the second-line options can be considered. Those who continue to have persisting side effects or who do not respond to any medication may require ongoing behavioural management at home and at school. A referral to a child psychiatrist or developmental paediatrician is indicated in these cases. Parents need to be aware of the risks associated with taking their child off

medication during the weekend and vacation periods. Their participation in the treatment process is very important.

Dysphoria and rebound

Dysphoria and emotional flattening in the middle of the day are often related to the dose. Older patients should be advised about how to recognize if they might be on too high a dose, such as feeling "wired," irritable, or "too serious" during peak drug periods. This side effect may subside over time, but if it persists, the dose should be decreased.

If the feelings of dysthymia (crying and irritability) occur later when the medication should be wearing off, the child is likely experiencing the "crashing" rebound effects of quickly decreasing drug levels. Children may also demonstrate rebound hyperactivity with exacerbation of ADHD symptoms in the afternoon when the dosage is wearing off, so that the child is fine at school but becomes unmanageable at home. Both of these issues are often addressed by either choosing the longer-acting stimulants, which wear off more gradually, or by giving a small afternoon dose of a short-acting stimulant as a "taper-off dose." Some children may develop this dysphoria after being on the medication for three to four months.

Cardiovascular risk

Stimulant medications have generally been considered safe, although reports of adverse events—including cases of sudden death, myocardial infarction, and stroke—have raised levels of public concern. All medications for the treatment of ADHD are

Table 15–2 Medical Treatment for Uncomplicated ADHD in Adolescents

Brand name (active chemical)	Dosage form	Starting dose	Titration schedule every 7 days		Maximum per day[1,2] (>40 kg)	
			Per product monograph	Per CADDRA board	Per product monograph	Per CADDRA board*
FIRST-LINE AGENTS – long-acting preparations						
Adderall XR® (amphetamine mixed salts)	5, 10, 15, 20, 25, 30 mg cap	5-10 mg q.d. am	↑ 5-10 mg	↑ 5-10 mg	20-30 mg	50 mg
Biphentin® (methylphenidate HCl)	10, 15, 20, 30, 40 50, 60, 80 mg cap	10-20 mg q.d. am	↑ 10 mg	↑ 10 mg	60 mg	80 mg[3]
Concerta® (methylphenidate HCl)	18, 27, 36, 54 mg tab	18 mg q.d. am	↑ 18 mg	↑ 18 mg	54 mg	90 mg (54 + 36 mg)
Strattera® (atomoxetine)	10, 18, 25, 40, 60, 80 100 mg cap	0.5 mg/kg/day	Maintain dose for a min. of 7-14 days before adjusting 0.8 mg/kg/day then 1.2 mg/kg/day for patients <70kg[4]	Maintain dose for a min. of 7-14 days before adjusting 0.8 mg then 1.2 mg; 70kg: 60 then 80mg/day[4]	lesser of 1.4 mg/kg/day or 100 mg/day	lesser of 1.4 mg/kg/day or 100 mg/day
Vyvanse® (lisdexamfetamine dimesylate)	20, 30, 40, 50, 60, mg cap	20-30 mg q.d. am	By clinical discretion	↑ 10 mg	60 mg	70 mg

CB * Doses per CADDRA Board that are over product monograph maximum doses should be considered off-label use. A consensus decision has been made based on clinical use and research data.

SECOND-LINE/ADJUNCTIVE AGENTS – short-acting and intermediate-acting preparations

CB **Indications for use:** a) p.r.n. for particular activities; b) to augment long-acting formulations early or late in the day, or early in the evening and c) when LA agents are cost prohibitive. To augment Adderall XR® or Vyvanse®, short-acting and intermediate-acting dextro-amphetamine products can be used. To augment Biphentin® or Concerta® short-acting MPH products can be used. b.i.d. refers to qam and qnoon and t.i.d. refers to qam, qnoon, and q4pm.

Brand name (active chemical)	Dosage form	Starting dose	Per product monograph	Per CADDRA board	Per product monograph	Per CADDRA board*
Dexedrine® (dextro-amphetamine sulphate)	5 mg tab	2.5-5 mg b.i.d.	↑ 5 mg	↑ 5 mg	40 mg	30 mg
Dexedrine® Spansule[5] (dextro-amphetamine sulphate)	10, 15 mg cap	10 mg q.d. a.m.	↑ 5 mg	↑ 5 mg	40 mg	30 mg
Ritalin® (methylphenidate HCl)	10, 20 mg tab	5 mg b.i.d. to t.i.d.	↑ 5-10 mg	↑ 5-10 mg	60 mg	60 mg
Ritalin® SR[6] (methylphenidate HCl)	20 mg tab	20 mg q.d. am	↑ 20 mg (add q2pm dose)	↑ 20 mg (add q2pm dose)	60 mg	80 mg

[1] Maximum off label doses have been published in the AACAP Practice Parameters[14] but the off label maximums are either the same or lower in the CAP-G based on CB

[2] The maximum daily dose can be split into once daily (q.d.), twice daily (b.i.d.) or three times daily (t.i.d.) doses except for once a day formulations

[3] While the theoretical maximum off label dose for Biphentin® could be 100 mg, clinical practice currently suggests that 80 mg is the maximum that is used

[4] For adolescents greater than 70 kg, use the adult dose titration schedule

[5] Dexedrine Spansule® may last 6-8 hours

[6] Ritalin SR® may help cover the noon period but clinical experience suggests an effect similar to short-acting preparations.

Source: The Canadian ADHD Resource Alliance (CADDRA). Canadian ADHD Practice Guidelines, version October 2011. Reproduced with permission. Refer to www.caddra.ca for updates.

(Continued)

Table 15–2   Medical Treatment for Uncomplicated ADHD in Adolescents (continued)

Brand name (active chemical)	Dosage form	Starting dose	Titration schedule every 7 days		Maximum per day*	
			Per product monograph	Per CADDRA board	Per product monograph	Per CADDRA board
GENERIC MEDICATIONS						
PMS® or Ratio®-methylphenidate	5, 10, 20, mg tab	5 mg q.d. a.m. and noon	↑ 5 mg	↑ 5 mg	60 mg	60 mg
			(add q4pm dose)			
Novo-MPH ER-C® (methylphenidate)	18, 27, 36, 54 mg tab	18 mg q.d. a.m.	↑ 18 mg	↑ 18 mg	54 mg	90 mg

THIRD LINE AGENTS
These medications (impramine, buproprion, modafinil, etc.) should be initiated or first prescribed only by a specialist. These are off-label products and described only in the members section of the CADDRA website.

Source: The Canadian ADHD Resource Alliance (CADDRA). Canadian ADHD Practice Guidelines, version October 2011. Reproduced with permission. Refer to www.caddra.ca for updates.

sympathomimetic and have stimulatory effects on the sympathetic nervous system. According to a recent retrospective cohort study, there were 3.1 serious cardiovascular events per 100,000 person-years (adjusted hazard ratio, 0.75; 95% confidence interval [CI], 0.31 to 1.85).(23) These events are extremely rare, and there is no compelling clinical evidence to demonstrate that the likelihood of sudden death is higher in children receiving medications for ADHD than in that of the general population.(24) It is recommended that clinicians carefully assess all children by using a targeted cardiac history to include previously detected cardiac disease, palpitations, syncope, seizures; a family history of sudden death in children or young adults; hypertrophic cardiomyopathy; or long Q-T interval syndrome. ADHD medications should not be used if a patient has symptomatic heart disease, moderate to severe hypertension, advanced arteriosclerosis, or hyperthyroidism. They are generally not used in patients with known structural cardiac abnormalities. A physical examination, including a careful cardiac examination, should always be carried out prior to the initiation of medication with periodic evaluation of their cardiovascular status. If family history, patient history, or physical exam suggests cardiac disease, either before or during the medical trial, then further evaluation is indicated, with input from a paediatric cardiologist. Routine ECGs are not indicated for most children.(25)–(29)

In October 2011, Health Canada issued warnings about cardiovascular side effects with atomoxetine.(30) Approximately 25% of patients treated experience an increase of blood pressure of 10 mmHg and 5% to 8% an increase of 20 mmHg, while 33% of patients experience an increase in heart rate of 10 bpm and 12% by 20 bpm. These increases could represent a risk for some patients. Atomoxetine is contraindicated in patients with symptomatic cardiovascular diseases, cardiovascular disorders, and moderate/severe hypertension. It should be used with caution in patients with hypertension, tachycardia, cardiovascular disease, congenital or acquired long QT interval, or a family history of QT prolongation. Heart rate and blood pressure should be measured before starting treatment, after increasing the dose, and periodically to detect clinically important increases.

Suicide risk

There is a black-box warning on atomoxetine for the possibility of suicidal ideation, including thinking about self-harm and/or increasing agitation with the initiation of treatment. If there are concerns about suicidal ideation after treatment with atomoxetine, the parents should be instructed to notify the physician immediately, and further evaluation and reconsideration about the use of this medication is indicated. A referral to mental health services should be made.

Nutrition and appetite suppression

Stimulant medications can suppress appetite and lead to weight loss. Families can shift the timing of meals and food intake to a period when the effect of medication is wearing off. This usually means children will want to eat later in the day, especially for those on the longer-acting formulations. Parent and child education about the importance of good nutrition for learning and attention is an important part of ADHD follow-up care.

There is ongoing interest in the role of the stimulant effects of appetite suppression leading to poor nutrition and growth delay. The concern is greater in those with low weight, small stature, or picky eating habits. A recent study revealed persistent effects of stimulants on growth velocity in the range of 1 to 2 cm, especially in those given higher doses delivered on a consistent basis. Children who receive stimulant medication showed growth deceleration compared to those who did not for up to three years.(31) By the third year of treatment the effects diminished, and there was no rebound growth, so that children on stimulant medication may end up somewhat shorter than control children upon reaching maturity.(32)(33) The clinical significance of this is unclear, but parents need to be aware of the possibility. Parents may benefit from seeing the growth charts at each visit so they can be aware of any changes over time. They should be reassured that early weight loss usually stabilizes.

It is important to address the general nutrition of children on medications and provide families with information on the Canada Food Guide, along with supplemental strategies. Aim for three meals and three snacks daily. Teach children that their brain needs fuel to pay attention, and that skipping meals will not help them do well in school. Let the child engage in food selection and meal preparation, and encourage a solid breakfast high in protein. Switch to whole milk, and offer nutritious snacks that a child can graze on at times when appetite is decreased. Offer high-protein-/calorie drinks for lunch, and allow meals to be spread out during the evening when rebound appetite occurs. Children should be encouraged to eat when they are hungry, especially early in the morning and in the early evening. Gorging in the evening and midnight snacks should be discouraged, however.

Headaches

Headaches are a common side effect, occurring in approximately 3% of children. They tend to be tension headaches accompanied by nausea or gastric irritation that occur within the first two to three hours of taking the medication. The nausea is often addressed by giving the medication with food. Treatment includes mild analgesics and rest. Headaches usually disappear after one to three weeks. Occasionally they may lead to discontinuation of the medication, especially in children with pre-existing migraine or a family history of migraine.

Sleep problems

Problems with sleep should always be addressed with a careful sleep history and good sleep hygiene. A regular bedtime routine, even on weekends and holidays, and avoidance of caffeinated beverages and screen time after supper can go a long way to helping a child settle. Details related to the behavioural management of sleep are outlined in Chapter 14. As stimulants may induce insomnia in some children, it is important to administer medication as early as possible in the morning. If sleep continues to be a problem after adjusting dose timing and after putting into place appropriate sleep hygiene measures, consider melatonin treatment, which has demonstrated efficacy. Melatonin at a dose of 3 to 6 mg can be administered at least thirty minutes (up to two to three hours) before the desired bedtime. There is no information available on the long-term safety and efficacy of melatonin use in children.(34)

Use of drug holidays

Parents often ask whether the child should take medication on weekends and over extended breaks from school. With our growing appreciation of

ADHD as a chronic condition with executive functioning and emotional dysregulation that affect many areas of life, there has been a move toward continuing medication seven days a week for children whose symptoms are severe and interfere with functioning in all settings. However, we have also become more aware of potential effects on growth over the long term.(35) In addition, there are the issues of managing the common side effects which, while not medically serious, still affect quality of life and are frequently cited as the reason that so many parents choose to discontinue medication(36)(37), even when it is still effective for ADHD symptoms.

Little in the current medical literature exists to guide physicians with regard to the issue of taking time off medication.(38) Most of the research has focused on the issue of linear growth with the statement that the small decrease in long-term height attainment is not clinically significant and that the increased risks of not treating children with significant ADHD symptomatology shift the risk-benefit in favour of a seven-day schedule.(39)–(42) Children with severe hyperactivity and impulsivity might be more at risk for injuries (to themselves and others) off medication, and in these children it has been recommended that medication be given daily.(43) For children with milder and/or primarily inattentive type ADHD, the picture is less clear-cut, and a recent double-blind study demonstrated some benefit of weekends off medication, especially with regard to managing other side effects (anorexia, insomnia) without worsening of teacher-reported ADHD symptoms on return to school on Mondays.(44) At this point in time, evaluating the risks and benefits for each child in the face of the child's type and severity of ADHD symptoms and side effects seems to be the most prudent approach.

Enhancing compliance

Noncompliance with psychoactive medications is frequent.(45)(46) Many parents and teachers have strong prejudices against their use, often based on misinformation from the Internet and various media, and amplified by well-intentioned but ill-informed friends and relatives. Many myths about methylphenidate arose when poor diagnosis, indiscriminate use, and high dosages were common. Ask the child's

caregivers what they have heard about medication; counter misinformation by demonstrating your knowledge of the medical literature regarding medication management. Be alert to information in the media about medication use, as discussion is needed whenever a parent raises concerns. Caregivers should feel you are being completely open with them. Sufficient appointment time must be made available for optimal information-sharing. This can be shortened if well-prepared patient education handouts are available; however, always be familiar with the content of any materials that you use.

The very idea of psychoactive drugs is frightening to many parents and even some professionals. Many people have strong moral convictions against their use, even though the same individuals may have no difficulty accepting a prescription for a much more toxic medication for a so-called "physical" ailment. People often shrink from the use of behavioural medications because of a deep-seated conviction that children "ought" to be capable of controlling themselves. In discussing ADHD medication with families, a comparison with diabetes may be helpful. People with very mild diabetes may be able to control symptoms with effort: they can watch their weight, diet, and exercise schedule. However, many diabetics have so little insulin that they cannot control their blood glucose until oral medication or insulin is added. One would never expect such persons to just "try harder" while denying them their medication. Many children with moderate to severe attention difficulties behave as though they have a neurotransmitter deficiency, so dramatic is their response to medication. As there is evidence for this mechanism, using this analogy not only helps change attitudes, it also provides the parents with a way of describing the medication's role to relatives and friends.

If the child's evaluation was initiated by the school, some parents may question the teacher's motives for the referral. Stories in the media about the overuse of ADHD medications may insinuate that medicine is being used to maintain classroom discipline or to save money on special education. It is not surprising that some parents feel a bit suspicious. In such cases, a physician may be looked upon as an objective outsider who will confirm or refute the suggestions of the teacher or other school personnel. Such parents are often skeptical of the teacher's objectivity in reporting on their child's behaviour before and after medication. Helpful strategies include having both parents and teachers complete behavioural rating scales and commenting on their consistency.

In general, teachers should be aware that a medication trial is taking place. Children might exhibit side effects (or overdose effects) such as sedation at school, which might otherwise be attributed to fatigue or illness. As well, some teachers feel affronted if they are blind to the initiation of drug therapy, and parent-teacher-physician communication can be adversely affected. There is some evidence that teachers' impressions can be influenced by placebo effects. If there are concerns about objectivity, a double-blind crossover trial can be done using placebos; none of the involved parties will know when the child is receiving the active drug, but all know that a trial is taking place.

Children may also have heard all sorts of things about medications from friends and relatives or media. Instead of stories and misinformation, children need to know what their medication is supposed to do and how it works. Using analogy and metaphor may help in explaining medicine's function to school-aged children. Many children are highly suggestible where possible side effects are concerned, and some may even conveniently report side effects to avoid taking medication. If you suspect that this may be the case for a particular child, be careful about discussing possible side effects in front of the child and document pre-existing symptoms and behaviours that could later be attributed to a medication side effect (e.g., headaches, irritability after school).

If parents feel unable to give consent for a medication trial at the first visit, consider giving them educational material and information on the medications to read and inviting them to return for further discussion. With separated or divorced parents with joint custody and decision-making, educational materials and the opportunity to return and discuss the medication decision should be provided to both parents, especially if one parent did not attend the initial visit. Although such

extra visits may seem time-consuming, there is a longer-term gain in improved compliance and a trusting physician-patient relationship, which will also lead to more efficient and effective follow-up visits down the line.

A final point to be emphasized to the parents and the child is that a trial is only a trial, not a commitment for life. If the medication is not beneficial, if the side effects are too troublesome and cannot be handled by dose adjustments—whenever the risks outweigh the benefits—the medication will be stopped and the child's symptoms reassessed. Set up a specific appointment time or schedule a telephone call to make a formal decision to continue or discontinue medication. Specifying a decision point ensures that medicine that is ineffective or causing significant side effects will not be given indefinitely.

Following a child on medication

The AAP clinical practice guidelines for the diagnosis, evaluation, and treatment of ADHD have recommended primary care clinicians should recognize ADHD as a chronic condition. This means two things:

- The condition will continue to cause symptoms and dysfunction over long periods of time, even into adulthood.
- Treatments will address symptoms and function but are not usually curative.

Physicians should consider children and adolescents with ADHD as having "special health care needs" (SHCN). Management should involve a regular physician responsible for long-term coordination of the child's health care needs and emerging medical concerns, otherwise known as a "medical home." Research indicates that treatments are not always sustained over time, and this places children with ADHD at risk for significant problems. A medical home with strong family-school partnerships provides bidirectional communication with family, school, and mental health clinicians involved.(47)(48)(49)

During the first year on medication, it is suggested that the child be seen every three months to measure weight, height, and blood pressure. This can later be decreased to two visits per year if the child has been doing well on a stable dosage with no side effects, and there are no other significant ongoing problems that need to be addressed. During these follow-up visits, compliance, side effects of medications, supports required, and recommendations for school programming can be reviewed. Regular visits are reassuring to parents, enhance compliance, and allow opportunities for the physician to provide anticipatory guidance. Long-term compliance with any medication is challenging. *Never assume a child is taking medication or that the dose and type are the same as what was recorded at the last visit.* Specifically review the name, dose, and times of administration; ask if medication has ever been forgotten and if so, how many times in the past month that has happened. Help parents to problem-solve why medication might be missed and suggest solutions (e.g., using a pill-minder or checking administration off on a calendar).

The points of view of the child, the parent, and the teacher should be sought, and, as with the initial history, this can be facilitated by the use of questionnaires, although follow-up questionnaires do not need to be as lengthy as the initial ones. The most recent report card and results of any interim testing are also helpful.

Physical examination for those children on medication may be limited to height, weight, vital signs, and a cardiac exam unless there are particular concerns. The physician may wish to do a repeat reading screen or obtain a writing sample or have the child draw a person for monitoring co-existing learning problems.

Discontinuing medication

Patients on medications for treatment and management of ADHD are advised not to discontinue medication before consulting with their physician. Most children with ADHD will continue to need medication to manage symptoms well into adolescence and adulthood. Although the hyperactivity may have subsided, we are now more aware of significant impairments in executive functions that continue into adolescence in two-thirds of patients.

Because many parents hope that ADHD will be outgrown and their long-term commitment to medication is often half-hearted, especially early in the course, medication use is best addressed one

academic year at a time. If the child has had a positive response to a medication trial, it should be continued for the rest of a school year, unless problems occur. Periodic efficacy checks should be made at appropriate times during the school year, avoiding the months of September and June and the weeks immediately before and after the winter and spring breaks, which are full of excitement and schedule changes. (Worsening of attention and behaviour at these times is very common, which complicates interpretation of the effects of any changes that are made in the child's medication regimen.) These efficacy checks frequently confirm the ongoing need for medication for parents (and teachers) and can enhance overall compliance.

For the one-third of children and youth with ADHD whose symptoms may indeed fall below the clinical cut-off in adolescence, you may consider taking the child off medication "for good" if:

- The child has had a prolonged period with no significant impairment from ADHD symptoms.
- There are well-developed compensatory skills that are demonstrably effective during a trial without medication.
- Child and parents are committed to monitoring ADHD symptoms over time.

TREATING ASSOCIATED MEDICAL CONDITIONS

Somatic complaints, bowel and bladder problems, and sleep disorders are very common among children with any kind of developmental disorder, including those presenting with school learning problems.

Headaches, abdominal pain, or limb pain, as identified during your medical assessment and not accompanied by any worrisome features or physical findings, usually do not need specific interventions, but they serve as a measure of the child's level of stress. They tend to improve when the source of the stress (e.g., the child's difficulty with reading) is appropriately addressed.

Encopresis with daytime soiling usually should be treated if the child is functioning at a cognitive level for which bowel continence would normally be expected, because soiling can be a major social disadvantage for a child who already may have difficulty fitting into a peer group. Both the child and the parents should be given an explanation of the causes of encopresis. A bowel cleanout, maintenance stool softeners, and a formal toileting regimen may then be instituted with a fair degree of success.

Children with attention problems may have a difficult time sitting on the toilet long enough to relax the sphincter and pass a stool. Setting up an interesting sedentary activity (such as reading or drawing if these are easy and pleasant for the child) with materials available in a basket or container in the bathroom may be helpful. Many children enjoy dot-to-dot activities, word-find puzzles, and hand-held electronic games. Use of a kitchen timer can be helpful. The child's compliance with the toileting regimen can be charted on a behavioural record sheet, and the child may be awarded stickers or points. The end point should not be success with a bowel movement but success with sitting, as that is often the limiting factor. Attention to the child's diet and use of stool softeners usually ensure that if the child sits long enough, he or she will pass whatever stool there is to pass.

Nocturnal enuresis is a less visible problem, and the decision to treat is more variable, depending on the child's developmental age, the frequency of wetting, and how much the child and/or parents are distressed by the condition. The medical approach to treating enuresis in children with learning problems is similar to that of other children, with the caveat that developmental levels should be considered.

Sleep problems can be a major contributor to poor school performance. The first step to intervention here is a good sleep history, which will identify most issues, including problems with sleep hygiene that can be addressed behaviourally. Please see the reference in Chapter 14 to an excellent physician resource for managing sleep problems.

Remember that physicians often serve as the gateway to other specialists, and **developing collaborative relationships and directing referrals** is important. Referrals will be based on the physician's assessment and may be directed toward other medical specialists or to the allied health professions. Be familiar with what services accept self-referral and what ones need a written referral from you.

SUMMARY

Medication should be used to treat symptoms where there is good evidence of its efficacy. For example, there is both good evidence and sufficient information about the safety of stimulants to treat ADHD. Physicians can counsel parents about risks and benefits, so that parents can make informed decisions for their children.

While stimulants will be effective for most children with ADHD, child and parent preferences are important to consider. Guidelines support a combined approach, using medication with behavioural strategies. As children get older, longer-acting forms of medication are appropriate choices to avoid the need for taking medication at school, which can be stigmatizing.

Despite efficacy, compliance with medication for ADHD is often poor. Critical to effective treatment are regular follow-ups, patient education and attention to troublesome side effects, as well as a strong parent-physician alliance.

REFERENCES

1. Canadian ADHD Resource Alliance (CADDRA). Canadian ADHD Practice Guidelines (CAP-Guidelines), 3rd Edition. Toronto: CADDRA, 2011; 55–84. <www.caddra.ca>
2. American Academy of Pediatrics, Subcommittee on Attention-Deficit/Hyperactivity Disorder, Steering Committee on Quality Improvement and Management. ADHD: Clinical practical guideline for the diagnosis, evaluation, and treatment of attention-deficit/hyperactivity disorder in children and adolescents. Pediatrics 2011; 128(5): 1007–22.
3. American Academy of Pediatrics, Subcommittee on Attention-Deficit/Hyperactivity Disorder, Steering Committee on Quality Improvement and Management. Process of Care Supplemental Appendix. Implementing the key action statements: An algorithm and explanation for process of care for the evaluation, diagnosis, treatment, and monitoring of ADHD in children and adolescents. Pediatrics 2011; 128(5) Suppl: S11–S121.
4. Op. cit. Reference 1 (CADDRA).
5. Op. cit. Reference 2 (American Academy of Pediatrics).
6. Op. cit. Reference 3 (American Academy of Pediatrics).
7. Op. cit. Reference 1 (CADDRA).
8. Op. cit. Reference 2 (American Academy of Pediatrics).

9. Op. cit. Reference 3 (American Academy of Pediatrics).

10. Kollins S, Greenhill L, Swanson J, et al. Rationale, design, and methods of the Preschool ADHD Treatment Study (PATS). J Am Acad Child Adolesc Psychiatry 2006; 45(11): 1275–83.

11. The MTA Cooperative Group. A 14-month randomized clinical trial of treatment strategies for attention-deficit/hyperactivity disorder. Multimodal Treatment Study of Children with ADHD. Arch Gen Psychiatry 1999; 56(12): 1073–86.

12. Pelham W, Fabiano GA. Evidence-based psychosocial treatments for attention-deficit/hyperactivity disorder. J Clin Child Adolescent Psychology 2008; 37(1): 184–214.

13. Sonuga-Barke E, Daley D, Thompson M, Laver-Bradbury C, Weeks A. Parent-based therapies for preschool attention-deficit/hyperactivity disorder: A randomized, controlled trial with a community sample. J Am Acad Child Adolesc Psychol 2008; 37(1): 184–214.

14. Op. cit. Reference 2 (American Academy of Pediatrics).

15. Op. cit. Reference 3 (American Academy of Pediatrics).

16. Op. cit. Reference 1 (CADDRA).

17. Op. cit. Reference 1 (CADDRA).

18. Op. cit. Reference 2 (American Academy of Pediatrics).

19. Op. cit. Reference 3 (American Academy of Pediatrics).

20. Op. cit. Reference 1 (CADDRA).

21. Op. cit. Reference 10 (Kollins).

22. Perrin JM, Friedman RA, Knilans TK; Black Box Working Group; Section on Cardiology and Cardiac Surgery. Cardiovascular monitoring and stimulant drugs for attention-deficit/hyperactivity disorder. Pediatrics 2008; 122(2): 451–3.

23. Cooper WA, Habel LA, Sox CM, et al. ADHD drugs and serious cardiovascular events in children and young adults. N Eng J Med 2011; 365(20): 1896–904.

24. Op. cit. Reference 11 (The MTA Cooperative Group).

25. Op. cit. Reference 1 (CADDRA).

26. Op. cit. Reference 2 (American Academy of Pediatrics).

27. Op cit. Reference 22 (Perrin).

28. Op cit. Reference 23 (Cooper).

29. Canadian Paediatric Society, Canadian Cardiovascular Society, Canadian Academy of Child and Adolescent Psychiatry. Cardiac risk assessment before the use of stimulant medications in children and youth, App. 2: Screening tool for the identification of potential cardiac risk factors for sudden death among children starting stimulant medication. Paediatr Child Health 2009; 14(9): 584.

30. Health Canada. STRATTERA (Atomoxetine)—Association with Increased Blood Pressure and Increased Heart Rate—for the Public, October 24, 2011. <http://hc-sc.gc.ca/dhp-mps/medeff/advisories-avis/public/_2011/strattera_2_pc-cp-eng.php> (Version current at April 30, 2012.)

31. Spencer TJ, Faraone SV, Biederman J, Lerner M, Cooper KM, Zimmerman B; Concerta Study Group. Does prolonged therapy with a long-acting stimulant suppress growth in children with ADHD? J Am Acad Child Adolesc Psychiatry 2006; 45(5): 527–37.

32. Op. cit. Reference 31 (Spencer).

33. Pliszka SR, Matthews TL, Braslow KJ, Watson MA. Comparative effects of methylphenidate and mixed amphetamine salts on height and weight in children with attention-deficit/hyperactivity disorder. J Am Acad Child Adolesc Psychiatry 2006; 45(5): 520–6.

34. Canadian Paediatric Society, Community Paediatrics Committee (Principal author: Carl Cummings). Melatonin for the management of sleep disorders in children and adolescents. Paediatr Child Health 2012; 17(6): 331–3.

35. Op. cit. Reference 11 (The MTA Cooperative Group).

36. Op. cit. Reference 10 (Kollins).

37. Op. cit. Reference 22 (Perrin).

38. Martins S, Tramontina S, Polanczyk G, Eizirik M, Swanson JM, Rohde LA. Weekend holidays during methylphenidate use in ADHD children: A randomized clinical trial. J Child Adolesc Psychopharmacol 2004; 14(2): 195–206.

39. Op. cit. Reference 2 (American Academy of Pediatrics).

40. Op. cit. Reference 3 (American Academy of Pediatrics).

41. Op. cit. Reference 31 (Spencer).

42. Op. cit. Reference 33 (Pliszka).

43. Op. cit. Reference 1 (CADDRA).

44. Op. cit. Reference 23 (Cooper).

45. Hugtenburg JG, Griekspoor JE, De Boer I, Heerdink ER, Tso YH, Egberts AC. Methylphenidate: Use in daily practice. Pharm World Sci 2005; 27(3): 197–201.

46. Hazell PL, McDowell MJ, Walton JM. Management of children prescribed psychostimulant medication for attention deficit hyperactivity disorder in the Hunter region of NSW. Med J Aust 1996; 165(9): 477–80.

47. Op. cit. Reference 1 (CADDRA).

48. Op. cit. Reference 2 (American Academy of Pediatrics).

49. Op. cit. Reference 3 (American Academy of Pediatrics).

16

Complementary and Alternative Therapies for Learning and Attentional Disorders

William Mahoney

Complementary and alternative medicine (CAM) is defined as a group of diverse medical and health care systems, practices, and products that are not currently considered part of conventional medicine.(1) *Complementary* medicine is used together *with* conventional medicine, and *alternative* medicine is used *in place of* conventional medicine. In this chapter we review some of the reasons parents explore CAM for their children with learning problems, as well as how to evaluate the evidence about CAM and discuss this with families.

CAM is often suggested as a solution to or treatment for difficult symptoms and disorders, advocated by colleagues, other health professionals, media, and consumer groups. The supportive rationale and documentation appear logical, and there are increasing reports of clinical trials of specific CAM interventions.(2) Testimonials from proponents and recipients of various interventions, through print and broadcast media, help bolster considerable support for these therapies. Parents are often in a vulnerable position, hoping for the best outcomes for their children, who may improve slowly when receiving conventional interventions.

The CAM issue is further complicated by the declining perceived credibility of conventional medical approaches to some chronic disorders for which there is no existing "cure." Many of these problems are related to central nervous system (CNS) function and are particularly difficult to deal with, both for those affected by the disorder and those providing care. The high prevalence and chronicity of many learning problems, together with the absence of any medical cure, have resulted in a number of unproven approaches. Over the past ten years, some good research trials have actually demonstrated

responses to supplements, such as melatonin for improving sleep latency and omega-3 fatty acids to improve attention. These interventions would no longer be considered controversial or alternative, although there is concern about the quality of the supporting literature.(3)(4)(5)

EVALUATING RESEARCH ON CAM

Physicians need to know about CAM for a number of reasons. Patients and families may ask for advice or information, or they may need medical referral to another resource to ensure insurance coverage or tax subsidies. If physicians are concerned about the evidence for a particular therapy, careful review of the available information at credible and up-to-date websites (like www.pedcam.ca) and the literature can help in decision-making.

Some of the recommended therapies for children with learning and behaviour problems include, but are not limited to, the following:

- dietary supplementation and restrictions
- dichotic listening techniques
- chiropractic therapy
- anti-motion-sickness medication
- physical exercises
- developmental optometry and other visual modalities, including different coloured lenses

There are periodic reviews of these therapies(6)(7)(8), which need to be continually updated, as new therapies appear regularly. Physicians are often asked for an opinion about therapies or for a referral to a CAM practitioner. Colleagues in tertiary care centres are often aware of what is "around town," and academics should be familiar with the research literature that covers a particular approach, in addition to the suggested web resources at the end of this chapter.

In evaluating the evidence in support of any intervention, reasonably high standards of methodological rigour are required. There is no reason why the highest standards of evidence-based medicine should not be applied to the field of learning problems and to the methods offered to help children with school-based difficulties. With time, more appropriately designed trials of interventions—educational, behavioural, and psychopharmacological—are being completed and published.

The highest standard for research involves the randomized controlled trial (RCT). With other types of study design, the conclusions drawn must be considered tentative. The least supportive type of design is the testimonial, where the authors simply claim that their treatment works. It is important to review the details of each study, as a number of issues can produce bias and result in a misleading conclusion.

A current approach to evaluating research evidence on a particular topic is to perform a systematic review and/or meta-analysis, where results from different studies of appropriate quality are brought together. However, even the results of such reviews published in high-quality journals may differ, and results can change over relatively short periods of time. As noted, some of these trials and reviews have actually led to certain therapies now being considered conventional.

It is useful to become proficient in performing literature searches for quality publications, as reviews can become outdated very quickly. Become familiar with reputable websites that review CAM treatments and refer to them often. One useful Canadian resource is the Pediatric Complementary and Alternative Medicine Research and Education Network, which has links to many useful databases (www.pedcam.ca/resources/databases).

DISCUSSING CAM WITH PARENTS

Parents may bring up current CAM use during the medical history, but are more likely not to disclose unless they are specifically questioned. Due to the known frequency of CAM use in the population, particularly with chronic conditions, it is appropriate to inquire at each visit.(9) Here are some suggestions for physicians:

- Adopt an open, inquiring stance to CAM and volunteer to find out information if needed.
- Encourage parents to be good medical consumers and help them understand what makes for good research.
- Use a "risks versus benefits" approach and suggest that they think about long-term safety. Many of the substances parents use do not have clear information about risks with long-term use. This may also be true of some conventional medical therapies.

When discussing specific CAM interventions with parents, the following framework in Figure 16–1 may be helpful.

Ideally, any medication should be *efficacious* (i.e., it should work for the condition or symptom for which it is being prescribed) and *safe* (i.e., it should not cause any adverse effects). Judgments of efficacy and safety should be based on evidence, i.e., by reviewing the studies and tests done to evaluate CAM treatments. If the CAM treatment being considered has evidence for both effectiveness and safety, then the physician may support the family in its use (upper-right quadrant of Figure 16–1). Regular discussion of evidence also allows families to compare the treatment they are considering with other more generally accepted treatments for which the specific information for efficacy and safety is well known. They may then realize that the physician is not as much being resistant to CAM as preferring to recommend more efficacious and/or safer options.

Use of treatments for which there is evidence for efficacy but not for safety (lower-right quadrant of Figure 16–1) should be carefully monitored for side effects if the parent wishes to proceed. Schedule follow-up visits as you would for any medication, and monitor the literature on the particular treatment used.

For CAM medications for which there is insufficient evidence of efficacy (upper-left quadrant of

Figure 16–1 Evaluation Framework for Complementary and Alternative Therapies

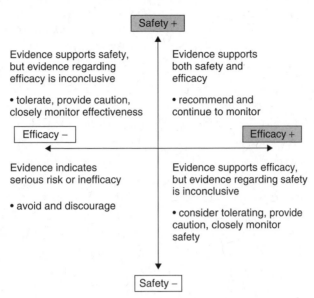

Source: Cohen AM, Eisenberg DM. Potential physician malpractice liability associated with complementary and integrative medical therapies. Ann Inter Med 2002; 136(April): 596–603. Adapted and used by permission.

Figure 16–1) but support for safety, monitor efficacy carefully if the parents choose to proceed with the treatment. For example, you could have the parents and teacher fill out questionnaires such as the Vanderbilt or SNAP-IV Rating Scale questionnaires (see Chapter 7), which are typically used to monitor the use of stimulant medications. This practice helps the family to understand the need for rigour in assessing whether a treatment works and may reassure them that you will carefully monitor any treatment given to their child.

Finally, if there is insufficient evidence for efficacy, or if there is evidence for non-efficacy (we know the treatment does not work) *and* there are safety concerns (lower-left quadrant of Figure 16–1), parents should be actively discouraged from pursuing that treatment.

Using the diagram in discussions with parents and reminding them that you want their child's treatment to work and not cause side effects can help strengthen your therapeutic alliance with families.

SUMMARY

Many people turn to CAM for treatment of chronic conditions for which there is no cure, encouraged by testimonials and case reports. There is an increasing body of evidence evaluating CAM therapies, and physicians must know where to find good information both for themselves and the families they see. Using a risk versus benefit approach that weighs what is known about safety and efficacy can assist families who are trying to decide about using CAM for their children.

RESOURCES

Pediatric Complementary and Alternative Medicine Research and Education Network, University of Alberta. <www.pedcam.ca>

National Institutes of Health, National Center for Complementary and Alternative Medicine. <www.nccam.nih.gov>

REFERENCES

1. National Center for Complementary and Alternative Medicine. What is Complementary and Alternative Medicine? <http://nccam.nih.gov/health/whatiscam>
2. Lawson ML, Pham B, Klassen TP, Moher D. Systematic reviews involving complementary and alternative medicine interventions had higher quality

of reporting than conventional medicine reviews. J Clin Epidemiol 2005; 58(8): 777–84.

3. Raz R, Gabis L. Essential fatty acids and attention-deficit-hyperactivity disorder: A systematic review. Dev Med Child Neurol 2009 Aug; 51(8): 580-92.

4. Bloch MH, Qawasmi A. Omega-3 fatty acid supplementation for the treatment of children with attention-deficit/hyperactivity disorder symptomatology: Systematic review and meta-analysis. J Am Acad Child Adolesc Psychiatry 2011 Oct; 50(10): 991–1000.

5. Vohra S, Moher D. Complementary and alternative medicine in Canadian children: A call for action. J Paediatr Child Health 2005; 10(3): 154–56.

6. Kemper KJ, Vohra S, Walls R. The Task Force on Complementary and Alternative Medicine, the Provisional Section on Complementary, Holistic, and Integrative Medicine. The use of complementary and alternative medicine in pediatrics. Pediatrics 2008; 122(6): 1374–86.

7. Galicia-Connolly E, Shamseer L, Vohra S. Complementary, holistic, and integrative medicine: Therapies for learning disabilities. Pediatr Rev 2011; 32: e18–e24. <http://pedsinreview.aappublications.org/content/32/2/e18.extract>

8. Canadian Paediatric Society, Psychosocial Paediatrics Committee (Principal author: Bernard-Bonnin AC). The use of alternative therapies in treating children with attention deficit hyperactivity disorder. J Paediatr Child Health 2002; 7(10): 710–8. <www.cps.ca/english/statements/PP/pp02-03.htm>

9. Op. cit., Reference 6 (Kemper).

Part IV: Trajectories

CHAPTER 17

Supporting the Adolescent with Learning Problems

Elizabeth Mickelson

Adolescence is a time of complex change affecting the student's physical appearance, physiology, neurological and behavioural functioning, and sense of self as an autonomous individual. In this chapter, we discuss some of the issues for adolescents with learning problems as they try to cope with these changes and adjust to a school system that has also significantly changed.

THE CHALLENGES OF TRANSITION: JUNIOR HIGH AND HIGH SCHOOL

Middle school or junior high school may start in Grade 6 or 7, and high school in Grade 8, 9, or 10 depending on provincial public education and local school board organization. Regardless of the grade at entry into secondary learning, the student faces many challenges. The nature of work and learning becomes more complex and demanding; the volume of work assigned increases, the language demands increase, and there is also the need for increased written output in terms of tests and assignments both timed and untimed. Speed, automaticity, and fluency of academic skills become increasingly important for success. Such expectations as timed tests pose additional challenges for students with learning disabilities, in particular those with written output problems or developmental coordination disorder (DCD). Accommodations, such as a scribe or extra time allowances, may only be made for major examinations such as provincial exams if the student has been identified by the educational system or has an individual education plan (IEP). Students with executive function problems, e.g., ADHD, often struggle with negotiating a class

schedule where there is not one teacher but many, each of whom operates independently of the others, requiring the student to discover how to organize study time and assignments and still have time for the increased opportunities for extracurricular and social activities that junior high and high school provide.

Often teens do not have an isolated learning disability. For example, some 25% to 40% of individuals with DCD also have learning disabilities and/or attention problems that further challenge learning and socialization. Adolescents with nonverbal learning disabilities may not be able to read the nonverbal cues used socially by their peers and miss out on the intent of a facial expression or gesture, as well as having problems with executive skills.

Elementary school is the optimal time to identify learning problems because the child is well known to the teacher and supports, and strategies can be reinforced both at school and at home. Early identification helps to facilitate social development and self-esteem, which is critical in the pre-teen and teen years. It is hoped that interventions will empower the student. This in turn will enable students to advocate for themselves during the junior high and high school years as, appropriately, parental involvement in schooling is diminishing.

Ideally students will have been identified as having learning problems prior to junior high school. Without elementary school intervention and support, the greater expectations of junior high and high school may impact significantly on students who have been marginally coping until this point. Typically, for students with identified learning problems, there is some form of a transition planning process. The information from the elementary school team to be shared with the receiving school's intake team would include current information regarding academic achievement; current school-based psycho-educational testing (as required); specialty consultants' recommendations; and the IEP. Transition planning to high school is generally well established for teens with intellectual disability (ID) for whom a life skills program is a key curriculum requirement. This type of specialized program may not be offered at every community high school. Children with mild ID may be referred to a *vocational school* (see the Glossary). Supervised work experience is often an important part of such programming.

Once a transition plan is in place, high school learning resources and support may take on several forms. These include, but are not limited to, adjustments to assignments; decreased volume of homework (such as answering every other math question); alternate ways to present assignments (for example, performing a skit, writing a song, creating a model); second-language study exemptions; and supervised, facilitated study periods during regular school time. With assistive technologies, the possibility for accommodations increases significantly for those students with problems in memory, organization, and written output challenges. Tools like electronic tablets, laptops, and "smart boards" (for visual learning and printing off homework assignments and notes) are being increasingly used, and students are often trained in their use prior to starting high school. Assistive technologies also fit well with the developmental phase of adolescence, as adult support systems decrease given the student's increasing responsibility for the learning process. These tools can also be less stigmatizing than having a scribe or in-class support. Peer acceptance is paramount to most teens, and this need can pose a barrier for the teen in accepting an accommodation or learning strategy. The ultimate goal of any accommodation is to offload the "extra weight" the student with learning disabilities is carrying, while still meeting the academic rigour and building the student's knowledge base. It is important to recognize, however, that even with comprehensive testing, planning, and services, just getting through high school for those with learning problems can be daunting.

WORKING WITH TEENS WHO HAVE LEARNING PROBLEMS

Adolescents with learning problems may conceal their disabilities by using specific learning styles or face-saving strategies. This again relates to teens wanting to fit in with their peer group. A classic example of peer influence is seen in young teens dressing in a similar fashion or adopting a hairstyle to show their individualization, frequently to the dismay of their family. For those students with motor difficulties, learning a current dance style or grooming one's hair in a certain manner can be difficult.

Depression and anxiety, possible affective components or consequences of having learning problems, are of increasing significance in adolescence, often becoming main areas of concern requiring clinical intervention. The normal developmental process of identity formation may be hindered due to a self-perception of being "damaged" and leading to poor self-esteem. Learned helplessness may be the result of previous, well-intentioned attempts by parents and teachers to buffer the child from repeated negative experiences related to learning difficulties. This may result in the teenager being too dependent on external assistance and special education supports to cope.

Circumstances may have led to an adversarial relationship between parents and school system that is quite entrenched by adolescence and results in communication difficulties among parents, professionals, and school personnel. Physicians should adopt a neutral stance with all these parties and act as the adolescent's advocate, remaining nonjudgmental. Direct contact either in person or by telephone, with permission, between the physician and appropriate school personnel is critical to ensure that the physician's suggestions are understood and taken in proper context. Similarly, obtaining direct information via a phone call, letter, or meeting with the school about the teenager in question may help clarify the issues. Building the community team is key to successfully supporting the adolescent, whether there are mental health concerns, learning disabilities, or intellectual disabilities.

Physicians are frequently questioned about the prognosis for a student's learning problems. There is no reason to automatically assume that learning problems will be outgrown, although their manifestations may be attenuated and modified with increasing age, in large part because the individual learns to build on strengths and circumvent or use bypass strategies for areas of weakness. Specific, appropriate, and sufficient educational interventions coupled with family and peer support offer the best chance for optimal adult functioning. Life as an older adolescent or adult with learning problems is addressed in Chapter 18. The teen's optimal progress relies on a team approach involving the student, the family, the school-based team, and the clinician(s). While this is no different from during the elementary years, there now needs to be direct discussions with the adolescent. The teen needs to be involved with program planning and consent to any communication between the physician and school-based team. Consent legislation varies from province to province, but, in general, appropriate, informed, written consent from the adolescent should be obtained prior to exchange of information.

STRATEGIES AND SUPPORTS FOR HOME AND SCHOOL

At home, it is important that the student continues to be exposed to an environment that models the enjoyment of reading and writing and is one that encourages the student to take the initiative for learning. Finding a key contact person in the secondary school—a guidance counsellor, homeroom teacher, or resource teacher who is available, dependable, and trusted by all parties—is also important. This person can act as a facilitator for communications with the many teachers with whom an adolescent has to interact. For adolescents with learning problems, such help is particularly critical so that *accommodations* (see the Glossary) and compensatory strategies being taught to the student are supported within *all* the learning environments (i.e., different classes and teachers) at school. The teacher may need to be supported to integrate new educational strategies or a new technology. Typically, teachers are eager and supportive of techniques that support their students and allow for a dynamic and well-functioning class. Teacher professional education can focus on

a number of behavioural and developmental topics. At some point, teachers will encounter students with differing disabilities (ranging from learning disabilities, medical conditions, and mental health conditions to developmental-specific conditions, like fetal alcohol spectrum disorders).

For the adolescent with learning problems, alternative secondary school settings may need to be examined more closely. These include work-school programs, independent (supervised) study programs, online and distance education, residential/therapeutic programs, and specific schools with interest in and expertise with adolescents with learning difficulties. The main objective is to keep the adolescent connected with a school system in order to prevent dropout and its negative prognostic consequences.

Academically, teenagers with LDs may read slowly, resulting in the student spending excessive time on home reading assignments. Learning foreign languages may be difficult or impossible for the teenager with LDs or, conversely, a student for whom English is a second language (ESL) may have considerable difficulties with all language components of their subjects (particularly social studies and English). In some cases, consideration of an alternative program or negotiating the elimination of the requirement for a course credit (for example, French) may be necessary. It is also important to ensure that practical study and organizational skills are taught.

EVALUATING TEENS WITH LEARNING PROBLEMS

When assessing teenagers with school problems, there is an extra layer of assessment in addition to the many other viewpoints needed, and that is direct input from the teen. This can be done by using a questionnaire or interview format that generates the student's own description of strengths and weaknesses, interests and problems. Recognize that teenagers as a group tend to under-report their symptoms. Building a rapport with the teen over a period of time will facilitate this type of information gathering.

Self-report inventories are available to help teenagers give their own perception of their development and performance. These include the self-administered student profile of the ANSER system, which is a more open-ended descriptive form, and the Achenbach System of Empirically Based Achievement, including the Child Behavior Checklist, Teacher Rating Form, and Youth Self-Report (see Chapter 7). Many self-report inventories are based on the more advanced cognitive development of adolescents and their consequent ability to develop personal insights into their strengths and weaknesses, and may not be as useful in students with ID or severe LD. Be sure to compare the developmental age of your patient with the suggested age range of such self-report questionnaires, and be sensitive to reading level. Helpful information can be found in web-based resources (see the list at the end of this chapter) targeting information respectively for the individual, family, community, and school.

Both family and individual interviews (with the student and/or parents) are important to understand the perspective and dynamics of the teenager's situation in the family as well as his or her perceptions and affective status. Language checklists specific to secondary-school-aged students can be used to collect further information from teachers as an aid to understanding the student's difficulty. Psycho-educational testing can help clarify the adolescent's learning profile and facilitate educationally based interventions. This information may also help with vocational planning.

The physical examination is used to identify evolving medical disorders of importance, such as possible thyroid dysfunction, evidence of an eating disorder, or new onset of hearing or visual impairment. Unless the history has suggested a change or deterioration of function, serious neurological conditions such as a brain tumour are exceedingly rare. A previously unrecognized genetic condition like 22q11.2 deletion syndrome may be a potential etiology for the LD profile, and as always, an analysis of environmental/psychosocial factors should be reviewed. The HEADDSSS acronym is useful: home, education/school, activities/peers, drugs/substance use, dieting, sexual activity/sexual identity, safety, suicide/mental health (see Grant et al. in the resources at the end of this chapter, and Chapter 9 for guidelines and investigations).

Further evaluation, using a neurodevelopmental assessment tool (see Chapter 10), formal psycho-educational testing, and/or psychosocial/emotional evaluation are often essential in developing an appropriate formulation and plan. However, there may be barriers to completing full testing, including wait-lists for assessment; costs incurred, whether by the family or school/school board; and the availability of skilled professionals to do the evaluation. For older teenagers, specific assessment of aptitudes, vocational skills, and interests offers very practical and helpful information in guiding post-secondary and career directions. Be cautious about the limited predictive validity of specific vocational testing.

MANAGEMENT ISSUES WHEN FOLLOWING ADOLESCENTS

The physician's role in management may include reviewing the findings of formal testing with the teen and family, counselling, advocacy, and referral to appropriate mental health and community supports, special educational, or vocational services. Physicians also play a critical role in managing medication for students with ADHD and monitoring adherence; the consequences of poorly controlled ADHD symptoms may be significantly more severe when the adolescent is behind the wheel of an automobile or exposed to peers who may be experimenting with tobacco, alcohol, other substances, or sexual activity. Please see the section on special issues for adolescents in Chapter 15 on medication management.

As physicians may continue to be an important connection between the student and family and the school, communicating with teachers (with the appropriate permission) to encourage and build on the teenager's strengths will support appropriate programs and promote good self-esteem. Help parents to emphasize "today" issues and to look for short-term gains, always ensuring appropriate follow-up to accomplish whole assignments and tasks. Encourage parents to facilitate close and regular communication among resource personnel, the student, and classroom teachers. Schools also have counsellors, multicultural workers, First Nations workers, school nurses, and other staff who can be valuable resources for the student. Encourage each teen to be involved with co-curricular activities, too. Often, the student derives the most social enjoyment and self-esteem building from these endeavours. A positive environment will help teens see their "disabilities" more as differing strengths and abilities, and help them embrace their skills to connect in a positive manner to their community and school during adolescence. A positive sense of self and completing high school are the ultimate goals.

SUMMARY

Adolescents with learning problems may have specific issues that affect assessment and management as compared to younger, elementary-aged children. A good transition plan, awareness of how junior high and high school differ from primary school, and attention to the adolescent's emerging identity and independence issues are all important in following this group of students with learning problems.

RESOURCES

Alberta Learning and Information Services has information for parents and students on transitioning to adulthood for youth with disabilities. <http://alis.alberta.ca>

Canadian Attention Deficit Hyperactivity Disorder Resource Alliance (CADDRA). Canadian ADHD Practice Guidelines, 3rd Edition. Toronto: CADDRA, 2011. See Chapter 4: Specific Issues in the Management of Adolescent ADHD.

CanChild Developmental Coordination Disorder. <http://dcd.canchild.ca/en/>

D.O.O.R. to Adulthood is an Ontario resource that aims to improve the transition to adulthood for youth with disabilities, their families, and service providers. <www.hollandbloorview.ca/door2adulthood/TransitionGuides.htm>

Government of Alberta, Transition Planning Protocol for Youth with Disabilities. <www.seniors.alberta.ca/disabilitysupports/documents/TransitionPlanning-Protocol.pdf>

Grant C, Elliot AS, Di Meglio G, Lane M. What teenagers want: Tips on working with today's youth. Paediatr Child Health 2008: 13: 15–18.

Paquette H, Gerson C, Gerson P. Learning Disabilities: The Ultimate Teen Guide. Scarecrow Press, 2003.

Kirby A. The Adolescent with Developmental Coordination Disorder (Foreword by Professor David Sugden). Jessica Kingsley Publishers, 2004. London, England, and New York, NY.

Learning Disabilities Association of Canada. <www.ldac-acta.ca>

Learning Disabilities Association of Canada. A literature framework to guide the research study: Putting a Canadian face on learning disabilities (PACFOLD). 2005. <http://www.pacfold.ca/download/Supplementary/Framework.doc>

18

Learning Problems from Adolescence into Adulthood

Mervyn Fox

Ultimately, children grow up, leave school, and enter the workforce. In this chapter we review how the different learning problems and their effects can continue to be clinically important through this transition and into adult life.

Many learning problems are lifelong conditions for which there are no definitive cures. Neither the child nor the adolescent will "grow out of it"—indeed, the first intimations of the diagnosis, which may be quite tenuous, must be taken seriously while the child "grows into" the full-fledged syndrome. Although permanent, the effects of a learning problem on an individual do change with age, environment, and experience, and many individuals are able to develop effective coping strategies and avoid severe disability. Although learning problems are usually recognized as impeding academic progress, their social and neurobehavioural implications remain generally significant throughout a person's lifespan. A recent review of the literature(1) on learning disabilities, intellectual impairment, and attention deficit hyperactivity disorder provides detailed information on outcome, especially emphasizing the important long-term consequences for this population. However, recommendations for practice are geared to American more than Canadian settings and legislation.

Paediatricians are expected not only to recognize and participate in management but also to prognosticate and assist parents in planning for their child's future. A properly taken family history will, in many cases, reveal that a parent suffered through school experiences that were very similar to their child's current circumstances, usually coping somehow and often denying underachievement or attributing it to not being interested in academics. A parent's poor organizational skills may be secretly acknowledged within the family circle, and his or her infamously poor spelling is identified, perhaps, as the only obvious sequela.

Family physicians may recognize LD in many patients for whom life never seems smooth or easy, who seem constantly to underachieve, yet for whom no obvious neuropsychiatric diagnosis can be made. Some patients become familiar visitors to the doctor's office—with psychosomatic complaints. Others are the parents of children experiencing academic or behavioural difficulties in school.

Learning problems may produce significant comorbidities associated with a wide range of psychiatric diagnoses, and may also directly contribute to an interpersonal, emotional, or behavioural problem. All too often, the adult with learning problems must endure not only the social and economic consequences of low academic achievement but also an abiding sense of frustration or the need for undue effort to accomplish many of life's generally pleasant and routine activities. The accumulated social humiliations and self-abasements of a lifetime may produce what has been referred to as the "wilted flower syndrome" (2), predisposing individuals to low self-esteem, unassertiveness, dependent relationships, and apparently inadequate personalities. The development of self-esteem is discussed in Chapter 14.

FACTORS CONTRIBUTING TO QUALITY OF OUTCOME

Because many individuals with learning problems make satisfactory adaptations to their individual patterns of strength and weakness, even in childhood, the physician's task is often to identify factors that prevent successful coping or precipitate decompensation in a particular case, rather than to make a neurological diagnosis. Such factors may be observed within the individual's life experience, in the family context, or in the classroom. In adulthood, the workplace and social milieu impose their own challenges. Just as knowledge of local resources is essential for physicians dealing with students, familiarity with the (often meagre) facilities available to support adults with learning problems can be invaluable. Being alert to the presentation of symptomatology in adult life, in this population, can change a patient's life.

As a group, adults who were identified as having learning difficulties while in school differ very little on quantitative measures from adults in whom the diagnosis is not suspected until later. However, individual prognosis is highly variable and influenced by such factors as parental socio-economic status, compensatory areas of intellectual strength, the presence of accompanying neurological problems(3) or co-morbid psychiatric disorders, in addition to the potential benefits of interventions. Persistence in the neurological examination of markers of neuromaturational delay (so-called neurological "soft" signs) has been associated with a less benign outcome.(4) As in all chronic neurobehavioural disorders, the ongoing commitment of a supportive and intact family is crucial for optimizing the innate compensatory potential of the individual.

Maturation tends to bring improvement in some areas: mathematical skills tend to improve after puberty, especially in women, and behavioural inhibition generally increases with age, usually resulting in less intense episodes of inappropriate behaviour than may have been experienced in childhood. The neuropsychological profiles and relative academic strengths and weaknesses of adults, however, are probably similar to those found in children.(5) Just as no specific test profile is absolutely predictive of actual life experience, some individuals transcend the difficulties to which others are unable to adapt.(6) Studies have pointed to self-awareness, perseverance, a proactive attitude, striving for appropriate goals, and utilizing social supports, along with emotional stability, good physical and mental health, and strong motivation as powerfully associated with better outcomes among adults with learning disabilities.(7)

Studying the ways that particular individuals have coped with their LD may be more fruitful than labelling and dissecting the difficulties themselves. Physicians need to be familiar with the pantheon of successful adults with LD: Hans Christian Andersen, Thomas Edison, Nelson Rockefeller, Auguste Rodin, General George Patton, Woodrow Wilson, Albert Einstein, and even Leonardo da Vinci. An ability to identify with such outstanding people may be therapeutic. Of course, poor handwriting is said to be characteristic of physicians. Harvey Cushing, despite his severe difficulties with spelling, won the Pulitzer Prize for literature.(8) Citing examples of positive outcomes for other individuals with learning disorders can be encouraging.

The concept of goodness of fit(9) among an individual's capacities, motivations, and behavioural or cognitive style, and the properties, demands, and expectations of the social, vocational, or academic environment, is very useful. Optimal development can occur when there is congruence between the capacities of the person and the values and expectations of parents, teachers, and employers. The ability to recognize and build upon the unique qualities of any individual is obviously important. Rigid belief systems, with implicit assumptions that there is only one way of achieving any particular goal and only one style of behaviour that is appropriate in a given situation, will produce dissonance and distortion over the course of personal development, perhaps manifesting as maladaptive behaviours.

There are wide-ranging character traits that reduce vulnerability to adverse experiences for people living with or without learning problems. Strongly expressed desires to succeed and to gain control over life's ups and downs, persistence, goal orientation, adaptability (with creative coping mechanisms), and a strong personal support system were identified as salient in one study.(10) Also, an ability to reconceptualize features of the problem itself as reflecting strengths as well as weaknesses (*reframing*) is considered important.

Counselling can assist the process of reframing, and intervention programs can reinforce character traits that contribute to success. However, Western society also has counter-tendencies that might label a person's quest for control in life as noncompliant or oppositional, or perceive persistence as stubbornness.

Far more than children, adults who have achieved even minimal academic attainments are able to seek out environments that match well with their own temperament and abilities. This ability may account for the personal "blossoming" that so often seems to occur when the constraints of a rigid school system are left behind. Unfortunately, as minimal academic standards inevitably rise and our complex technological society encounters periods of economic decline, adults with learning problems become increasingly vulnerable, despite their personal achievements.

ADULTS WITH LEARNING DISABILITIES

In contrast to the wealth of personal experience recorded by individuals with LDs and involved professionals, and the many published reports of small or biased samples that sustain the concept of persistence of symptoms into adult life, generally with a gloomy prognosis, methodologically satisfactory studies are rather few. For example, deficits in methodology and research include the absence of a generally agreed upon operational definition of LD; insufficient diagnostic criteria and biological markers; a lack of standardized assessment measures for diagnosis and outcome; extreme variability in modes of expression and severity (from poor spelling to suicide, from illiteracy to social incompetence); a reluctance in many individuals to be identified or to self-identify; an absence of control groups; attrition; inadequate follow-up; and the reluctance to fund longitudinal population-based studies of a condition that is perceived as common but non-serious.

Choice of outcome measure further influences prognosis. Using real-life success and adaptation as measures paints a better picture than psychometric or attainment tests (which are stable over time) or estimates of behavioural or emotional function (which reflect the heavy toll exacted by living with a learning problem).(11)

A British Columbia survey(12) suggested that some type of LD exists in 15% of adults, with very much higher prevalence in selected groups, such as recipients of adult literacy programs and basic-level

job entrants.(13) Adults with learning problems tended to live at home longer than individuals in the study's control group, but were less pleased than the controls with the family support provided. Job finding and retention are comparable to controls but job satisfaction is lower. One Canadian study(14) of adults suspected of having an LD (because of observable discrepancy between potential ability and current performance not due to sensory loss, physical or intellectual impairment, or emotional disorder) revealed a small preponderance of males (sex ratio 1.5:1), a finding that is in line with current literature and a long-standing history of these academic difficulties. One in six persons reported no school problems before the junior to intermediate levels (Grades 7 to 10). Only one-quarter of them had post-secondary education. Unemployment was much higher than in the general population. The great majority had significant difficulties in at least one activity of daily living, such as banking, using maps, making notes, and time or home management. Major problems were reported in self-expression, particularly in writing, reflecting academic learning difficulties in communication areas.

Poor communication skills range from immature spelling and handwriting through persistent misunderstanding of the meaning of words and phrases and an inability to recognize jokes (no sense of humour) to inability to articulate ideas in public. Filling in forms and taking telephone messages may provoke phobic anxiety, while the avoidance of these tasks is interpreted as evidence of general incompetence or worse. Applying and being interviewed for a new job creates special anguish.

Verbal difficulties may be exacerbated by problems in analyzing nonverbal messages (body language), leading to the repeated misunderstanding of social situations, involuntary social isolation, and even unpopularity (e.g., being unable to make friends). Aside from difficulty with following directions or reading a map, driving a motor vehicle may be rendered hazardous by difficulties judging speed and distance. Poor organizational skills are the most pervasive of all findings, reflected not only in fearfulness, inefficiency, and unpredictability in everyday pursuits, but also in pervasive slowness, poor punctuality, untidiness, and procrastination. Many individuals with learning problems are consistent only in their inconsistency.

Being accident-prone or clumsy are unwelcome in the workplace. Difficulty with learning sequential tasks is seen as evidence of intellectual dullness. Poor organizational skills predispose spouses, offspring, and workmates to develop negative, intolerant, and ultimately unsupportive attitudes because disorganized behaviours are interpreted as laziness or poor motivation, rather than as signs of neurological abnormality. Job dissatisfaction is rife even among those who overcome or hide their disabilities sufficiently to remain employed. The strategies used to conceal symptoms can also generate stress, and people who self-identify as learning-disabled sometimes meet with negativity or disbelief.(15)

ADHD IN ADULT LIFE

Although the criteria for diagnosing hyperactivity have evolved considerably in recent years, the identification of children with this behavioural syndrome provides more homogeneous cohorts for longitudinal follow-up than the less discriminating rubric of LD. ADHD is associated with reduced vocational and social success.(16) Young adults with ADHD tend to indulge in risky behaviours (including unsafe sexual activity and reckless driving), and they use significantly more health care resources when compared with their peers.(17) It is appropriate that physicians offer anticipatory guidance in these areas and ensure continuity of pharmacological and psychological treatments.(18)

Attention problems, like other manifestations of LD, may be "forever." However, both symptom and disability levels can change with maturity and experience, and success stories are common. Neuropsychological measures change little with age, but they are less effective for showing impaired attention in adults than in younger people. Most boys who are hyperactive demonstrate the full syndrome until around age fifteen; 25% to 30%(19) will demonstrate a conduct disorder some time during adolescence (although about one-third of adolescents have no diagnosable psychiatric illness). A marked diminution of impairment occurs in late adolescence, but many boys who were hyperactive continue to manifest ADHD, antisocial personality, and substance abuse during adult life. Deficits in executive function in children with ADHD are predictive of corresponding behavioural and emotional difficulties in adult life.(20) ADHD alone seems not to predispose to criminality, but when an antisocial personality disorder co-exists, arrest rates are double the rate in controls. It remains extremely difficult to predict an individual outcome.(21)

Features of ADHD that were unacceptable in childhood may, when attenuated by age, be turned into assets in adult life. The minimal need for sleep, early rising, high energy levels, and an imperative need to start the day are positive endowments in many occupations. Being satisfied with superficial social interactions, rapidly repeated, is advantageous in some vocational settings. An over-willingness to take risks may "reappear" as physical courage.

ADULTS WITH INTELLECTUAL DISABILITY

The parents of children diagnosed with an ID are often afraid to ask for information about the future, information they need to establish reasonable expectations for their child and to allow family participation in forward planning. A health care provider who cannot provide windows on the future may, inadvertently, be making parents more anxious and less able to cope or plan ahead. While it is easier and more accurate to prognosticate for groups than individuals, there is information that allows for some specificity when looking to the future.

Life outcomes for people with ID are closely related to the severity of their disability. Severity can be measured by individually administered psychometric tests in middle childhood; standardized measures of adaptive skills; a review of co-morbidities; and an appraisal of the number and intensity of supports and resources that a child requires for optimal function.

The majority of individuals with ID (about 85%) fall into the "mild" category. Communication and many adaptive skills have developed by school entry, and despite slower academic progress, skills around the Grade 6 level are acquired during adolescence. In good economic times, about half this group seems to merge into the population at large, functioning in unskilled or semi-skilled occupations with varying needs for supervision. Extra guidance and support become necessary when this group must face social or economic challenges. During tough times, or in places where requisite supports and guidance are unavailable, vocational success will elude many in this group. Often people with an intellectual disability appear to lead normal lives, with varying degrees of support, more frequently living at home with parents than their peers. Many will marry and have children, and most report being satisfied with their social lives, although their social circle tends to be somewhat circumscribed.(22)

Although vocational performance and outcome correlate highly with the severity of intellectual disability, there are other influential factors that can be nurtured through childhood and adolescence. The ability to form and keep positive interpersonal relationships predicts vocational success in later life, as does an individual's motivation to procure employment and to work hard. Self-knowledge—especially of one's own strengths and weaknesses—recognizing when extra support is required, and the ability to ask for learning or other supports and adaptations ("self-advocacy") are collectively known as "self-determination." Independent of IQ scores, there is a strong association between self-determination and rates of employment and remuneration.(23)

About 10% of the population with ID falls into the "moderate" range. Communication and many self-help skills, including basic hygiene and the ability to travel over familiar routes, are acquired during middle childhood. Academic learning is unlikely to surpass the Grade 2 level, and support is required for unskilled or semi-skilled employment. Eventually, a group-home placement usually becomes appropriate.

Persons with severe and profound ID together account for only about 6% of the whole group. Speech, basic self-help skills, and participation in social routines are the learning objectives of the school years. Those with severe disabilities may be able to perform simple, often repetitive tasks under close supervision, and perhaps learn to recognize a few essential "survival" words in print. Supervised living accommodation will become desirable.

In adult life, individuals with ID are at increased risk for a variety of medical problems, including obesity, osteoporosis, and mobility difficulties, unrecognized seizures and sensory impairments, digestive problems, and sexually transmitted diseases.(24) Health maintenance programs should acknowledge their high-risk status and take the additional time required for clinical diagnosis. Parents and other caregivers also need to be familiar with the increased risks for this group. Mental health and behavioural disorders also occur much more frequently among these individuals than in the general population ("dual diagnosis"), with a prevalence of psychiatric disorders of around 40%, and the co-morbidity rate increasing with the severity of ID.

It is important for paediatricians and family physicians to be familiar with local lay and professional resources for people with ID and with supportive organizations in their community. It also helps families to become acquainted with, and share information about, current legislation that can directly affect daily life for this population in particular, such as their provincial/territorial school act (see Chapter 5).

DELINQUENCY AND LEARNING PROBLEMS

The greatest fear expressed by many parents of children with LDs is that their child will end up in jail, perhaps following in the footsteps of the family black sheep. There is no question of the correlational link between criminality and LD.(25) Youth with LD and young offenders share many common characteristics, and there are two to three times as many adolescents with LD among young offenders as in the population at large. While academic failure is common among delinquents, this is not always due to LDs, and research suggests that academic delays as such are not the main reason for the association between LD and delinquency. There is evidence that, rather than committing more criminal acts, the learning disabled are more likely to be detected and prosecuted.(26)

School failure, with concomitant negative labelling within the community, limits access to employment and may lead to criminal activity as an easier way to acquire the material goods thought to be necessary for peer-group respect and self-esteem.

The young person with a learning problem, easily led into trouble and scapegoated by peers, is less likely to plan an escape route or to make a favourable impression on police or judicial authorities.(27)

The physician caring for young people with learning problems is sure to encounter, sooner or later, the justice system on a patient's behalf. While determining competence may require a psychiatric assessment, the paediatrician or general practitioner can help by documenting behavioural features associated with a diagnosis and by explaining that certain personality traits have a neurological basis. Police officers are increasingly aware of the significance of learning problems, and a physician's willingness to affirm a diagnosis may be therapeutic.

A note on a physician's or clinic's letterhead stating that a patient has a behavioural disorder may prove invaluable if it is carried on the person. Young people with learning problems and a propensity for poor choice of friends, impulsivity, and material acquisitiveness also need "street-proofing." By contrast with peers who have a diagnosed conduct disorder, the adolescent with a learning problem generally lacks "street smarts" and will often commit a criminal act clumsily, almost inviting detection. When arrested, this youth may admit to more than the act in question and communicate with law officers in ways that are inappropriate and likely to make a negative impression.

LDs are never an excuse for delinquency. However, by advocating for remediation rather than incarceration, physicians may serve both their patients and society well. If possible, effective management might involve combining a behaviour-modification program directed toward appropriate social behaviours, with remedial academic instruction and counselling, cognitive training involving problem-solving strategies, more recreational activity, and improved nutrition.(28)

LEARNING PROBLEMS AND ADULT PSYCHIATRIC DISORDERS

LD may complicate or co-exist with a multitude of child and adult psychiatric disorders, and these always must be considered during differential diagnosis and formulation.

A strong association exists between childhood LDs and childhood depression and suicide: one study of suicides younger than fifteen years of age found that 50% had been diagnosed to have an LD.(29) Feelings of worthlessness, hopelessness, and unhappiness (often expressed by young people with LDs) usually indicate co-existing affective disorders.

A more specific link has been postulated between so-called "nonverbal LD" (NVLD)(30) and adult depression and suicide. Characteristics of NVLD include left-sided tactile perceptual deficits and clumsiness, deficits in visual-spatial-organization and nonverbal problem-solving, difficulty adapting to novel and complex situations, poor social skills, internalizing emotional disorders, relative weaknesses in arithmetic allied to superficial proficiency in written language, and verbosity that is accompanied by poor social language use. Without insight, language is employed to excess by such individuals to develop social relationships and to deal with anxiety.(31) It has been suggested that these symptoms are consistent with diffuse anomalies or dysfunctions of right hemisphere white matter, and have been observed in a variety of neuropathologies, including high-functioning autism. However, NVLD is infrequently diagnosed, and its clinical utility in practice is controversial.(32)

Physicians should recognize that individuals with any type of LD may lack some cognitive opportunities for coping with emotional disturbance. It is appropriate to probe for mood disorders and suicidal ideation.

INDICATORS OF LEARNING PROBLEMS IN ADULTS

Many of the following characteristics are shared by individuals without learning problems, and no one trait is pathognomonic.(33) However, an individual who is experiencing significant underachievement, dissatisfaction, or stress-related symptoms, and who displays a cluster of these behaviours, deserves consideration as potentially having a learning problem.

- **Performance inconsistency.**
- **Clumsiness.**

- **Poor academic skills.** A person avoids reading or writing; writes much better than she or he speaks or vice versa; reveals poor and inconsistent spelling and handwriting skills; and/or has difficulty with the mathematics of everyday life (e.g., one's share of a restaurant bill or gratuity, making change, estimating costs).

- **Poor organizational skills.** A person has difficulty organizing time and space; habitually procrastinates, with a long list of unfinished projects; seldom meets deadlines (always too late or too early); forgets or loses materials necessary for projects; does everything too slowly and seemingly over-carefully (or does everything twice); repeatedly gets lost; cannot plan ahead; or cannot say "no." This can be evidence of continued difficulties with executive function.

- **Poor communicative skills.** A person may have unclear speech; have poor auditory discrimination; confuse similar sounds and words; have poor listening skills; have an inability to hear when there is loud background noise or when in a crowd; have a habit of repeating utterances to him/herself; have a tendency to lose the thread of conversation; have a voice that is too loud or too soft; use language that is inappropriate for social situations (e.g., often missing the point of a discussion or story, consistently losing track of her/his own stories, often seeming confused, making inconsequential comments, "answering the last question but one," seeming humourless, and taking sarcasm, irony, or exaggeration literally); and daydream frequently.

- **Hyperkinetic behaviour.** A person continuously fidgets, cannot sit still, speaks too quickly, is impatient, has little need for sleep, tries to do two or three things at a time, and avoids long contacts or sessions.

- **Poor social skills.** A person has few friends, avoids social gatherings, cannot interpret feelings or the body language of others, "comes on too strong," "makes people feel uncomfortable," stares at others, is quick to take offence, easily loses his/her temper, and seems to have low self-esteem.

RESOURCES FOR ADULTS WITH LEARNING PROBLEMS

Many adults with LDs make the transition from high school to the workforce with relief and, for the first time, are able to actualize their personal goals. For others, just as the move from elementary to high school uncovers organizational or social difficulties not previously apparent—making academic difficulties and inappropriate grade advancement the more obvious—so entry into the workforce or tertiary education can precipitate a crisis. Problems may arise in finding and maintaining employment or in meeting adult expectations of independence, organizational skills, interpersonal skills, and literacy. Reactive stress may contribute to psychosomatic or emotional symptoms, inappropriate behaviour, or mood disorders. Other adults may be recognized by the physician only because they are the parents of children with LDs.

Comprehensive rehabilitation programs for adults exist, but they may be difficult to access. Quality programs include academic remediation, vocational guidance, stress management, social skills training, and cognitive retraining. It may be necessary to refer an individual to different agencies, but the first step usually should be to ensure contact with an appropriate self-help group, such as the Learning Disabilities Association of Canada (www.ldac-acta.ca), its provincial/territorial branches, or local chapters. A number are mentioned in Chapter 5. Through this network, an adult with an LD may, perhaps for the first time, encounter others who are coping with similar difficulties.

Increasing numbers of adults with learning problems are being recognized, in part because the academic and cognitive requirements for jobs in growth areas are higher than ever before. Of course, not all adult illiteracy is due to an LD, and appropriate assessment is required, just as it is in childhood.

Rehabilitation counselling, retraining, and adult education can help to overcome past academic inadequacies. New technologies make drill and practice easier. The adult who has achieved success in one area of life or work may be more motivated to develop new skills in an area of weakness, and less ashamed of a past or present inadequacy, than the child living with an LD.

Job accommodation strategies can offer a second chance at desirable employment: computer programs designed for the visually impaired may be equally helpful for a worker living with dyslexia. Electronic organizers can improve organizational skills and punctuality. Calculators and word processing (notably the spell-check feature) are increasingly ubiquitous, and many communication technologies are also effective "work-around" and social tools for people living with LD.

SUMMARY

Children with learning problems often grow into adults who continue to manifest a similar profile of strengths and weaknesses. Some of their challenges can continue to be seen as "character flaws," while others reappear as assets. Some people are only identified as having LD for the first time in adult life. There are resources and coping strategies that can be accessed, and the physician can be uniquely helpful in recognizing the nature of these problems and for providing support and direction.

Once away from the school environment, many adults are able to find and be successful in their work. Many also carry the burdens of childhood into later life. Appropriate supports in childhood go a long way to mitigate negative effects, such as low self-esteem, and can help lead toward a fulfilling and successful adult life.

REFERENCES

1. Stein DS, Blum NJ, Barbaresi WJ. Developmental and behavioral disorders through the life span. Pediatrics 2011; 128(2): 364–72.
2. Smith BK. The "wilted flower" syndrome. Paper presented at the 23rd Annual Conference of the Association for Children and Adults with Learning Disabilities. New York; 1986: Mar 12–15.
3. Spreen O. Prognosis of learning disability. J Consult Clin Psychol 1988; 56: 836–42.
4. Spreen O. Learning Disabled Children Growing Up: A Follow-up into Adulthood. New York: Oxford University Press, 1988.
5. McCue PM, Shelly C, Goldstein G. Intellectual, academic and neuropsychological performance levels in learning disabled adults. J Learn Disabil 1986; 19: 233–6.
6. Bruck M. The adult outcomes of children with learning disabilities. Annals of Dyslexia 1987; 37: 252–63.
7. Raskind MH, Goldberg RJ, Higgins EL. Patterns of change and predictors of success in individuals with learning disabilities: Results from a twenty year longitudinal study. Learn Disabil Res Pract 1999; 14(1): 35–49.
8. Hornsby B. Overcoming dyslexia: A straightforward guide for families and teachers. Scarborough: Prentice-Hall Canada, 1984.
9. Henderson LJ. The Fitness of the Environment. New York: Macmillan Company, 1913. Cited in: Thomas A, Chess S. Temperment and Development. New York: Brunner/Mazel, 1977.
10. Gerber PJ, Ginsberg RJ, Reiff HB. Identifying alterable patterns in employment success for highly successful adults with learning disabilities. J Learn Disabil 1992; 25: 475–87.
11. Horn WF, O'Donnell JP, Vitulano LA. Long-term follow-up studies of learning-disabled persons. J Learn Disabil 1983; 16: 542–55.
12. Advisory Committee on Educational Opportunities for Adults. A Design for Learning for Adults with Learning Disabilities. Victoria: British Columbia Department of Education, 1984.
13. Woods Gordon Management Consultants. Evaluation of Literacy and Basic Skills Initiatives: Report for Ministry of Skills Development. Toronto: Ministry of Skills Development, 1988.
14. Malcolm CB, Polatajko HJ, Simons J. A descriptive study of adults with suspected learning disabilities. J Learn Disabil 1990; 23: 518–20.
15. Kroll LG. LD's—What happens when they are no longer children? Academic Therapy 1984; 20: 133–48.
16. Safren SA, Sprich SE, Cooper-Vince C, Knouse LE, Lerner JA. Life impairments in adults with medication treated ADHD. J Atten Disord 2010; 13(5): 524–31.
17. Leibson CL, Katusic SK, Barbaresi WJ, Ransom J, O'Brien PC. Use and costs of medical care for children and adolescents with and without attention deficit hyperactivity disorder. JAMA 2001; 285(1): 60–6.
18. Op. cit., Reference 1 (Stein).
19. MTA Cooperative Group, Molina BS, Hinshaw SP, Swanson JM, et al. The MTA at 8 years: Prospective follow-up of children treated for combined-type ADHD in a multisite study. J Am Acad Child Adolesc Psychiatry 2009 May; 48(5): 484–500.
20. Biederman J, Petty CR, Doyle AE, et al. Stability of executive function deficits in girls with ADHD:

A prospective longitudinal follow-up study into adolescence. Dev Neuro-psychol 2008; 33(1): 44–61.

21. Klein RG, Mannuzza S. Long-term outcome of hyperactive children: A review. J Am Acad Child Adolesc Psychiatry 1991; 30: 383–7.

22. Hall I, Strydom A, Richards M, Hardy R, Bernal J, Wadsworth M. Social outcomes in adulthood of children with intellectual impairment. J Intellect Disabil Res 2005; 49(part 3): 171–82.

23. Wehmayer ML, Palmer SB. Adult outcomes for students with cognitive disabilities three years after high school: The impact of self determination. Educ Train Dev Disabil 2003; 38(2): 58–68.

24. Van Schrojenstein Lantmann-de Valk HM. Health in people with intellectual disabilities: Current knowledge and gaps in knowledge. J Appl Res Intellect Disabil 2005; 18(4): 325–33.

25. Cooper SA, Smiley E, Morrison J, Williamson A, Allan L. Mental ill-health in adults with intellectual disability: Prevalence and associated factors. Br J Psychiatry 2007; 190(1): 27–35.

26. Op. cit., Reference 1 (Stein).

27. Crealock CM. The relationship between learning disabilities and delinquent behavior. Learning Disabilities Magazine: Fiftieth anniversary of the Learning Disabilities Association of Canada. 1987; 1: 55–8.

28. Crealock CM. The Learning Disabilities/Juvenile Delinquency Link: Causation or Correlation? Ottawa: Solicitor General Canada, Ministry Secretariat, 1987.

29. Peck ML. Crisis intervention treatment with chronically and acutely suicidal adolescents. In: Peck ML, Farberow NL, Litman RE, eds. Youth Suicide. New York: Springer, 1985; Cited in: Guetzloe E. Suicide and depression: Special education's responsibility. Teaching Exceptional Children 1988 (Summer); 25–8.

30. Clayton MC, Dodd JL. Nonverbal neurodevelopmental dysfunctions. Pediatric annals 2005; 34(4): 321–27; Rourke BP. Syndrome of non-verbal learning difficulties: The final common pathway of white matter disease/dysfunction? Clinical Neuropsychol 1987; 1: 209–34.

31. Op. cit., Reference 30 (Rourke).

32. Spreen O. Non-verbal learning disabilities: A critical review. Child Neuropsychol 2011; 17(5): 418–43.

33. Learning Disabilities Association of Canada (LDAC). Learning disability indictors. Adapted from LDAC information sheet.

C H A P T E R

19

Encouraging Reading

Debra Andrews

Most physicians are familiar with anticipatory guidance relating to physical health, for example, diet and lifestyle counselling, or accident prevention and safety issues. They may feel much less well equipped to discuss or promote literacy, because they have always thought that it was the teacher's job. However, as with nutrition, good and bad habits are established early in life, and intervention may be more difficult if delayed until the child presents with a problem.

How much physicians do to promote reading will depend on the strength of their conviction that it is worthy of promoting and that they are truly able to make a difference. In response to the first concern, the statistics on reading disability and illiteracy speak for themselves. For example, from 5% to 15% of school-age children have a significant delay in their reading skills. This prevalence is higher than such common childhood conditions as congenital heart disease or diabetes. As for the second concern, there is ample evidence in the literature for the effectiveness of literacy intervention done through physicians' offices.(1)(2)

Enhancement of literacy skills may be regarded as a significant preventative intervention for many child and adult emotional and behavioural problems and as a meaningful contribution to young patients' eventual quality of life. This chapter provides some practical office suggestions to physicians for encouraging reading. Many of the strategies are directed toward children who are at risk for or have learning disabilities (LDs) and other developmental conditions affecting literacy attainment, for whom the task of reading may be particularly aversive after years of failure in school. There are suggestions and resources for promoting literacy with all children, including those who have been struggling.

WHAT CAN PHYSICIANS DO?

Ask about reading. Physicians are taught to ask questions about developmental milestones during well-baby visits, but developmental histories tend to become sketchy in school-aged children. Taking a good developmental history for the child presenting with poor school performance is discussed in Chapter 6, and will not be repeated here, but even with children whose academic performance is not a cause for concern, the physician should ask about school, and specifically about reading.

- Is the preschooler interested in books? Does the child wish to be read stories? Does the child "pretend" to read?
- Is the child in early elementary school making appropriate progress in reading? Does the child enjoy it? (A "no" answer often is an early clue to reading difficulties.)
- Does the middle-schooler or adolescent read for fun? If so, has the student read any good books lately? How many? What are the student's favourite books?
- If the child is not doing any recreational reading, why not? Is it because reading is a problem or because reading is not a preferred activity among important role models (parents, older siblings, peers)?

By putting such questions on the agenda, you are also telling the parent and the child that these are important issues, important enough for their physician (often a person whose opinion is valued) to discuss with them.

Take a "screen time" history. Just as it is important to ask about reading, you should ask about all the activities that compete with reading for the child's (and family's) time. With myriad easy ways to be entertained in our digital world, books, even electronic ones, have a lot of competition. Limiting screen time frees up time for other more developmentally enriching activities, especially reading. Many parents have been led to believe that television and computers are inherently "educational" and do not realize that unlimited screen access has drawbacks. Well-child visits are a great opportunity to discuss this.(3)

Make suggestions for developmentally appropriate activities that encourage literacy and discuss ways in which parents can model literate behaviour. The CPS website has many resources to help promote literacy.(4) CPS "Read, Speak, Sing" materials and a parent handout for promoting reading in school-aged children can be accessed from this website. You may wish to participate in a formal literacy promotion program such as Reach Out and Read, which provides books at no cost to babies and young children at each well-child visit and has been associated with improved literacy outcomes in longitudinal research.(5)

Be familiar with resources on children's literature. If you take the time to talk about the importance of reading, parents may ask for recommendations of specific books. Although the temptation is great to say "anything so long as the child reads," it is even better to be able to make suggestions appropriate to the particular child and the goals for that child's reading. The body of children's literature is vast, but there are excellent guides to selecting children's books and most public libraries will provide age- and stage-related suggestions. (See the section about choosing books for children at the end of this chapter for some additional resources.) Encourage parents to ask teachers for suggestions of good books for their child.

Have good books available in the waiting room. Books should be selected carefully to reflect the best in children's literature and to promote positive social values. Waiting-room books should be short enough to read in an average wait, but many preschool and other early readers will fit easily into this category. You might also consider examples of books for specific reading purposes or set out a few good medium-length novels in hopes that if a child

found the first chapter engaging, the book could be obtained at the local library or bookstore to finish it.

Be aware of risk factors for reading problems. As outlined in Chapter 1, risk factors for literacy problems can be identified in preschoolers, and these children need added vigilance as they start school. Children whose parents are weak readers or nonreaders form another high-risk group. Many parents who are not recreational readers may themselves have had problems in school and may still read slowly and with difficulty, lacking the fluency and expression that is necessary if the excitement of the printed page is to be shared with the young listener. Such adults do not model literate behaviour, and they may avoid reading to their children because they are embarrassed at their own mistakes when reading aloud.

Socially disadvantaged children may be at risk because reading may not seem to be a priority compared with "real" concerns about having enough to eat, a roof over one's head, and sufficient warm clothing. Moreover, there are often no books to read in the household. If you work in an area where there are many such children, a program that provides books to low-income families can be helpful. One example, the Reach Out and Read program developed in the United States, has over twenty years of outcome data supporting effectiveness in improving literacy skills.(6) In Canada, there are some similar programs: the Read to Me program in Nova Scotia provides all newborns with a bookbag containing three books selected for infants, and the Canadian Children's Book Centre provides all Grade 1 students in the country with a free book.

WHAT CAN PARENTS DO?

Read *to* children. Even very young babies are fascinated by books. They enjoy flipping the pages and looking at the pictures. Parents can provide picture books made of tough baby-proof materials in formats such as cloth books or board books.

Toddlers are able to name what they see in picture books, and they will attend to rhymes or short stories, often requesting familiar ones over and over again as they commit them to memory. They will take a book and recite the story to themselves, pretending to read it.

Older toddlers and preschoolers will sit and listen to longer stories and will often discover that the letters and words on the page have importance in and of themselves. Children of this age group should be exposed to a wide variety of books, from fairy tales and poetry to short "chapter books" that cannot be read in one sitting, depending upon the child's attention and memory—thus encouraging them to follow a longer and more complex plot.

Parents should continue to read aloud to their child, even when the child is able to read alone, choosing material somewhat above the child's reading level but within his or her range of interests and understanding.

Read *with* children. As the child begins to learn to read, it is important to practice this new skill. Many classrooms have home reading programs, in which children are able to bring home short books of appropriate difficulty to read with their parents in the evening. Nightly home reading is a chance for the child who is doing well to show off. For the child who is having difficulty, home reading offers a safe way to practice with a trusted family member who will encourage effort and not ridicule mistakes.

Turn off the television and limit screen time. This is a critical feature of any home reading intervention. In many households, television and computers are the main after-school, evening, and weekend entertainments, encroaching not only upon reading but upon other leisure activities such as interactive games and pastimes, physical activities, and just plain "doing nothing." Many screen-based activities are passive, with little stimulus to creative thought, careful listening, and active visualization.

Families should practice critical appraisal of television and other screen-based media content. (Many communications courses in schools now emphasize media awareness.) To make time for reading, parents should analyze the screen habits of the whole family, including the adults, and then set some firm household guidelines. Limiting screen time forces children to be selective in what they do watch or play, and also frees up time for homework and recreational reading.

Model literate behaviour. *One of the most important things parents can do is to be seen enjoying reading.* Children tend to model their own behaviour on that of important others, and if they see

those important people with books, newspapers, and magazines they will internalize the idea that reading is important and valuable. If there are more books than toys in the house, the child is much more likely to pick up a book when there is nothing to do.

Each child should have a library card from an early age. Visits to the library should become a regular routine, and visits to the bookstore may reward for good behaviour instead of going to the toy store. Books make excellent gifts.

Parents also demonstrate the value of the written word by using lists and notes in everyday life, by writing letters and postcards, and by encouraging children to write their own news and stories.

Take advantage of others' expertise in choosing reading materials. Ask teachers and librarians for suggestions on books for different purposes, ages, reading levels, and themes. Some bookstore personnel are very knowledgeable. Parents may also use one or more of the many excellent indexed children's booklists. (See the end of this chapter to help parents get started.)

Choose books rich in context for children with poor reading skills. Look for familiar stories and relevant experiences, and select literal illustrations in lieu of more abstract ones.

Choose books with movement for impatient readers. Short chapters, especially those with cliffhanging chapter endings, encourage the reader to continue on rather than stop reading.

Be aware that books offer more than just "reading." Children who don't especially like stories may enjoy books and other print materials (e.g., magazines, text on websites) that give information on how to do something. Books tell how to make chocolate chip cookies, where to find the nearest shoe repair, when to set tomato plants out in the garden, and how soon it will be possible to eat the crop. Reading tells the name of streets, what breakfast cereal is made of (in English and French), and what football or hockey team leads the standings.

Parents should read signs and boxes and newspapers and instructions, and let their children see them doing it. Recipes are especially good choices for reading for detail (as well as following a sequence)—if they are not read carefully, an essential ingredient may be omitted with disastrous results. The reward for careful reading and full understanding of a recipe is obvious, relatively immediate, and delicious.

Supervise safe Internet searching for something the child wants to learn about. This demonstrates the need to know how to spell what's wanted and how to read the results. Print out some of the text that is found for the child to reread later or save as a text document "report."

Give children some *choice* among books. Children seldom like to be told what to read; however, left to their own devices, they often will make inappropriate selections, picking a book because it is the biggest (or the smallest) or has the most attractive cover. They may neglect many books that would be better choices and that they would enjoy.

Students who are behind in their reading level may not want to be seen with a book perceived as too "babyish," and therefore they may end up choosing books that are beyond their ability. Sometimes materials for older students with low reading levels may be boring.

Librarians often can advise on high-interest, low-difficulty texts that are also relevant for the reading-impaired adult. In general, students with reading problems have the same interests as their peers, and they may resent being made to read stories that are not relevant to their lives.

A good strategy is for the parent or teacher to say, "You choose one; I choose one."

Give children some *control* over who reads and when. Struggling readers often complain that reading is too hard, and they give up after reading only for a very short period of time. Left to themselves, many settle for short books with simplified text. Such readers rarely experience the excitement and satisfaction of bringing a longer tale to a close, and they are deprived of the linguistic richness of much good children's literature.

- Be sure to provide support when children decide to tackle a longer work.
- Take turns reading, perhaps alternating paragraphs or pages or use a paired-reading approach. The child may also help act out the story by being assigned to read the dialogue of one or two of the characters while the parent acts as the narrator and the rest of the cast.

Help parents set up reading incentive programs. Reading is a skill that takes practice. Regular reading helps build fluency and gives needed rehearsal for rapid retrieval of sight word vocabulary. Poor readers often avoid practicing reading because it is unpleasant, and lack of practice leads to an ever widening gap between good readers and weak readers. For elementary school-aged children, a minimum of fifteen minutes per night is recommended to develop and maintain skills.

Because practice may not be intrinsically motivating, poor readers may need outside incentives to persist. A behaviour modification approach may be used, the child receiving tokens or stickers for daily reading practice, starting with only five or ten minutes but later increasing to a whole chapter or short book. The child can be encouraged gradually to set his or her own goal for the number of sessions or books needed to gain the agreed upon reward. This approach has been successful in classrooms and library reading programs. The child also may help choose the reward, but rewards that are meaningfully related to reading are suggested (for example, allowing the child to select for purchase a special book, going to see a movie made about a book recently read, or having the parent promise to read aloud a book that may still be too difficult for the child to tackle).

When giving assistance, focus on *meaning*. The essential task of reading is not the ability to attach sounds to symbols, but to extract meaning from text. Reading for the sake of decoding alone becomes a mere exercise, a rote skill.

Help the child to think about more than "sounding it out" by talking about the text, asking questions, and looking for answers together. Direct the child to contextual clues from previous passages or illustrations, or suggest that the child try to read ahead and come back to the difficult section if needed.

Limit corrections to those that impair the child's ability to comprehend what he or she is reading. Suggest that the child go back to where a passage last made sense, and let him or her know that this is what fluent adult readers do when they get stuck.

Work on *comprehension*, using shared reading and Cloze exercises. A shared reading approach encourages the reader to make use of all the information available in a text, including the title, chapter names, and illustrations, and also to make predictions about what will happen next from what has already occurred. The parent guides the child through the passage, asking questions about the story and modelling appropriate skills. When the story is finished, they discuss what they thought about the story.

Phrasing questions about the story in the form of asking for an emotional response (e.g., "What did you like about the story?") is often more successful in initiating a meaningful discussion than interrogating the child with comprehension questions, which frequently elicit nothing but silence.

The Cloze method involves leaving a word or words out of a passage and having the child try to use the context to guess at what has been omitted. Many parents are already using a variant of this method when they leave the endings off phrases in familiar books, waiting for their child to fill in the blanks. This works particularly well with rhyming books.

Work on fluency, using paired or assisted reading. This choral reading technique involves a skilled reader (or helper) and a learner reading aloud simultaneously from text that is at an appropriate instructional reading level for the learner. One method suggests that the helper first read the passage to the learner. When the passage is read a second time, words or phrases may be left out, using a Cloze procedure. After that, the helper and learner read together with one of them using a finger to track the text. When the learner feels confident to read alone, he or she may touch the helper's hand as a signal for that person to drop out. If the learner begins experiencing difficulty, he or she may then signal for more assistance; if the learner is struggling badly, the helper simply starts reading along without making a specific correction. The idea is to keep the flow of the story going throughout. Many children like this approach because it gives them some control over how much correction they get and how soon they get it.

Encourage word play to increase meta-linguistic awareness, phonic skills, and vocabulary.

- Tell jokes with puns in them and play games involving words, for example, Scrabble, Boggle, and hangman.

- Do crossword puzzles and word searches together.
- Invent games using the Cloze technique, for example, requiring the child to fill in the blank with rhymes.
- Play "I spy" using beginning letter names or sounds instead of colours.
- Provide opportunities for word play through poems and lyrics to songs.

Use text media judiciously to encourage reading and writing. Being able to send and receive a text message or e-mail from a friend or relative can be a great incentive to learn to type and read, but must be monitored in young children. Older students may need to remember that the informal style they use for texting may not be appropriate for a book report or a social studies assignment. For young children, an old-fashioned "snail mail" letter that they can hold in their hands and reread can be a potent concrete reminder of the importance of reading.

Keep a record of what is read. This can be done on an incentive chart or may take the form of a reading diary or simple book list (of the books and their authors). In a reading diary, one would also note down one's impression of the book and other comments. As soon as they are able, children can be encouraged to take charge of keeping the list themselves, which also gives them practice in writing.

Writing and reading are complementary tasks, and **parents can encourage writing**, such as keeping a journal, making lists, cataloguing collections, and corresponding with friends and relatives. The parent can send a note daily in the child's lunch and encourage written responses, if the child wishes to do so.

Have fun! To reiterate, *one of the most important things parents can do is to be seen enjoying reading*, in whatever form that activity is being delivered, whether it's indulging in a novel, reading a newspaper, or sharing a story with their children. If reading together has become an unpleasant or stressful chore, parents should let the teacher (or physician) know and try to problem-solve how to improve the quality of the interaction. For some families, it is better for parents not to try to "teach" reading skills but simply focus on enjoying the process of sharing a book or story together. This may create the kind of pleasant memories that motivate a weak reader to continue to work hard to be able to read on his or her own during formal school hours.

CHOOSING BOOKS FOR CHILDREN

The following is a list of books that contain information about children's books, both for reading aloud with children and for children to read by themselves:

Baker D, Setterington K. A Guide to Canadian Children's Books in English. Toronto: McClelland and Stewart, 2003.

Kirkpatrick W, Wolfe G, Wolfe SM. Books That Build Character: A Guide to Teaching Your Child Moral Values Through Stories. New York: Simon and Schuster, 1994.

Lansberg M, Baker D. Follow That Broomstick! A Guide to the Best Fantasy Literature for Young Readers. Toronto: McClelland and Stewart, 2005.

Lipson ER. The New York Times Parent's Guide to the Best Books for Children, 3rd Edition. New York: Three Rivers Press, 2000.

Silvey A. 100 Best Books for Children: A Parent's Guide to Making the Right Choices for Your Young Reader, Toddler to Preteen. New York: Mariner Books, 2005.

Trelease J. The Read-Aloud Handbook, 6th Edition. New York: Penguin Books, 2006.

READING RESOURCES

Canadian Paediatric Society (CPS) has resources and materials to help physicians promote literacy in their communities. Visit the CPS website and follow the links to Focus Issues, Literacy. <www.cps.ca>

Caring for Kids is the Canadian Paediatric Society's website for parents and has handouts on encouraging literacy and limiting screen time. <www.caringforkids.cps.ca>

Reach Out and Read is a U.S. evidence-based organization that promotes early literacy and school readiness in paediatric exam rooms by giving new books to children and advice to parents about the importance of reading aloud. <www.reachoutandread.org>

Read to Me! is a hospital-based program in Nova Scotia developed to help families enrich their child's early years with books and reading. <www.readtome.ca>

Canadian Children's Book Centre. <www.bookcentre.ca/resources_parents>

Toronto Public Library, KidsSpace. <http://kidsspace.torontopubliclibrary.ca/genCategory15785.html>

SUMMARY

Health professionals are one of the most trusted sources for information about enhancing child development for parents. Physicians can do much to promote literacy and help all children get off to a good start with reading, starting with awareness of the issue. The strategies in this chapter can be used in a physician's office, both for children who struggle with reading and as part of anticipatory guidance in paediatric primary care.

REFERENCES

1. Zuckerman B. Promoting early literacy in pediatric practice: Twenty years of Reach Out and Read. Pediatrics 2009; 124(6): 1660–65.
2. Reach Out and Read, 2011. Reach Out and Read: The Evidence. <www.reachoutandread.org/FileRepository/Research_Summary.pdf>
3. Canadian Paediatric Society, Healthy Active Living Committee (Principal authors: Lipnowski S, LeBlanc CMA). Healthy Active Living: Guidelines for physical activity for children and adolescents. Paediatr Child Health 2012; 17(2): 209-10. <www.cps.ca>
4. Canadian Paediatric Society. Community Paediatrics Committee (Principal author: Shaw A). Read, speak, sing: Promoting literacy in the physician's office. Paediatr Child Health 2006; 11(9): 601-6. <www.cps.ca>
5. Op. cit., Reference 1 (Zuckerman).
6. Op. cit., Reference 1 (Zuckerman).

20

Illustrative Cases

Barbara Fitzgerald and Wendy Roberts

The following cases comprise four of the most common developmental presentations to a general paediatrician's office for children with academic difficulties. A method is suggested whereby a differential diagnosis is considered based on the presenting concerns, and the clinician is directed how to rule in/out the various possibilities as the rest of the history, physical exam, and developmental assessment are done. Clinical tools that are helpful in the diagnostic process are presented.

CASE I: DEREK
ATTENTION WEAKNESS AND
ACADEMIC DELAY

Presenting concerns

Derek is a six-year-old boy referred because of inattention and delay in beginning reading skills in Grade 1.

His parents are concerned because Derek has had difficulty remembering letters and numbers, and he is described as very inattentive and restless during group lessons and discussions in class. He has had to sit in the "time-out chair" several times, especially when he is disruptive during circle time. The teacher's aide in the classroom often has to sit behind Derek at circle time to keep him on task. At home he often "doesn't listen" to instructions.

He is more comfortable playing with children in junior kindergarten or with a four-year-old boy at home. He is doing well on his soccer team on game day, but his coach finds him a bit of a handful at practices. His teacher has sent a completed SNAP-IV rating scale, which indicates significant difficulties with inattention and mild features of impulsivity.

Differential diagnosis

- attention deficit hyperactivity disorder
- learning disability
- intellectual disability
- speech-language delay
- family issues
- hearing impairment

Developmental history

For children with school problems, the investigation of the chief complaint is also the developmental history of the cognitive domain. The remaining developmental skill areas should be systematically explored.

- **Gross motor:** Gross motor milestones were age-appropriate. Derek was walking at fifteen months and riding a tricycle at three years of age. He is already riding a two-wheeled bicycle without training wheels.
- **Fine motor:** He feeds himself using a knife and fork. He holds a pencil with a mature grasp and draws at an appropriate level for his age. He has just learned to tie his shoelaces. He likes to do puzzles and builds intricate Lego constructions.
- **Speech-language:** His language development was slower with single words at two years and only simple phrases at three and a half years. At two and a half years he was referred for speech therapy. The speech-language pathologist said that he had mild to moderate delays in expressive and receptive language abilities. Family members attributed this to his being a boy with two older sisters who were very verbal. Full

sentences were not heard until age four years. Strangers could not understand him until age five years, and some words are still difficult to comprehend. He did not seem interested in rhymes or songs.

- **Adaptive:** He dresses himself. He has been fully toilet trained for daytime since age two years and for nighttime since age five years.
- **Social:** Derek is sensitive to other people's feelings and seeks out comfort appropriately when he needs it. He has had some conflicts with peers where he has gotten a bit physically aggressive and frustrated in the classroom at certain times, but in sports he gets along well with his friends.
- **Behaviour, attention, and mood:** Parents were also concerned that Derek did not want to sit and listen to stories unless they were very short and familiar. When playing with blocks or Lego, Derek can sit for an hour and is quite happy to play alone. He is aware of danger and is careful crossing the street. He takes turns in games and lines up well in class.

Medical history

- **Prenatal:** Derek was born after thirty-seven weeks gestation with spontaneous onset of labour. Caesarean section was performed for fetal distress, and the Apgar scores were 8 at one minute and 10 at five minutes. Derek was a "very good" infant (easy temperament) who was breastfed until nine months of age. His mother was at home with him until he was three years of age.
- **Health:** Derek has been healthy except for recurrent otitis media between one and three years of age. The episodes resolved quickly and he did not need myringotomy tubes. Audiology last year was normal. The only hospitalization was for a typical febrile seizure at two and a half years of age. There were no sequelae and no subsequent seizures.

Family history

Derek's mother and father presented as concerned and very involved parents who wanted to understand and help him as much as possible. Both are only children. His mother completed high school and went on to do a college degree. She works as an administrative assistant. She had no academic difficulties. His father says that he wasn't really an academic and didn't have a lot of interest in school. After graduating from high school, he started his own company as a general contractor and is successful at that. Derek's father doesn't read for pleasure, but his mother is an avid reader.

Derek is the youngest of three children and the only boy. His sisters are in Grade 5 and Grade 3 and are doing very well academically and socially.

How does this information inform your differential diagnosis?

- His developmental milestones have been typical with the exception of speech-language delay. By history, he has good nonverbal and visual-spatial problem-solving skills. This makes an intellectual disability less likely.
- He may still have language difficulties that are impacting him in the classroom and with peers.
- His attention is good for nonverbal activities and poor for language-based activities, making a diagnosis of ADHD less likely.
- Early speech-language delay is a risk factor for language-based learning disabilities.
- Hearing impairment has been ruled out.
- The family is caring and intact and psychosocial factors don't appear to play a major role in his presentation.
- His social skills are good when the language factors are taken into account, and no concerns have been raised about social reciprocity, making an autism spectrum disorder very unlikely.

Observations

As you are taking the history, make observations about the child. Note his attention level and play. How does Derek play with the toys in the room? Does he choose age-appropriate toys or does he limit himself to those more suitable for younger children? Does he engage in a sequence of play or does he just briefly explore one and move on to another? Does he show adults his accomplishments when doing a puzzle, drawing a picture, etc. (joint attention)? Does he play imaginatively with the toys? What is the quality of his fine and gross motor skills? Does he appear clumsy? What about expressive language—does he speak in full sentences? Can you understand him? Give him an instruction without a visual cue and see if he follows it (e.g., "Please put the trucks on the shelf." Don't point or give other visual cues). Can he follow a two-part instruction (e.g., "Please put the puzzle on the shelf and choose a book to look at.")?

Child interview

Derek was quiet when his parents left the room, but he warmed up after starting to play with Lego. He concentrated well on various tasks, including drawing and puzzles, but he became fidgety and restless when he was asked many questions. He printed his name, but there was inconsistent recall and recognition of many letters. He had number sense up to ten but lost one-to-one correspondence with larger quantities. He discussed his favourite cartoons and his enjoyment of playing ball with his dad. Derek's grammar was often poor and he omitted small words in conversation. He tended to use short three- to four-word sentences. He appeared to misunderstand, even when paying attention, and his answers were frequently off-topic. He had a lovely social smile and he was an engaging child.

Physical exam

- **Growth parameters:** all at 50th percentile
- **General physical exam:** normal, no dysmorphic features
- **Neurological exam:** cranial nerves II-XII intact, muscle bulk, strength, and tone all normal and symmetrical, balance normal

Developmental assessment

- **Gross motor:** He demonstrated typical walking and running gaits, threw and caught a ball underhand and overhand, hopped, balanced on one foot for ten seconds, walked on heels, walked on toes.
- **Fine motor/graphomotor:** He used mature pencil grasp, drew a circle, square, triangle, picked up small objects adeptly.

- **Visual problem-solving:** He did an age-appropriate puzzle quickly and built a fairly complex car with Lego.
- **Speech-language:** He has mild articulation difficulties, struggles to answer any comprehension questions when you read him a story, speaks in short sentences, can't relate a story about an event at school, can't rhyme simple words.
- **Memory:** He has normal auditory and visual memory, repeated four digits back to you, was able to copy a pattern of five objects that you pointed to on the table.
- **Social skills:** He makes normal eye contact, responds normally to his name. He also demonstrated joint attention, interactive and imaginative play, social reciprocity in conversation, social gestures and expressions.

Areas of concern following history and examination

- Expressive and receptive language skills are areas of concern; articulation is weak but is improving.
- Attention is poor for verbal activities but normal for nonverbal activities.

Formulation

Derek has a history of delayed language development, which interferes with his readiness for the academic challenges of Grade 1. (Boys don't talk later than girls, and boys with older sisters don't have delayed language development.) Receptive language skills appear weak, and therefore it is expected that listening/comprehending would be difficult for him, especially in a group. Following instructions is challenging, and his failure to understand leads to poor task engagement and disruptive behaviour at circle time. When he doesn't comprehend, he looks inattentive and overactive. Reading readiness problems are predicted by inability to rhyme, and other indications of poor phonological awareness suggest that he is not ready for understanding phonics and sound-symbol associations. This is not ADHD. His inattention is related to language comprehension difficulties.

Since oral language has been slow to develop, the ability to predict words and anticipate sentence structure in context when reading is likely to be slow. Listening to stories may be more tiring and less enjoyable. Parents should persist, however, keeping to simple texts about subjects he likes, with visual cues.

Derek's social problems in relating to same-age peers are most likely related to his discomfort in understanding and communicating as quickly and easily as other children his age. By age five, children's indoor games become more language-based, and children with language delays who socialized well in preschool, doing things like playing cars, find themselves at a disadvantage with their more verbal peers. He does better in sports situations when there isn't as much language.

Derek should be encouraged in his areas of strength: building, drawing, and puzzles. Keyboard experience would help letter recognition. Derek needs help in language development. Consultation from a speech-language pathologist would provide suggestions for his parents and teachers to work on. Reassessment after the first term in Grade 1 is suggested, since Derek is at high risk for a language-based learning disability.

Careful monitoring for signs of frustration or distress is required, particularly sleep disturbance or other somatic complaints. Derek's history of academic difficulties increases the risk of school refusal. In addition to reading to Derek, parents may find that oral discussions of situations, problems, and feelings will help Derek to learn to use self-talk (*internalized scripts*) to problem-solve and resolve conflicts. It is especially important for his teachers to know that he has weak language comprehension skills and that not following instructions and inattentive behaviour may just be signals of not understanding what is being asked of him. Visual cues for classroom schedules and other visual teaching methods will be helpful. He should be given lots of opportunity in class to demonstrate his strong visual skills so that he and his classmates see him as a competent student.

A psycho-educational assessment should be considered if he does not learn to read in Grade 1, as he is at high risk for a language-based learning disability. If his parents can afford it, he may benefit from outside tutoring that uses a multimodal approach to learning.

Derek has had a normal hearing test. He needs to have his vision tested. There are no indications that his learning problem is part of a syndrome or more global picture, and therefore blood tests are not indicated. This learning style is often seen to run in families, and there is possibly a genetic basis; by history his father may have had a similar learning style.

CASE II: PARMINDER
READING DIFFICULTIES AND ENGLISH AS A SECOND LANGUAGE (ESL)

Presenting concerns

Parminder is a nine-year-old boy, seen for consultation in June, after his Grade 3 year. His parents were concerned because, despite two years of remedial help within his regular class, he is still unable to read. He does well in art, music, and physical education but is struggling academically because of his poor reading skills. There have been no concerns related to socialization or behaviour. He is well liked by both peers and teachers. Punjabi is the first language at home, and Parminder was not exposed to English until kindergarten.

Differential diagnosis

- specific reading learning disability
- ESL issue
- intellectual disability
- visual impairment

Academic history

- **Kindergarten:** This was Parminder's first real exposure to English. He played well with his peers and gradually learned to speak English.
- **Grade 1:** Parminder liked school that year. He had a very understanding and supportive teacher who had a well-structured program, but by the third term he still could not consistently identify all the letters or simple words and could only print his first name. The resource teacher began some extra reading activities with him, taking him out of the class for three half-hour sessions each week. When his parents expressed their concern about his difficulty reading, they were reassured that it was "just because he is ESL."

- **Grade 2:** Parminder had two good friends at school and was active in soccer and baseball. Although he continued to say he liked school, he was asking his parents why he could not read the way his friends could. Resource help continued for three half-hour sessions weekly, and his parents were encouraged to be patient. They were anxious about Parminder maintaining his positive self-esteem and requested that the school do a full psycho-educational assessment. The school psychologist was reluctant to do this because of the ESL factor, but his parents persisted and it was done in the second term of Grade 3.
- **Grade 3:** Parminder continued to struggle with reading in Grade 3, and, as word problems were introduced in math, he struggled with them as well. He started to talk about not wanting to go to school and asking why he wasn't "smart like the other kids." More intensive help was begun, with the resource teacher assisting Parminder and two other children in his class for one hour each day. The teacher's report indicated they spent ten minutes on letter recognition, ten on sounds of letters, ten on word families, and thirty minutes on worksheet activities that were completed for homework. In spite of this help, Parminder could still recognize only about ten words and was becoming very discouraged about his lack of reading skills.

Psycho-educational assessment

- **Cognitive:** average intelligence with strengths in nonverbal, visual-spatial areas and relative weakness in language-based and sequential tasks. The difference was considered "statistically significant," and a full-scale IQ score was not computed.
- **Achievement:** Parminder was below the 1st percentile in reading and spelling and was at the 50th percentile in math. Writing was at the 5th percentile.

Developmental history

- **Gross motor:** He walked at one year, rode a bike at age five, and is a good athlete.

- **Fine motor:** He was doing buttons and zippers by age three and has always been good at manipulating small building toys.
- **Speech-language:** He was a bit late to talk in Punjabi. His parents feel that he communicates well now. They speak Punjabi at home. By Grade 2, he was answering in English when the parents spoke to him in Punjabi.
- **Social:** There have never been any concerns regarding social skills.
- **Behaviour, attention, and mood:** Parents have no real concerns here, although they are worried that Parminder's continued lack of progress is making him feel discouraged.

Medical history

- **Prenatal:** He was the product of a normal pregnancy with no exposure to substances. Born eight weeks prematurely, he weighed 2,300 grams, and he needed oxygen for one day. He subsequently gained weight well and was an infant with an easy temperament. He settled well into routines and had no feeding problems.
- **Health:** Parminder has been healthy with only a couple of ear infections as a preschooler and no hospitalizations. He has no known allergies. Vision and hearing assessments have been normal.

Family history

His parents immigrated from India in their twenties, and Parminder was born in Canada. They both graduated from university in India. His father is a computer technician and his mother works as a unit clerk at a hospital. There is no family history of learning difficulties or intellectual handicap. The family lives in a house and has no significant financial concerns. Parminder is cared for after school by his maternal grandparents, who also live with the family. There are no marital issues.

How does this information inform your differential diagnosis?

- Parminder presents as a child with no obvious developmental delays except for difficulties learning to read. The history and psycho-educational assessment is compatible with a specific learning disability in reading and written expression and not with an intellectual disability.

- Speaking English as a second language (ESL) does not explain his reading difficulties. Children who learn two languages at the same time may show some confusion in both languages initially, and ESL children will take some time to learn English in school. By Grade 1 or 2, children for whom English is a second language are at least as competent in English as in their native language. ESL is commonly used to explain why children don't learn to read at the expected time, and this can be a cause of unnecessary delays in providing targeted assistance.
- Sensory examinations have been completed and are normal.

Observations

While you are taking the history you observe that Parminder plays quietly with some Lego and then draws a picture at your request. He shows no signs of hyperactivity or inattention. He is polite and has an obvious bond with his parents.

Child interview

Parminder tells you that he is really discouraged at school. He feels like he is really "dumb." He loves his soccer and baseball teams and hopes to be a professional athlete. He gets down about school but he has never considered running away or harming himself. He describes things at home as good and he likes to go into his dad's shop and work with him on carpentry projects. He loves it when he and his dad play soccer with his cousins.

Physical exam

- **Entirely normal:** no dysmorphic features and the neurological exam is normal.

Developmental assessment

- **Gross motor:** He is well-coordinated, has good ball skills, and a normal running gait.
- **Fine motor/graphomotor:** Parminder has a normal pencil grasp, needed to be reminded

about the formation of some letters, used vocalization to recall the alphabet when he printed it.
- **Visual problem-solving:** While you were talking to his parents, he created an intricate structure from Lego. He drew a detailed picture of his family.
- **Language:** He struggled to rhyme words. When you gave him a phonological awareness task, asking him, "What word do I get when I change the 'b' in ball to a 't'?" he really struggled. He could follow instructions and showed good comprehension when you read him a story and asked him questions. His expressive language skills were normal.
- **Memory:** He could recall five digits forward and could repeat back sentences. When you put a series of objects on the table and pointed to them, he was able to remember six items.
- **Academic:** He was unable to read the Grade 1 paragraph (from this manual). He wrote a few words but he didn't want to write a paragraph, saying that it was "too hard for me." Arithmetic skills were much stronger. Two-column addition and subtraction and one-digit multiplication were all done accurately and with obvious pride and enjoyment.
- **Social:** Parminder is a quiet boy who interacted in a typical way during the assessment. There were no concerns.

Formulation

Parminder has significant learning disabilities in reading and written expression. His achievements in reading and writing are significantly lower than would be predicted based on his average cognitive abilities and despite intensive traditional reading instruction. The resource support hasn't worked because the teacher has used the same form of instruction that is being used in the classroom, without accommodating Parminder's visual style of learning. He will benefit from direct, individualized instruction that uses a multimodal approach to learning. If his parents can afford it, private tutors who use this approach may prove helpful. An individual education plan (IEP) needs to be put into place. It is important to explain to the parents that he is an intelligent boy and that there is a difference between being "slow" or intellectually disabled and having a learning disability. Parminder also needs to have an explanation as to how his brain is wired differently compared with other children. Draw attention to his many strengths, and give him examples of other successful people's strengths and weaknesses. His parents' approach at home of engaging him in things that he does well is a good one. They should continue to read with him at home as well, but the focus should be on an enjoyable experience. Parminder could be asked to read to his younger brother from simple board books as part of his responsibilities at home. Children with learning disabilities who are engaged in their school and community and feel good about their strengths are less likely to drop out of school or engage in risky behaviours.

CASE III: JEWEL
ACADEMIC DELAY, BEHAVIOURAL CONCERNS IN THE CONTEXT OF PRENATAL ALCOHOL EXPOSURE

Presenting concerns

Jewel is a ten-year-old girl in Grade 5. She was referred to you for academic difficulties, behavioural issues, and social-emotional concerns. She just came to the referring school in Grade 4, and it was clear that she was very behind academically. In math and reading, she is estimated to be at a Grade 1 or early Grade 2 level. She has been in six different schools and has never stayed long enough for any formal testing to be done. She has an unusual pattern of learning where she seems to forget things from one day to the next, only to be able to do them again later without being retaught. She is a wonderful artist and loves to sing. Her attention span is very weak, and she really doesn't get much work done without one-to-one assistance. She is very impulsive and has very poor organizational skills. Her concept of time is very poor. She has become attached to her teacher very quickly and always wants to stay in at recess and lunch to help with classroom chores. Her teacher has had to talk to her about not hugging teachers and other adults in the school. Jewel makes friends quickly but has

a lot of conflict with them and doesn't maintain friendships. She gets along better with her kindergarten reading buddy. The teacher finds her to be very immature, more like a six- or seven-year-old child. Jewel has to be reminded of routines and doesn't seem to understand simple things like how to dress warmly for the cold. She tries to trade belongings to make friends and is very vulnerable to being taken advantage of.

Differential diagnosis

- intellectual disability
- learning disability
- fetal alcohol spectrum disorder (FASD)
- ADHD
- psychosocial issues
- mental health concerns (e.g., depression or anxiety)

Developmental history

- **Gross motor:** Jewel walked at one year and rode a trike at three years. She is a very active child but doesn't play any team sports. She didn't ride a two-wheeled bicycle without training wheels until she was nine years of age.
- **Fine motor:** There were no early concerns.
- **Speech-language:** She was late to talk, and at the Healthy Start toddler daycare program they enrolled her in speech therapy through the community health clinic. She attended daycare and had speech therapy up until kindergarten. She was discharged with a final evaluation indicating that she had made significant progress but still had mild delays in both expressive and receptive language.
- **Adaptive:** Her mother has no concerns, but her teacher finds that Jewel is like a much younger child.
- **Social:** She is a very social girl. Her mother is concerned that she is too friendly with strangers. She will approach people on the bus and chat with them.
- **Behavioural rating scale:** Her teacher completed a SNAP-IV rating scale that indicates significant symptoms of inattention, hyperactivity, and impulsivity.

Medical history

- **Birth history:** Jewel was the product of an unplanned pregnancy when her mother, Annette, was sixteen years old. Annette found out about the pregnancy when she was four months along. Up until then she had been going out on weekends with her friends and drinking alcohol and smoking pot. She had a fairly high tolerance and could drink eight to ten beers in an evening. She smoked half a pack of cigarettes per day. When she discovered the pregnancy, she stopped all substances. Jewel was born in hospital at term by spontaneous vaginal delivery. Her birth weight was at the 10th percentile, height was at the 15th percentile, and head circumference was at the 10th percentile. There were no neonatal complications. She was breastfed briefly and then bottle-fed.
- **Health:** Jewel has been a healthy child with no serious medical illnesses or accidents. She is on no medications.

Family history

Jewel's mom, Annette, is a single mother. Annette grew up in various foster homes. Her own mother was an alcoholic and couldn't care for her. Annette has since reunited with her family, and they are all much healthier. Annette has had a series of relationships with violent men, and this is why she has moved so much. When Jewel was eight years old, Annette was reported to Social Services due to a domestic dispute and was required to go into an alcohol and drug treatment program by her social worker. She did that and has been clean and sober for two years. She completed her Grade 12 equivalent last year and is now in a community college program to become a daycare worker. She doesn't recall any academic problems and dropped out of school when she became pregnant. Jewel's father is not involved and does not help with child support. He has been in and out of jail for theft to support his cocaine habit. He dropped out of school in Grade 8. He grew up with his alcoholic parents in a violent home.

There is no family history on either side of intellectual disability. Jewel has two cousins who also struggle in school.

How does this information inform your differential diagnosis?

This is a complicated history. We know that Jewel was exposed heavily to alcohol for the first four months of pregnancy in a binge-type pattern. This puts her at risk for FASD. By history, she has many features compatible with that condition: poor academic achievement, immaturity, poor executive function, and other qualitative things, like her vulnerability, poor sense of time, over-friendliness with strangers, etc. She also has a number of environmental risk factors: her early years were with an alcoholic mother; she lives in poverty; she has likely witnessed domestic violence. At this point, it is still not clear whether she may have an intellectual disability versus severe learning disabilities, or whether her behavioural issues relate to psychosocial concerns or may reflect ADHD.

Child interview

Jewel was happy to talk to you privately. She told you about school and how much she likes her teacher. She says she has "lots of friends." She admits to getting sad sometimes but says that things are much better now that it is just her and her mom at home and that her mom isn't drinking anymore. She feels close to her mom now. She denies wanting to run away or harm herself. She says that she has a hard time understanding things at school sometimes but her resource teacher gives her work that is at the right level for her. She likes going with her mom to the community centre, where she takes swimming lessons. She doesn't have a boyfriend and giggled when you asked her that question. At home she likes to play Barbies or on the computer. She denies ever having been the victim of physical or sexual abuse (see Chapter 6 for an approach to asking these questions). She does recall witnessing violence between her mom and one of her partners and remembers how frightened she was by that.

Developmental assessment

- **Gross motor:** Jewel demonstrated a normal gait. She had average ball skills. Her balance was very poor and she could not stand on one foot for more than a few seconds.

- **Fine motor/graphomotor:** Her printing was neat and legible. She forgot the alphabet sequence and had to be prompted. She drew the Gesell diagrams (see Tools 10–4 to 10–6 in Chapter 10) up to a nine-year-old level.
- **Visual problem-solving:** She did much better on this task. She worked on a puzzle while you were talking to her mother. She was able to do a word search without difficulty.
- **Speech-language:** She spoke in full sentences with a reasonable vocabulary. She wasn't concise about answering a question and took a long time to get to the point. She wasn't able to "read between the lines" of what you said. The language assessment for higher-level skills, Tool 10–6 in Chapter 10, was too challenging for her.
- **Memory:** She followed simple directions but her working memory was poor.
- **Academics:** She had difficulty answering comprehension questions from a story that you read to her. She read the Grade 2 paragraph with difficulty.
- **Attention:** Her attention span was poor. You needed to constantly redirect her back to the task, whether it was verbal or nonverbal.

Physical exam

- **Growth:** Weight at the 10th percentile; height at the 25th percentile; head circumference at the 25th percentile.
- **Dysmorphology:**
  - Her palpebral fissures are short (>2 SD below the mean). (See Figure 20–1, Figure 20–2, and Figure 20–3.)
  - Her philtrum is 4/5 and her lip is 4/5 on the lipometer lip and philtrum guide. (See Figure 20–4.)
  - Lipometer for recording lip and philtrum ratings on a Likert scale out of 5. (See Figure 20–3.)
- ENT, chest, cardiovascular, abdominal, and skin exams are normal.
- **Neurologic exam:** CN II-XII normal, muscle tone low-average and symmetrical, bulk and strength normal and symmetrical, balance poor, dysmetria with bilateral intention tremor, deep tendon reflexes +2 bilaterally. Babinski reflex negative. Romberg negative.

Formulation

Jewel is a ten-year-old girl in Grade 5 with academic delay and behavioural issues in the context of prenatal alcohol exposure and psychosocial stressors. Your assessment shows that she is delayed but not severely enough to explain her extremely weak academic achievement. In addition, she is showing signs of executive and adaptive function weakness. Her physical exam shows facial features compatible with prenatal alcohol exposure, and her poor balance and other cerebellar signs are also commonly seen in this population. Your provisional diagnosis at this time is FASD. You will need the help of other specialists to confirm the diagnosis and to assist you in advocating for her at school. You refer her to a developmental clinic.

Jewel has likely suffered neglect in her early years when her mother was drinking, and Jewel has witnessed partner violence. The social worker can help refer her to therapeutic programs for children who have witnessed violence. Her mother should be supported in the incredible work she has done to get her life back on track and commended for seeking help for her daughter.

Several months later, you get the results from the developmental clinic:

The developmental paediatrician agrees with your provisional diagnosis, and, using the Canadian Standards and Guidelines for the Diagnosis of Fetal Alcohol Spectrum Disorder (1), has diagnosed Jewel with "partial fetal alcohol syndrome and ADHD, combined type."

The report from the psychologist states that Jewel has low-average cognitive skills, with her verbal skills falling in the borderline range. Her visual problem-solving is relatively better developed. Her achievement in reading, writing, and math are all well below what would be expected for her cognitive abilities and she was diagnosed with severe learning disabilities in reading, math, and written expression. Her adaptive skills are low and, overall, she is more like a child of six to seven years old. Her executive function is problematic in all areas. It is recommended that she receive classroom support for

Figure 20–1 Canadian Norms (Mean and SD) for Girls Aged 6 to 16 Years

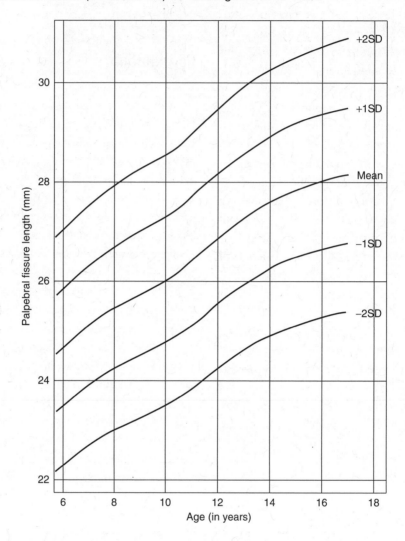

Source: Sterling KC, Chudley AE, Wong L, Friesen J, Brant R. Normal distribution of palpebral fissure lengths in Canadian school age children. Can J Clin Pharmacol 2010; 17(1): e67–78. Reproduced by permission.

learning and small group or individual support several times weekly. An IEP has been recommended. The speech-language pathologist finds that Jewel has low-average vocabulary and expressive language skills. Her higher-level language skills are impaired and she has poor social use of language.

Follow-up

You meet with Annette a couple of weeks after she has received the reports from the developmental assessment. She is teary and tells you how guilty she feels about the diagnosis of FASD. You talk to her about all the positive things she is doing for Jewel now

and how to move forward. Jewel's inattentiveness is interfering with her ability to reach her cognitive potential. The teacher has written a note outlining this. You tell Annette that your first approach will involve lifestyle and behavioural changes and outline community resources that are available for parents of children with FASD and ADHD.

Recommendations

- **ADHD:** Recommendations and resources are available for free download and are updated regularly on the Canadian ADHD Resource Alliance (CADDRA) website at www.caddra.ca.

Figure 20–2 Canadian Norms (Mean and SD) for Boys Aged 6 to 16 Years

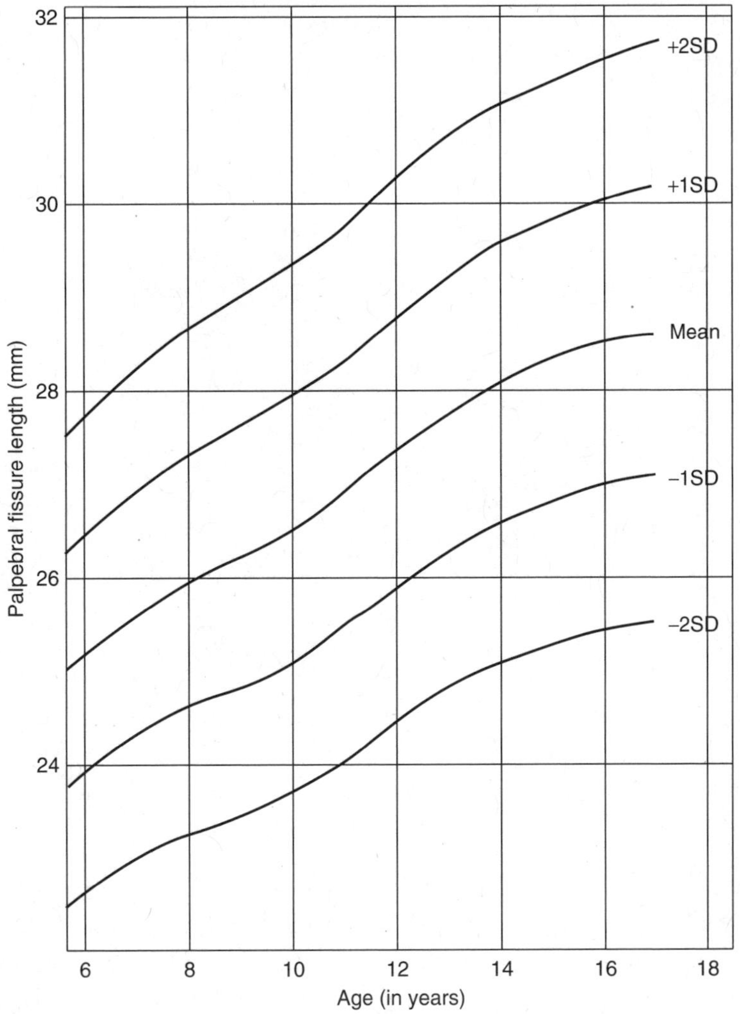

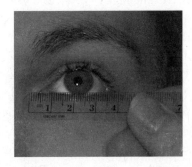

Source: Sterling KC, Chudley AE, Wong L, Friesen J, Brant R. Normal distribution of palpebral fissure lengths in Canadian school age children. Can J Clin Pharmacol 2010; 17(1): e67–78. Reproduced by permission.

Figure 20–3 The Palpebral Fissure Length (Distance from Inner Corner to Outer Corner of the Eye) Being Measured with a Small Plastic Ruler

Source: © 2012, Susan Astley, PhD, University of Washington. Used by permission.

Figure 20–4 The Three Diagnostic Facial Features of FAS: (1) short palpebral fissure lengths, (2) a smooth philtrum (rank 4 or 5 on the Lip-Philtrum Guide), and (3) a thin upper lip (rank 4 or 5 on the Lip-Philtrum Guide). Lip-Philtrum Guides 1 and 2 are used to rank upper lip thinness and philtrum smoothness. The philtrum is the vertical groove between the nose and upper lip. The guides reflect the full range of lip and philtrum shapes, with rank 3 representing the population mean. Ranks 4 and 5 reflect the thin lip and smooth philtrum that characterize the FAS facial phenotype. Guide 1 is used for Caucasians and all other races with lips like Caucasians. Guide 2 is used for African Americans and all other races with lips as full as African Americans.

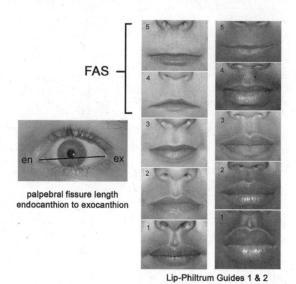

palpebral fissure length
endocanthion to exocanthion

Lip-Philtrum Guides 1 & 2

Source: © 2012, Susan Astley, PhD, University of Washington. Used by permission.

There is an emphasis on psychosocial, family, and behavioural strategies as first-line therapies in conjunction with stimulant medication. Chapter 14 outlines the steps to develop a behaviour management program and Chapter 15 provides a discussion of the approach to medication management. Parent training is very helpful for developing skills in adults for the ongoing management of behavioural challenges. It should be noted that in children with FASD, where cause-and-effect reasoning is impaired, reward systems may not be as effective but should still be tried. The biggest difference between children with FASD and ADHD and children with ADHD alone is that the problems in FASD tend to become more challenging over the long term. The behavioural strategies work while they are being used, but need to be continued or the effects fade. Like all children with ADHD symptoms, Jewel will benefit from educational strategies such as short chunks of work with movement breaks. There

have been many other treatments explored in the treatment of ADHD. Parents will ask you about them and it is important to consider the evidence base—many have been discounted and there is no evidence to support them at this time (e.g., gluten-free and other restrictive diets, energy-balancing bracelets). Further information regarding an approach to these therapies is found in Chapter 16. Many families want to explore interventions other than prescription medication. Research is emerging that offers other possibilities for managing this condition. On the positive side, they are modalities that do not have serious side effects and offer other potential health benefits. Some of these are listed, and references including available reviews(2)(3)(4) are provided at the end of this chapter:

- **Nutrition:** Jewel could be started on an adult dose of omega-3 fatty acids once daily. There is some evidence that this may be beneficial for the symptoms of ADHD.

- **Aerobic exercise:** Emerging evidence points to enhanced neural activity in children who have daily aerobic exercise. There is emerging evidence from trials that children with behaviour problems benefit from time in nature and that this exposure can also help symptoms of ADHD.
- **Relaxation and mindfulness training techniques:** There is emerging evidence that mindfulness training techniques can be beneficial in children with ADHD. There are many free guided examples of this on the Internet. Mindfulness training and other relaxation techniques are advocated in the CADDRA guidelines.
- **FASD:** The concept of the "external brain" in FASD is important—structure, predictable routines, and adult assistance when Jewel is having difficulties navigating daily life are all essential. She will need adult support because she is a vulnerable child and her daily life skills are more like a much younger child's. The variability in function from one day to the next can be a particularly challenging feature for teachers and parents to adapt to. In children with FASD, it is important to predict which situations tend to be difficult for the child (e.g., big crowds that overwhelm the child) and avoid them. One resource that can be helpful to families is the University of Washington's FAS Diagnostic and Prevention website (http://depts.washington.edu/fasdpn/htmls/interv-research.htm). Other resources are listed at the end of this chapter. A number of communities have organized teams for assessing children with FASD.
- **Emotional support:** Jewel has had trauma in her life and may benefit from therapeutic interventions for traumatized children and the support of another adult, such as a Big Sister.
- **Academic support:** Jewel needs an individual education plan/individual program plan (IEP/IPP). She will learn more slowly than other children and is stronger as a visual learner. There may be days when she is not able to remember previously learned skills and that issue needs to be accepted and not interpreted as a character flaw. To accommodate her written expression

disorder, Jewel can be taught keyboarding and be allowed to do her work on the computer. The resource teacher might help her organizational skills by implementing daily and weekly schedules for homework and other assignments both at home and school. Using a computer program for this could be beneficial.
- **Social skills development:** The goal is to develop one friendship, perhaps with suggestions from a teacher or swimming instructor, then parental support to plan activities. She may benefit from social activities outside school that she could attend with a mentor.
- **Medication:** You can discuss with Annette that, in the absence of improvement with the interventions above, a trial of stimulant medication should be considered. This requires close communication between school and home. Excellent tables with regimens and dosing of recommended medications are available on the CADDRA website at www.caddra.ca. (More information about medication management is found in Chapter 15.)

CASE IV: TRISTAN
GROSS MOTOR AND FINE MOTOR SKILL CLUMSINESS, POOR ATTENTION, AND IMPULSIVITY
Presenting concerns

Tristan is a nine-year-old boy in Grade 4 who was brought by his parents because of behaviour problems. He forgets to bring home assignments and resists doing them if he does bring them home. He is always getting up and trying to go to the computer to play games. It often takes two to three hours per night and many fights with his mother before homework is completed. It takes him a long time to do any written work and he gets very frustrated by it. He loves playing on the computer and does not like the many sports activities his parents have enrolled him in. They had to take him out of soccer, as he was complaining that his teammates wouldn't pass the ball to him. He still cannot ride a bicycle despite lots of opportunity. His teacher has told his parents that he is very inattentive and a bit fidgety but not impulsive at school. She has also noticed how clumsy he is, often tripping over desks and things as he moves around the classroom. He has been teased on hot-dog day at school because of how messy he is when he eats. The teacher asked his parents to take him to a paediatrician to see if he might have ADHD. His parents state that he is much more disorganized than his sisters ever were and needs constant reminders to get anything done. They assumed that was "just how boys are." He is not doing very well in school, in part because he does not hand in his work or complete projects on time. His parents and teacher are wondering if he has a learning disability, but he learned to read in kindergarten, has good comprehension, and really enjoys reading for pleasure.

Differential diagnosis

- ADHD
- learning disability
- cognitive disability
- developmental coordination disorder
- family issues

Developmental history

- **Gross motor:** Tristan walked at fifteen months and has always been described as clumsy. His parents have put him into lots of sports and he is always the weakest on the team. He trips when he runs and his ball skills are poor. As sports became more competitive, he has asked to be allowed to quit.
- **Fine motor:** He has never had good fine motor skills. It took him a long time to be able to use a knife and fork. He still has difficulty manipulating small objects. He learned to tie his shoelaces when he was eight years of age, but now wears skate shoes that he doesn't need to tie or untie.
- **Communication:** Tristan spoke his first words at age one and was speaking in sentences by age three years. He had difficulties understanding, and he had speech therapy for articulation difficulties in preschool. There are no concerns now.
- **Social:** He has always been a friendly, likeable child. He has some good friends, and they play computer games together.

Medical history

- **Prenatal:** This was an unplanned pregnancy that was discovered early on. It was a healthy pregnancy with no exposures to substances. Tristan was born at term by elective C-section. There were no complications.
- **Health:** Tristan has been a healthy child with no serious illnesses or injuries. He has required stitches on several occasions for falls leading to lacerations. He is on no medications.

Family history

Tristan's parents both graduated from high school, and his mother went to college to train in home decorating. She works part-time. His father works full-time as an insurance agent. His parents were both average students with average athletic abilities. There is no family history of intellectual disability or specific learning disabilities. The parents report that their marriage is good. They disagree as to whether Tristan should be forced to continue in competitive sports. His dad thinks it is good for him, but his mother thinks he should be allowed to quit. Tristan has two older sisters, aged twelve and fifteen years, who are both average students and average athletes. Teachers have never remarked on any behavioural issues with them.

How does the history inform your differential diagnosis?

Tristan has weaknesses in gross and fine motor skills. He is having a lot of trouble with attention at school. This constellation of findings is common in developmental coordination disorder. He read early and has good comprehension, which indicates against a diagnosis of intellectual disability. A specific learning disability, such as a nonverbal learning disability, cannot be ruled out at this time. His behaviour does not seem to be reflecting a poor home situation, although the disagreement regarding how to approach competitive sports will need to be worked out.

Child interview

Tristan was an easy boy to establish rapport with. He said that he likes school well enough but that he gets blamed a lot by the teacher. She always says that he does not listen and does not do what he is told. He says that he tries his best, but that he often finds it hard to concentrate on what she is saying. He says he can understand her when he is paying attention; other things just distract him. He says that he is not worrying about anything. He loves his family but he does not like it when his parents argue about his sports. He loves to play computer games with his friends.

Developmental assessment

- **Gross motor:** Very immature gross motor skills. Tristan is very uncoordinated in terms of running gait and ball skills.
- **Fine motor/graphomotor:** Very weak skills. Letter formations immature. His drawings are very messy and he was discouraged by their appearance.
- **Visual reasoning:** He played a game of X's and O's with you at a typical level. He did a word search without difficulty. He was able to copy block designs without difficulty.
- **Language:** Tristan has appropriate expressive language skills. He is able to comprehend a story you read to him, although you had to read it twice because he wasn't focusing the first time and got all the answers wrong.
- **Academic:** He read to you from a Grade 4–level paragraph and showed good reading comprehension. He was able to do multiplication for you. He wrote out some sentences, but it was very laborious and his printing was like that of a child in Grade 1. He was able to tell you his ideas verbally when you told him he could stop printing.
- **Social:** He has typical social skills with you and when his parents are present.

Physical exam

- **Growth parameters:** normal
- **Dysmorpology exam:** noncontributory
- **General physical exam:** noncontributory
- **Neurologic exam:** normal and symmetric tone, strength, bulk, and deep tendon reflexes, Babinski downgoing, CN II-XII normal, difficulty balancing on one foot, awkward hopping, cannot do tandem gait. There were overflow movements and mild dysmetria.

Formulation

Tristan is a nine-year-old boy who is struggling academically and has weak fine and gross motor skills. Your developmental assessment does not give you any indication that his academic weakness relates to a specific learning disability or cognitive delay, with the exception of his very weak written output skills. His attention span is weak, and he acknowledged difficulties paying attention, even in the quiet one-to-one setting with you. He has only mild fidgetiness and no hyperactivity. He meets criteria for ADHD, inattentive type. His inability to express his ideas in written form, combined with his inattention, is leading to his academic difficulties.

Tristan also has significant gross motor and fine motor coordination problems. This combination of gross and fine motor skill weakness in a child, commonly accompanied by features of ADHD, is called developmental coordination disorder (DCD). DCD is sometimes accompanied by learning disabilities in other subjects, which Tristan does not appear to have. Your diagnosis will be informed by assessments from a psychologist, a physiotherapist, and an occupational therapist, but intervention does not need to wait for these assessments. The psychologist will formally assess his cognitive abilities and achievement to determine if there is a subtle learning disability that was not picked up on your assessment. Although a diagnosis of written output disorder will come from both the occupational therapist's and psychologist's assessments, many schools will accept the diagnosis of a developmental coordination disorder from a physician. The physiotherapist's and occupational therapist's recommendations for adapting physical education at school, recreational activities in the community, and written work at school will be very valuable. A child who is not writing with ease by Grade 3 should be taught to keyboard and should use a computer for the majority of his written work. Tristan could also receive notes and diagrams in electronic form for studying. It is important to allow Tristan to get credit for the knowledge and ideas that he has but cannot express with pen and paper. This can take the form of oral examinations, through the use of a scribe, or by keyboarding or voice-activated transcription. Children who struggle to this degree with written expression are unlikely to become fluent manual writers and will only become frustrated with not being able to produce written work at the level of their intellectual potential. Tristan's parents can be advised to listen to his desire to leave competitive sports and to consider enrolling him in other recreational, non-competitive activities. As always, his strengths should be emphasized at home and in the community.

From the information that has been gathered regarding his attention weakness, it is apparent that his inability to pay attention in class is affecting his performance. Standard recommendations for ADHD, including giving him smaller chunks of work to complete, movement breaks, seating near the teacher and away from distractions, and a rewards system for keeping him on track may be helpful. His parents would benefit from reading materials regarding management of ADHD and possibly by contacting CHADD (Children and Adults with ADHD) Canada. The Canadian ADHD Resource Alliance (CADDRA) has recommendations and resources for the management of ADHD available free of charge on its website at www.caddra.ca. Please see the previous case recommendations for consideration of strategies for which there is some supporting evidence with rigorous trials still underway. Close attention should be paid to Tristan's sleep hygiene. He may benefit from relaxation techniques such as mindfulness training. If these treatments, in conjunction with classroom adaptations for his DCD and the development of parent management strategies, are not effective, a trial of stimulant medication should be considered. (See Chapter 15 for an approach to medical management.) Close paediatric follow-up, and paying attention to this child's overall sense of self and well-being, are important. Children with DCD can suffer from feeling different and be left

out of sports and games, so it is very important to ensure that they also have activities and pursuits that they can feel good at.

RESOURCES
ADHD

CADDRA Canadian ADHD Guidelines, 3rd Edition, 2011 (updated annually). <www.caddra.ca>

Greenberg MT, Harris AR. Nurturing mindfulness in children and youth: Current state of research. Child Dev Perspect 2011; DOI:10.1111/j.1750 8606.2011. 00215.x:1–6.

Harnett PH, Dawe S. Review: The contribution of mindfulness-based therapies for children and families and proposed conceptual integration. Child Adolesc Ment Health 2012 DOI:10.1111/j.1475–3588.2011.00643.x.

Hillman CH, Erickson KI, Kramer AF. Be smart, exercise your heart: Exercise effects on brain and cognition. Nat Rev Neurosci 2008; 9(1): 58–65.

Richardson, AJ. Omega-3 fatty acids in ADHD and related neurodevelopmental disorders. Int Rev Psychiatry 2006; 18(2): 155–72.

Sinn N, Bryan J. Effect of supplementation with polyunsaturated fatty acids and micronutrients on learning and behaviour problems associated with child ADHD. JDBP 28(2): 82–91.

Taylor AF, Kuo FE. Children with attention deficits concentrate better after walk in the park. J Atten Disord 2009; 12(5): 402–9.

Taylor AF, Kuo FE. Could exposure to everyday green spaces help treat ADHD? Evidence from children's play settings. Applied Psychology: Health and Well-Being 2011; 3(3): 281–303.

FASD

Astley S. Clinical assessment of individuals with Fetal Alcohol Spectrum Disorders (FASD). The Encyclopedia of Child Development. <www.child-encyclopedia.com/documents/AstleyANGxp1.pdf> (Version current at February 9, 2011.)

Chudley AE, Conry J, Cook JL, Loock C, Rosales T, LeBlanc N. Fetal alcohol spectrum disorder: Canadian guidelines for diagnosis. CMAJ 2005; 172(5 Suppl): S1–S21.

Books for families

Kleinfeld J, Wescott S, eds. Fantastic Anton Succeeds: Experiences in Educating Children with Fetal Alcohol Spectrum. Fairbanks AK: University of Alaska Press, 2003.

Kleinfeld J, Morse B, Wescott S, eds. Fantastic Anton Grows Up: Adolescents and Adults with Fetal Alcohol Spectrum. Fairbanks AK: University of Alaska Press, 2000.

Malbin, D. Trying Differently Rather Than Harder: Fetal Alcohol Spectrum Disorders. Fetal Alcohol Syndrome Consultation, Education and Training Services (FAS-CETS), 2002.

REFERENCES

1. Chudley AE, Conry J., Cook J, et al. Fetal alcohol spectrum disorder: Canadian guidelines for diagnosis. CMAJ 2005; 172(5 Suppl): S1–S21.
2. Raz R, Gabis L. Essential fatty acids and attention-deficit-hyperactivity disorder: A systematic review. Dev Med Child Neurol 2009; 51(8): 580–92.
3. Bloch MH, Qawasmi A. Omega-3 fatty acid supplementation for the treatment of children with attention-deficit/hyperactivity disorder symptomatology: Systematic review and meta-analysis. J Am Acad Child Adolesc Psychiatry 2011; 50(10): 991–1000.
4. Millichap JG, Yee MM. The diet factor in attention-deficit/hyperactivity disorder. Pediatrics 2012; 129(2): 330–7.

21

A Resource Worksheet for Physicians Who Work with Students with Learning Problems

Debra Andrews

The following worksheet is meant to assist physicians who do not have immediate access to a multidisciplinary tertiary referral clinic for assessing children with school problems. Such physicians may wish to put together their own "teams" using local resources. In working through this form, physicians can get a feel for what resources are needed and the rationale. Once completed, the resource sheet serves as a reference document for recommendations and referrals.

The resource worksheet that follows may be reproduced without permission.

Item 1

What school boards are represented in my referral population?
- Public? Separate?
- Anglophone? Francophone?
- Home schooling? Other?

Who are the contact persons for each of these school boards?

In many areas, consultants involved in placement and program planning are the usual contacts. Depending on the size of the school district, there may be one special needs consultant or many, divided up by the age ranges of students served (preschool, elementary, junior high, high school) or the type of disabilities (physical disability, varying levels of intellectual disability, learning disability, gifted, sensory impairment, etc.).

What schools are included in each school board? Which are elementary, junior high, senior high? Which are English, French, bilingual programs, immersion programs? Which house the programs for children who are gifted, learning disabled, have multiple disabilities? How are home-schoolers served?

Often a school board will have information that lists its schools and the types of programs available, either as a brochure or website or both. A contact person as described above may be able to meet with you or discuss the allocation of resources in the school system with you over the phone.

For a given school, who is to be the contact person?

This may be the child's teacher, the principal, the special education or resource teacher, the guidance counsellor or school psychologist. Some questionnaires include a place for the school to designate a liaison person; check for this information.

Items 2 and 3

What types of programs does the child's school have available?

Recommendations should reflect services that the school can reasonably provide. Does the school have a resource room, self-contained special education or behaviourally based classrooms, speech therapy, occupational therapy, counselling?

Item 4

What are the criteria or standards for admission into special services?

These can often be found in documents on school board websites.

Item 5

What resources can be tapped from the allied health professions?

These types of services may be provided through the schools, the local board of health, or a nearby hospital or clinic. Some of these professionals may operate private practices. Consult the professional practice organization websites associated with a specific discipline to find qualified practitioners near you.

Item 6

What medical consultants are available?

Developmental paediatrics, paediatric neurology, and child psychiatry will likely be found at a local children's hospital, although some of these consultants may have private practices. Many general paediatricians have developed expertise evaluating school problems and are the logical next step for family doctors' referrals. In some areas, general psychiatrists and neurologists see children as well as adults, providing continuity of care across the transition to adulthood. Other consultants who may be helpful are in the fields of ophthalmology, ENT, and genetics.

Item 7

What services can be obtained through social service agencies, both government-funded and those supported by charitable or religious organizations?

Item 8

Are there parent support or advocacy groups such as a local chapter of the Learning Disabilities Association of Canada (LDAC) or Children and Adults with Attention Deficit/Hyperactivity Disorder (CHADD)?

Item 9

What private resources are available for counselling, tutoring, or other services?

Item 10

Where is the nearest multidisciplinary team? How are referrals made? Can you obtain a phone consultation?

SUMMARY

Taking the time to collect information about the people and resources needed for collaborative care of children with learning problems can help save time and expedite workup down the line. Be sure to update your resource sheet at least annually, as information may change. Websites of school boards, professional associations, and tertiary services such as children's hospitals can help you find the information and contacts you need quickly and efficiently.

Please refer to Chapter 2 for additional information about working with schools.

A RESOURCE WORKSHEET FOR PHYSICIANS
WHO WORK WITH STUDENTS WITH LEARNING PROBLEMS

1. School boards represented in referral population

Geographic area (city, county): _____

Name of board: _____

Designation (circle): public/separate,
anglophone/francophone, other (list): _____

_____

Website: _____

Address: _____

_____

Phone: _____

Name of contact person: _____

List schools in this school board's jurisdiction:

#	Elementary
#	Junior high (If offered)
#	Senior high

2. Sites for special programs (indicate board and contact person)

Other languages: _____

_____

_____

Gifted: _____

_____

_____

Learning disabled: _____

_____

_____

Behaviour disorder: _____

_____

_____

Mild intellectual disability: _____

_____

_____

Moderate-to-severe intellectual disability: _____

_____

_____

Autism spectrum disorder: _____

_____

_____

Physically handicapped: _____

_____

_____

Hearing impaired: _____

_____

_____

Visually impaired: _____

_____

_____

_____

3. Types of programs available (indicate board and school)

Resource room: _____

_____

_____

Self-contained special education classroom for children with learning disabilities: _____

_____

_____

Self-contained special education classroom for children with mild intellectual disabilities: _____

_____

_____

Life skills classroom for children with more severe intellectual disability: _____

_____

_____

Work/study programs: _____

_____

_____

Classroom for children with behaviour/emotional problems: _____

_____

_____

Programs for children with autism spectrum disorder: _____

_____

_____

Speech-language therapy: _____

_____

_____

Occupational therapy: _____

_____

_____

Counselling/Social worker: _____

_____

_____

_____

4. Criteria or standards for admission into special services (attach reference documents as needed)

Program/Board: _____

Classification/Diagnosis: _____

Criteria: _____

_____

_____

_____

Program/Board: _____

Classification/Diagnosis: _____

Criteria: _____

_____

_____

_____

Program/Board: _____

Classification/Diagnosis: _____

Criteria: _____

_____

_____

_____

Program/Board: _____

Classification/Diagnosis: _____

Criteria: _____

_____

_____

_____

Program/Board: _____

Classification/Diagnosis: _____

Criteria: _____

_____

_____

_____

5. Community allied health professions (location/phone/contact name/website)

Speech-language: _____

_____

_____

_____

Audiology: _____

_____

_____

_____

Physiotherapy: _____

_____

_____

_____

Occupational therapy: _____

_____

_____

_____

Psychology: _____

_____

_____

_____

Resources for children with developmental coordination disorder: _____

_____

_____

_____

Social services: _____

_____

_____

_____

Mental health services: _____

_____

_____

_____

6. Medical consultants (name/specialty/phone/website)

Developmental paediatrics: _____

Paediatric neurology: _____

Psychiatry: _____

Ophthalmology: _____

ENT: _____

Genetics: _____

Other: _____

_____

_____

_____

7. Public and private social service agencies (name/phone/website)

_____

_____

_____

_____

8. Parent support or advocacy groups—local chapters (phone/contact name/website)

Learning Disabilities Association of Canada (LDAC): _____

Children and Adults with Attention Deficit/Hyperactivity Disorder (CHADD): _____

Canadian Association for Community Living (CACL): _____

Other: _____

_____

_____

_____

9. Private or fee-for-service supports

Counselling (name/phone/website):_____

_____

_____

_____

Treatment groups, e.g., social skills, anxiety, anger management (name/phone/website): _____

_____

_____

_____

_____

Tutoring services (name/phone/website): _____

_____

_____

_____

_____

10. Nearest multidisciplinary team

Location: _____

Phone: _____

Contact: _____

Website: _____

Physician's letter needed?   ❏ Yes   ❏ No

Phone consultation available?   ❏ Yes   ❏ No

Glossary

AACAP   See **American Academy of Child and Adolescent Psychiatry**

AAP   See **American Academy of Pediatrics**

Accommodations   Accommodations are specific teaching strategies and assistive technologies that allow a student to be successful with achieving the knowledge and skills (curriculum content) for that student's grade. There is no change in achievement expectations; i.e., the student is expected to cover the same material as other students in the grade.

American Academy of Child and Adolescent Psychiatry (AACAP)   The professional organization of child and adolescent psychiatrists in the United States. The AACAP develops guidelines on the assessment and management of psychiatric conditions in children and adolescents, including ADHD.

American Academy of Pediatrics (AAP)   The professional organization of paediatricians in the United States. The AAP sponsors the journal *Pediatrics* and develops guidelines and position statements on many health issues affecting children.

Attention deficit disorder (ADD)   This was the term used in previous editions of the American Psychiatric Association's DSM (Diagnostic and Statistical Manual of Mental Disorders) and no longer officially exists. Some still use it synonymously with the inattentive subtype of ADHD.

Attention deficit hyperactivity disorder (ADHD) This is diagnosed using the criteria of American Psychiatric Association's DSM-IV. There are three subtypes, primarily inattentive, primarily hyperactive-impulsive, and combined—where the person meets criteria for both of the above subtypes.

Behavioural phenotype   Aspects of an individual's behaviour that are felt to be due to a specific biological or genetic condition such as Prader-Willi syndrome (overeating) or fragile X syndrome (gaze aversion).

CACAP   See **Canadian Academy of Child and Adolescent Psychiatry**

CADDRA   See **Canadian Attention Deficit Hyperactivity Disorder Resource Alliance**

Canadian Academy of Child and Adolescent Psychiatry   A national organization of child and adolescent psychiatrists and other professionals in Canada, committed to advancing the mental health of children, youth, and families through promotion of excellence in care, advocacy, education, research, and collaboration with other professionals.

Canadian Attention Deficit Hyperactivity Disorder Resource Alliance (CADDRA) A national Canadian alliance of professionals working in the area of ADHD and dedicated to research, education, training, and advocacy in the area of ADHD. CADDRA has developed a number of tools and guidelines for the assessment and treatment of patients with ADHD.

Canadian Paediatric Society (CPS) The professional association of paediatricians in Canada. The CPS produces position statements on a wide variety of child and youth health topics, including mental health and developmental disabilities; develops education for health professionals working with children and youth; and advocates for the health needs of kids. The official journal of the CPS is *Paediatrics & Child Health*.

Comparative genomic hybridization microarray (CGH) A method to measure copy number variants, both additions and deletions, in a person's DNA. Most tests measure at a resolution of 100 kilo bases, but it is becoming possible to increase the resolution as low as 200 base pairs. CGH is still a research investigation in many centres but is increasingly becoming available to clinicians.

Developmental coordination disorder (DCD) Evident when there is a marked impairment in the performance of motor skills and where medical causes of motor impairment have been ruled out. The marked impairment has a significant, negative impact on activities of daily living—such as dressing, feeding, riding a bicycle—and/or on academic achievement—such as through poor handwriting skills. Core aspects of the disorder include difficulties with gross and/or fine motor skills, which may be apparent in locomotion, agility, manual dexterity, complex skills (e.g., ball games) and/or balance.

Executive functioning The mental processes used to plan, organize, use feedback, problem-solve remembering different pieces of information, develop strategies, and manage time and space.

Fetal alcohol spectrum disorder (FASD) Used to describe the range of physical, neurological, and behavioural problems felt to be caused by a mother's ingestion of alcohol during pregnancy.

Fetal alcohol syndrome (FAS) Term used when a child has the combination of pre- or post-natal growth failures, typical facial features of being exposed to alcohol during gestation, and a significant cognitive impairment.

Gifted/giftedness A category that qualifies for special education services in some provinces. Usually based on evidence from a psychological assessment that a child's IQ is significantly above average, in the superior or very superior range.

ICD–10 The International Classification of Diseases (10th Edition). This was developed by the World Health Organization and articulates the criteria used for the diagnoses of the full range of human disease. It was published in 1994. The criteria for the diagnosis of ADHD, in particular, are different than in the DSM-IV.

Inclusion, inclusive education An approach to education where children with disabilities receive their program in a regular class with their age-appropriate peers. They participate as much as possible in the classroom program. They are provided with assistance in the regular classroom to reach the goals of their program.

Individual program plan (IPP), individual education plan (IEP), personal program plan (PPP) These terms refer to a written document developed by the school that outlines a child's needs and how these will be addressed. This type of document can be used to communicate to teachers and parents the strategies for assisting students.

Intellectual disability (ID) This is the current recommended diagnostic term for a person with significantly sub-average cognitive abilities accompanied by significant delays in adaptive functioning. Previous terms have included **mental retardation, cognitive impairment,** and **mental deficiency**.

Learned helplessness The belief of persons, having experienced chronic failure, that they are ineffectual and not able to control what happens to them through their own efforts. When approaching difficult tasks, they decrease efforts because they do not expect a positive outcome. They often rely heavily on others to give help, without which they believe failure will occur.

Lissencephaly Lack of development of gyri and sulci in the brain. This is due to an abnormality of neuronal migration, which occurs between week twelve and week twenty-four of gestation.

Locus of control (LOC) Locus of control is a concept referring to how much an individual believes he can control what happens to him. An internal LOC means a person feels that the things that happen to him are mostly a result of his own behaviour and that he has power or influence over the outcome of life events. People with an external LOC believe that powerful others, fate, or chance primarily determine what happens to them.

Mainstreaming, integration, least restrictive (most enabling, most appropriate) environment, normalization, non-categorical education Terms used to describe the approach to education where students with disabilities receive their education as much as possible in an environment with peers who are not disabled, while still having their needs met. This implies that students receive their education in regular or mainstream schools instead of special schools, with up to 100% of their time in a regular class.

Mental retardation This is an older diagnostic term for a person with significantly sub-average cognitive abilities accompanied by significant delays in adaptive functioning. Current preferred term is **intellectual disability**; however, the term **mental retardation** continues to be used concurrently, as it has been incorporated into many public laws and policies, particularly those related to eligibility for services..

Mild intellectual disability (MID) This term can be used in two ways. The first is to describe functioning at the upper end of the range associated with an intellectual disability. This would represent intellectual skills between 3 and 2 standard deviations from the mean of the test, between 55 and 70. For educational programs and services, the term refers to students with a general delay in their intellectual functioning, including children functioning in the borderline range or in the range that is sub-average. Assessments are often designed to discriminate between this group of children and children with a specific learning disability when setting educational programs and goals.

Modification Modifications are changes made to the grade-level expectations for a subject or course in order to meet a student's learning needs. Modifications may include the use of curriculum expectations at a different grade level and/or an increase or decrease in the number and/or complexity of expectations relative to the curriculum expectations for the regular grade level.

National Institute for Health and Clinical Excellence (NICE) An organization linked to the National Health Service in the United Kingdom that develops guidelines using the best available evidence.

Neuropsychological assessment An assessment of the cognitive, motor, behaviour, linguistic, and executive functioning of an individual. It can lead to the localization of organic abnormalities of the nervous system. This process is very difficult in young children.

NICE See **National Institute for Health and Clinical Excellence**

Operant conditioning An approach to changing behaviour or learning where voluntary or "operant" behaviour occurs because its consequences are reinforced. Consequences can be positive, where a consequence is delivered following a response, or negative, where something is withdrawn following a response. Reinforcement increases the occurrence of a behaviour, and punishment decreases the occurrence of a behaviour. If there is no consequence for a behaviour, it becomes less frequent. This is called "extinction."

Personal program plan (PPP) See **Individual program plan (IPP)**

Psycho-educational assessment An assessment of the psychological aspects of learning and of academic skills. The assessment evaluates intelligence and other learning skills as well as academic achievement.

Psychologist Licensed professional in psychology who can do psychological testing, diagnose mental illness, and provide psychological treatment. Each province designates the credentials necessary to be licensed as a psychologist. Most psychologists have a PhD in psychology as well as additional training in their specific field, such as neuropsychology or behavioural psychology.

Psychometrician/psychometrist A person who administers and scores psychological tests under the supervision of a licensed psychologist. A psychometrician/psychometrist is usually not able to make or convey a diagnosis without this supervision.

Resource teacher A teacher based in a school who provides assistance to students who are experiencing difficulty. They may be responsible for the development and monitoring of an individual education plan (IEP/IPP/PPP).

School board The governing body of the elected school trustees.

School board trustee An elected representative to the school board. The board of trustees is responsible for the operation of the school board and for the quality of education that the board offers. The board establishes policies that govern the administration of personnel. The board of trustees reviews the board's achievement of its goals and objectives.

Special educator A teacher who develops and advises regarding the education of students with special needs.

Temperament Refers to an individual's innate behavioural style as assessed by examining activity level, biological regularity (patterns of sleep, eating, and bowel movements), adaptability, initial approach, emotional intensity, quality of mood, persistence, and distractibility. Children's temperaments may affect their initial or longer-term adaptation to people, events, and experiences.

Theory of mind The ability to understand that others have thoughts and emotions that are different from one's own. It allows us to anticipate another's feelings and reactions. This is felt to be an area of weakness in persons with autism spectrum disorder (ASD).

Vocational school Also known as trade school; a secondary school where the focus of education is development of job skills as opposed to preparation for post-secondary education. Many students with a mild intellectual disability or severe learning disability are recommended to these programs.

Whole language, whole word, phonics, visual-auditory-kinaesthetic-tactile (VAKT), multisensory approach These are different approaches to teaching reading that have been used both for teaching regular students and students having difficulty acquiring reading skills. Whole language and whole word are based on recognizing the word as a whole, often relying on memory. Phonics is based on reading instruction focusing on the relationship between letters or graphemes and the sounds of the language they reproduce. VAKT and multisensory approaches use touch, tracing, seeing, and sound at the same time to teach reading. The greatest evidence is for techniques that are based on phonics, particularly for early intervention.

Index

Teacher Rating Scales (TSR), 56
telehealth technology, 150
television, 50, 140, 157, 212, 213
Test of Phonological Awareness Second Edition: PLUS
    (TOPA-2+), 156
text media, 215
textbooks, 158
The Explosive Child, 167, see also Ross Greene
"time-in," 68
time-out, 164, 167–68, 169
toxoplasmosis, 20
transition to formal education, 27
traumatic brain injury (TBI), 22, 24, 139, 145
tremor, 89, 145, 225
Triple P Positive Parenting Program, 166
tripod grasp, 28
Turner syndrome, 19

U

ungraded curriculum, 14

V

vaccination, 20
Vanderbilt NICHQ (National Initiative for Children's Healthcare
    Quality) Parent and Teacher Forms, 57, 195

Vineland Adaptive Behavior Scales, Second Edition
    (VABS-II), 46
viral encephalitis, 21, 22, 24
viral meningitis, 21
visual-auditory-kinaesthetic-tactile (VAKT), 15
visual-spatial skills, 20, 45, 139, 179, 207, 218, 221
vocabulary, 12, 45, 50, 88, 91, 102, 112, 119, 121, 123,
    125, 129, 131, 132, 138, 155, 156, 157, 158, 159, 160,
    214, 215

W

Wechsler, David, 45
Wechsler Intelligence Scale for Children, 45
Williams syndrome, 19
"wilted flower syndrome," 202
"word family" approach, 157
working memory, 3, 4, 20, 45, 95, 225
writing, 4, 5, 8, 37, 73, 90, 91, 104, 118, 131, 132, 140, 143,
    145, 155, 159, 161, 170, 171, 173, 190, 198, 199, 203,
    204, 208, 213, 215, 221, 222, 225, 231
written language, 1, 5, 150, 151, 207

Y

Youth Self-Report Form (YSR), 56
Yukon Territory, 43